NURTURING
YOUNG
MINDS

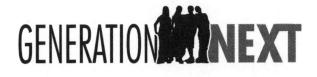

GENERATION NEXT

NURTURING YOUNG MINDS

Leabharlanna Poiblí Chathair Baile Átha Cliath
Dublin City Public Libraries

Ed. DR RAMESH MANOCHA and GYONGYI HORVATH

ROBINSON

ROBINSON

First published in Australia and New Zealand in 2017 by Hachette Australia

First published in Great Britain in 2018 by Robinson

A CIP catalogue record for this book
is available from the British Library.

ISBN: 978-1-47214-196-5

Typeset in Garamond by SX Composing DTP, Rayleigh, Essex

Printed and bound in Great Britain by CPI Group (UK) Ltd, Croydon CR0 4YY

Papers used by Robinson are from well-managed forests
and other responsible sources

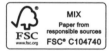

Robinson
An imprint of
Little, Brown Book Group
Carmelite House
50 Victoria Embankment
London EC4Y 0DZ

An Hachette UK Company
www.hachette.co.uk

www.improvementzone.co.uk

CONTENTS

FOREWORD

A friend once told me that the introduction is always the least-read part of any book. 'It's always skipped over as people rush to get to what you have to say,' she said. 'Never,' she advised, 'never waste your time writing an introduction!'

So here I am, living proof that advice may be listened to but is rarely followed.

The experience of many young people is that growing up is a bit like going on a wild roller-coaster ride. The aim of this book is to inform you so that you can help as many young people as possible to stay in the trolley car and not fall on the tracks.

From my days working in mental health crisis teams, I recall a wild-eyed young man I visited at home. I started to talk to him in his garden while he swung a machete back and forth. The machete looked sharp. As he looked at me with fear and desperation in his eyes, my overriding thought was, *What the hell do I do now?* In my career, this question has returned to me many times.

While many of the mental health challenges that we and the young people we care for will not be as extreme as this, the situation illustrates how out of our depth we can feel when trying to help a young person in their moment of need. Although no book can tell you exactly what to do now, or next, *Growing Happy, Healthy Young Minds* and *Nurturing Young Minds* go a long way towards helping. They contain sweat, fear, hope, dreams and the methods and experiences of many skilled experts to help you.

As I stood in that garden, the trickle of fear on the back of my neck told me I had only one chance to get it right. With every young person we work with, we also often get only one chance to shift things in a positive direction. That single opportunity, if taken, can have powerful effects. Effects that can last a lifetime.

This book will be important to anyone who is the parent of a young person or has an interest in working with people aged under twenty-five, such as youth workers, school support workers, social workers, child protection workers, psychologists, community workers, therapists, teachers and year-level coordinators. The type of work you do is variously described as counselling, assisting, mentoring, therapy and even 'hanging around with'.

Nurturing Young Minds is a bit like a single ride on a roller-coaster. We know we have only one chance to help parents and care givers and we want to get it right. I suspect you will delve into this book as you need, picking topics as they relate to young people in your family or who you are working with.

Every chapter of this book deals with an issue that, if tackled properly, can change a young person's life for the better. In some cases those chapters will not only be life-changing but quite possibly lifesaving.

We are proud of the accumulated wisdom collected in *Growing Happy, Healthy Young Minds* and *Nurturing Young Minds* and even more excited about how you might be able to use it to open up possibilities in the lives of the young people you work with.

On behalf of all of the clinicians, I would like to thank our teachers, especially those of you who thought you were our clients.

I would also like to thank the team at Generation Next: Dr Ramesh and Mrs Gita Manocha, Gyongyi Horvath, Ning Pruttivarasin, Bronte Baskin, Lisa Evans, Nick Chuah, Natalie Vo, Blake Galera-Holliss, Neil Harris, John Towner, Christie Ho, Shari Borodkin, Yvonne Diab, Paola Feliu and many others who have worked to support the development of this book.

Most importantly we need to acknowledge the team at Hachette Australia: Fiona Hazard, Publishing Director, and Sophie Hamley, publisher, for their wisdom in recognising the need for a book like this; and Sophie Hamley and Sophie Mayfield for going above and beyond the call of duty to get this information out for the benefit of young people. Each year Generation Next, as a not-for-profit charitable organisation, works to increase the skills and knowledge of many thousands of professionals and young people through its face-to-face events, live webcasts and free online resources. In doing so, it helps us all to create a better world for our next-generation leaders to inherit.

Andrew Fuller
Melbourne, 2017

HOW TO USE THIS BOOK

Nurturing Young Minds is designed to be read in separate bites. When you are concerned about a certain issue, look up the relevant chapter and read it. Each chapter is self-contained and does not assume that you have read any other section of the book. At the end of each chapter useful resources are included for you to access if you want more in-depth information, including resources, websites, articles and books, along with listing other chapters within this book that cover issues related to your main concern.

Nurturing Young Minds also has an excellent supporting website that you can access via www.generationnext.com.au by clicking on the book icon. Click on a chapter title and you will be taken to a page that will contain:

- Author photos, bios, and books and articles written by them.
- Where available the author's own website, in case you want to get in touch directly with them.
- Further reading, websites and resources with hyperlinks wherever possible.
- Where provided, the references used by the authors to write their chapters.
- Links to relevant lectures, interviews and short educational clips from the Generation Next YouTube channel.
- Updates to chapters as new developments and advances occur.

To continue to stay up to date on information and developments in this important field, you can also:

- Subscribe to the free weekly Generation Next newsletter, which provides a range of interesting news and information curated from around the world concerning the mental health and wellbeing of young people.
- Read the Generation Next blog, join our Facebook community and follow us on Twitter.
- Subscribe to our YouTube channel to receive a new video in your inbox each week.

USE THIS BOOK TO HELP OTHERS!

Are you a parent?

- Give a copy of this book to your child's grandparents, aunties and uncles.
- Buy a copy for your child's school or teacher.
- Encourage your school's PTA to host an event for fellow parents, focusing on youth mental health using resources and content from the book.
- Provide relevant sections of the book to your teen (recommended fourteen years plus) to increase mental health literacy.
- Use strategies and tips from the book to start conversations on tricky topics with your child/teen about issues affecting them.
- Use the resources directly to create a support services index to raise awareness of help-seeking avenues that you can post on your fridge – this can help your child/teen and can be used by them to help their friends.
- Recommend the book to others in your parent or community groups.
- Share the book with other parents or anyone who is concerned about a young person.

- **Are you a teacher or teacher-in-training?**
- Recommend this book to parents in your school community.
- Read chapters as part of your ongoing professional development and learning.
- Host professional development sessions for colleagues at school using content from the book to improve individual and organisational professional practice.
- Use some of the content for a mental-health-themed parent–teacher event, e.g. recognising common mental health concerns.
- Use relevant chapters in your lesson plans to meet relevant curriculum requirements (e.g. in PSHE).
- Pick an issue covered in the book and encourage your students to do a project or a peer-education initiative around it.
- Get the Student Representative Council or school to pick an issue(s) from the book and run a peer-education programme or an awareness day around it.
- Use the resources directly to create a support services index for your class or school to raise awareness of help-seeking avenues and so that students and staff know where they can go for help.
- Share warning signs and red flags about particular issues with parents of students you are concerned about.
- Use content to shape school wellbeing programmes, including induction programmes for new students and year levels.
- Use content from the book's supporting website (like videos and podcasts) for further professional development and learning.
- Order copies for your school library.

Are you a professional working with young people?

- Read chapters as part of your ongoing professional development and learning.
- Use some of the content for in-house professional development sessions for colleagues to improve individual and organisational professional practice.
- Share relevant content when working with young people or their parents, in particular relating to warning signs and red flags.

- Use the resources directly to create a support services index to raise awareness of help-seeking avenues that can be shared at work and put up in common areas.
- Use content from the supporting website (videos and podcasts) for further professional development and learning.
- Pick an issue and use the book's recommended resources to undertake further professional learning.
- Pick an issue and use the book's content as a springboard for undertaking research to improve the impact of your work with young people.
- Use content of the book to help inform your organisation's mental health policy/plan.
- Order copies for your organisation's library.

Advocate for a greater focus on mental health and help create environments that are supportive of young people's wellbeing.

Dr Ramesh Manocha & Gyongyi Horvath

WHERE TO GET HELP

If you or a young person you know needs to talk to someone anonymously, or needs help, the following services are available.

Samaritans

Samaritans operates a twenty-four-hour confidential telephone counselling line and information service, and can provide contact details for other help services.
Helpline: 116 123 (free)
Email: jo@samaritans.org
Hours: Helpline is available 24/7, 365 days a year

Childline

Childline operates a twenty-four-hour confidential telephone and online counselling service for anyone under the age of nineteen in the UK.
Helpline: 0800 1111 (free)
Online counselling and email: www.childline.org.uk
Hours: Helpline is available 24/7, 365 days a year

Emergencies

Phone: 999 or 112

THE DEVELOPING BRAIN

1. UNDERSTANDING TEEN SLEEP AND DROWSY KIDS

Dr Chris Seton

This chapter describes the common sleep problems seen in the adolescent years, the negative effects sleep problems have on physical and mental health, and how you, as a parent or professional, can rectify these problems. I will then explain when you can step in and help further if needed. You will read first about sleep problems, and then about sleep solutions.

AN EASY QUICK-CHECK METHOD FOR TEEN TIREDNESS

Are you wondering whether your own child, or a child you know, is sleep deprived? Below are the two key sleep questions that will give you the answer. We call these 'red flag' questions:

Q1. Does your teen have big weekend sleep-ins?
Q2. Is he/she very difficult to wake up and get out of bed on school mornings?

If the answer to either or both of these questions is 'yes', then you have a sleep-deprived teen on your hands. Big weekend sleep-ins represent 'catch-up sleep' from insufficient sleep on weeknights. Difficulties getting out of bed on school mornings reflect a lack of sleep, and possibly also a late body clock (see the section 'Wacky body clocks and "jet-lagged" teens').

INTRODUCTION

Adequate, good-quality sleep, healthy nutrition and regular exercise are the three pillars upon which health is optimised in adolescence. When these three factors are in place, teenagers are well protected from multiple physical and mental health problems. Additionally, resilient and good-quality sleep are important buffers against mood and learning problems, which are typically exacerbated by acute stress. Sleep deprivation is an important but poorly recognised health issue, particularly in young people. It results from inadequate and/or poor-quality sleep.

As our 24/7 world becomes busier, and increasingly electronically connected, our opportunity to sleep decreases, and so sleep deprivation is becoming more common. The tiredest group on our planet, by far, is adolescents. In fact, 70 per cent of Australian teens are chronically sleepy, so much so that the 'tired, grumpy, moody, monosyllabic' adolescent has been normalised. Australian teenagers are the third most sleep deprived in the world. Alarmingly, less than 2 per cent of sleep-deprived teenagers receive medical help, and in many of these cases, doctors and psychologists misinterpret sleepiness simply as a mood disorder, and thus sleep treatment is forgotten.[1] In order to increase awareness of this issue, US health authorities have recently officially listed adolescent sleepiness as a major public health issue. Australian health authorities, in contrast, have not given this key health issue the recognition it deserves.

The effects of sleep deprivation go way beyond simple tiredness, resulting in multiple physical and mental health problems. This long list of flow-on effects from sleep deprivation includes:

- impaired classroom learning;
- mood and behavioural disturbances;
- increased risk-taking behaviours;[2]
- emotional fragility;
- poor food choices;
- reduced sport performance;

- lowered self-esteem;
- poor coping with stress;
- reduced school attendance;
- increased alcohol and drug use;
- more infections; and
- elevated risk of anxiety, depression and suicidal ideation.

If some of these descriptions sound like your son or daughter, or a teenager you know, you will be keen to learn more about the underlying nature of these sleep problems and the solution pathways you can follow to solve sleep deprivation.

SO WHY ARE ADOLESCENTS SO TIRED?

Multiple factors conspire in a perfect storm to cause poor sleep in adolescence. Recognising and understanding how these factors sabotage sleep is a helpful first step in the pathway to good sleep. Let's now explore some of the key contributing factors to this perfect storm.

Too busy to sleep!

There is no doubt that being a teenager these days is a tough gig. There is so much to do each day, and there are only twenty-four hours in which to do it. School life extends increasingly beyond the classroom, into pre- and post-school extracurricular activities. Time is also needed for homework, socialising, meals, part-time jobs, sport, relaxation and down time. As these activities increase throughout high school years, and the time availability remains static at twenty-four hours per day, sleep time is shortened. Additionally, pressure to achieve all this may result in stress, and stress in turn leads to poorer sleep by causing insomnia – that is, difficulty in getting off to sleep. So pressure and stress shorten sleep, and shorter sleep means poorer coping with subsequent stress and pressure, and thus the negative spiral goes on, sometimes resulting in a crisis.

Interestingly, a disproportionately large number of sleepy adolescents who visit me at my sleep clinic attend schools where parent, teacher and student expectations and ambitions may be quite high. This is not unexpected given that parents who invest heavily in their child's education would typically have high expectations of good academic and other outcomes. Private schools typically offer and encourage a wide variety of extracurricular activities. This is all fine and good; however, there is some risk that all this may, in vulnerable students, result in a toxic mix of pressure, stress, anxiety and poor sleep, i.e. the wheels can fall off. The take-home message here is that in relationship to school, study and extracurricular activities, more is not necessarily better. I have included further information about how this axiom applies in relationship to learning later on.

In summary, the establishment of resilient sleep helps students cope better with the various pressures, stresses and anxieties associated with their busy lives.

The disconnect between society and science

The second reason teens are so tired relates to a difference between the amount of sleep teens (and parents) think they need, and the amount of sleep scientific research reveals they actually need. In humans, from babyhood onward, the amount of sleep we need reduces with age, and so bedtimes appropriately become progressively later during childhood. Not unreasonably, most teenagers, and their parents, think that this trend continues during adolescence. Typically in our society, school-night sleep time reduces by 1.5 to 2 hours across adolescence.[3] In distinct contrast, scientific research shows that sleep requirement remains static at an average sleep need of just over nine hours, right through teenagerhood. Stated another way, the amount of sleep one needs at twelve years of age and at eighteen years of age is the same. This sleep pattern, though, does not fit with our social and educational norms. For example, Year Twelve students have much more homework and study than Year Seven students, and educationalists assume that older students have more evening time available to complete this work, as their bedtime is later. Teenagers will often blame large study and homework loads on their inability to get to sleep on time. You can read more about the relationship between homework and sleep in the 'Ideal World Sleep Solutions' section to follow.

Progressively later bedtimes across adolescence explain why sleep deprivation becomes more common, and more severe, as teenagers progress through high school.

Wacky body clocks and 'jet-lagged' teens

The third factor in the tired teen equation relates to the sleep–wake body clock and how the teen body clock is misaligned with school scheduling.

The fact that we sleep at night is not a coincidence. Rather, our sleep patterns are carefully regulated by a clever brain body clock, which produces our sleep-inducing hormone, melatonin, predominantly during the evening and night. The natural sedative effect of rising melatonin in the evenings puts us to sleep, and keeps us asleep until morning, when melatonin production reduces, causing us to wake up.

In the lead-up to puberty the body clock starts switching on melatonin somewhat later at night, and switching it off later in the mornings. This results in some teens feeling more wakeful and energetic in the evenings, when they should be feeling more tired, and very sleepy on waking, when they should be feeling fresh. So these teens are the 'owls' (rather than the 'larks') of society. This is how we all feel when jet-lagged.

Around 15 per cent of, or one in every six, teenagers have a body-clock shift to a degree that causes them to have insufficient sleep (because they simply can't get to sleep at the appropriate time). They often lie in bed awake, become frustrated and stressed, and this compounds the problem and further delays sleep. Subsequently, they have great difficulty getting up on school-day mornings. Getting a teenager with a late body clock up, say, at 6.30 a.m. on a school morning is the same as you or me getting up at 3 or 3.30 a.m. It feels, to these teens, as if they are getting up in the middle of the night, as that is what their body clock is indicating. So it is understandable that they are often resentful about being woken. Even when they do get up, they are very slow to get moving, so showering, dressing, and breakfasting are all slow, and this often annoys and frustrates parents. Shouting at them to 'get moving' doesn't work. People have long assumed this is simply a teenage behaviour, but it is actually a physical rather than a psychological issue. The clinical name we doctors use for this condition is Delayed Sleep Phase Disorder, or DSPD, but when I talk to families about it, I simply call it a late body clock.

It is very important to understand the difference between choosing to have insufficient sleep by going to bed late (what I call 'won't sleepers') and having insufficient sleep because of a late body clock (what I call 'can't sleepers'). Trying to get a teenager with a late body clock to go to sleep at a reasonable time is futile. They just can't do it. Moreover, it may cause arguments with parents, stress and pressure, which result in further sleep delay and worsening sleep deprivation. Some teens become anxious when they can't get to sleep and this too compounds the problem.

If you have, or know, a teenager who perennially seems wide awake, full of beans and jumping out of their skin late at night, but then is pretty much impossible to wake and get out of bed on school mornings, he or she is highly likely to have a late body clock. We also sometimes refer to this as 'social jet lag'. The morning sleepiness and lethargy, and the inability to get up and get moving, are called 'sleep inertia'.[4] Unlike the temporary effect of travel jet lag, social jet lag is experienced on an ongoing and chronic basis. It can and should be fixed.

At weekends, if allowed, late-body-clock teens will have big sleep-ins, both because they have delay in getting to sleep and also because high morning levels of brain melatonin sedate them. A weekend sleep-in is okay in one way, as it allows them to catch up on missed weeknight sleep. Weekend sleep-ins are the repayment of a weeknight 'sleep debt'. The downside, however, is that sleep-ins teach the body clock to run even later than before, so getting to sleep on Sunday nights becomes a huge problem after Saturday and Sunday morning sleep-ins. Thus, Sunday night becomes the night of least sleep in the week. If you are a teacher, you can detect late-body-clock teens because they are the most tired, disengaged and poorly 'functioning' in the classroom on Mondays. This contrasts with the standard pattern of increasing tiredness as the school week progresses, with relative classroom alertness on Mondays, and 'maximum' tiredness on Fridays. Also, teens with late body clocks have higher levels of school lateness (because of morning tiredness resulting in slowness to get ready for school). As you would expect, school lateness is most likely on Mondays.

As a teacher, if you have suspicions about this you could ask your student if they have trouble getting to sleep at night. If the answer is 'yes', you have detected DSPD and then you should diplomatically pass on this information to the parent(s) and point them to the treatment solutions that follow.

MOODINESS, SLEEPINESS AND STRESS

Low moods and stress are potent triggers of sleep deprivation. In fact, the combination of sleepiness, moodiness and stress is very toxic because each of these factors makes the other two factors worse. For example, feeling anxious at bedtime may prevent one from getting to sleep. Equally, the inability to get to sleep may trigger anxiety. This is a 'bidirectional relationship'.

Sometimes teenagers are diagnosed with mood disorders such as anxiety or depression, when the key underlying trigger is sleep deprivation. Often these factors go together. Treatment should include both psychological treatment and sleep treatment, but the latter is often forgotten. Trying to fix depression or anxiety when sleep deprivation is present is futile, because good sleep is needed to improve moods and happiness in this situation.

Research has shown that the combination of acute stress and poor sleep in a teenager who is genetically vulnerable to a mood disorder will bring out or trigger the mood disorder. However, if the same stress occurs when sleep is optimal, the depression or anxiety will not manifest and moods will stay quite normal. Stresses of course are unavoidable in adolescence and genetic predisposition to abnormal moods is unchangeable. So good, resilient sleep protects teenagers from low moods and emotional fragility.

The take-home message here, therefore, is that the building of good-quality sleep is important in protecting a teen from mood decompensation in the face of stress. The second, equally important message is not to forget about sleep issues if your teenager is found to have a mood disorder. Remember, sleep problems and mood problems are fellow travellers.

'DIGITAL HEROIN' – HOW ELECTRONIC SCREENS SABOTAGE SLEEP

One of the major reasons teen sleep deprivation has reached epidemic proportions in recent years is the increasing nighttime use of portable electronic devices. A nation's rate of uptake of new electronic technology is very closely correlated to its rate of teen sleep deprivation. As rapid uptakers of digital technology, Australian teenagers now are the third most sleep deprived in the world. These devices are essential for social and peer interaction; they are very well marketed to young people, they are great fun, and they are increasingly affordable, but they are highly addictive. Sensible limiting of night usage of smart phones and other electronic devices is an important but sometimes difficult component of treatment.

Electronic screens cause sleep problems in four different ways. First, device activity late at night, like any other awake activity, takes up time that could be otherwise used to sleep, so sleep opportunity is reduced by nighttime screen engagement.

Second, as these devices have become more portable and multi-modal, they are increasingly used in and on the bed, rather than at a desk or table. With repetitive in-bed screen exposure, the brain begins to get mixed messages about where and when to sleep, and then begins to associate the bed as a place of wakeful activity, rather than a place of sleep. The somewhat quaint medical term for this problem is 'conditioned arousal'. This means the brain is trained to be awake in bed by repetitive screen exposure, and, in fact, begins to expect to be awake in bed. Thus, even on a night when there is no device use, difficulties getting to sleep occur because the brain is conditioned to be awake in bed, with resultant insomnia. On these nights, teens will then argue, 'See, it's not the smartphone that keeps me awake'. In fact, the smartphone is the chicken if you like, and conditioned arousal is the egg.

Third, screen activity, particularly gaming and texting, is excitatory to the brain, because it results in the release of wakeful and addictive neurochemicals like dopamine and adrenaline. This chemical surge increases wakefulness and reduces the brain's subsequent ability to get to sleep. The dopamine surge is thought by some to be similar to the effect seen with some types of illicit drug use, and so the Chinese press recently referred to this facet of electronic screen use as 'digital heroin'.

Fourth, and this is the BIG sleep saboteur, is the so-called 'blue light effect'. Blue light is at the right-hand end of the light spectrum, and is favoured by electronic screen developers because it results in better definition and screen clarity than any other light frequency. Unfortunately, though, blue light is also a potent inhibitor of our sleep hormone, melatonin. Bright light in general, and blue light in particular, sends a message to our brain that it is morning, and time to wake up. Morning sunshine helps to wake us up. As screen technology has advanced, screens have become smaller, and the intensity of light needed to maintain clarity increases, worsening the 'wake-up' effect. This is further compounded by the tendency to hold ever-smaller screens close to one's face. A small smartphone screen is much worse for sleep than a huge flat-screen TV. All this blue light at night is like having someone at the bedside shouting at you to stay awake. So if electronic screens are used frequently in or on the bed, teen brains get a mixed message about sleep.

The rapid development of digital technology has outpaced our ability to medically research the negative effects of ubiquitous screen exposure, particularly during critical teenage years of brain development.

FUTILE LEARNING AND THE LATE-NIGHT COGNITIVE TIPPING POINT

Any teacher will tell you that tired kids don't learn well. Research tells us that smart kids, who do learn well, have longer and better-quality sleep than poor learners. We all want the best academic outcomes for our kids, and good sleep is essential in achieving this aim.

Optimal learning requires good short-term memory and long-term memory

First, let's look at how sleep impacts on short-term memory. Just as your smartphone goes into low-power mode when the battery is almost flat, a fatigued teen brain goes into 'shutdown mode' and blocks out all attempts at new learning. Newly taught information is not absorbed if adequate sleep is not achieved on the night *prior* to any attempt at new learning. We all forget things when we are tired. Teachers and parents reporting that information or instructions go 'in one teenage ear and out the other' are in fact describing the impact of sleepiness (or, in some cases, selective deafness). So a failure of short-term memory through tiredness means that classroom learning on one day is totally forgotten pretty much immediately. Therefore, this learning is futile and wasted.

The second arm of good learning involves long-term memory acquisition. One of the many magical things about our brains is the ability to shift new learning from short-term memory into long-term memory. This shift, or 'filing', of memory only occurs effectively in REM (rapid eye movement) sleep, more commonly known as dream sleep. This shift from short- to long-term memory banks occurs on the night *following* a day of new learning. Many tired teens, particularly those with late body clocks, have inadequate amounts of dream sleep, and so the shift from short- to long-term memory is compromised. This missing information then needs to be re-learned at some other time. So, once again, learning time is wasted and new learning is quickly forgotten.

In summary, good-quality learning on one day requires two consecutive nights of good sleep.

Trying to learn late at night becomes increasingly difficult as we become sleepier. The processing speed of the brain slows down with late-night tiredness. There comes a point where the brain, craving sleep, shuts down all new learning processes. This is called the 'late-night cognitive tipping point' or, put more simply, the time at night beyond which no learning at all is retained in short-term memory. This non-retained learning is called 'futile learning'. Attempts at futile learning late at night then result in later bedtimes and reduced sleep. This means that a whole day of learning is at risk of being wasted if good REM sleep is not achieved, as this learning will not be shifted into the long-term memory bank. So all this can easily become a negative spiral.

Therefore, rather than continuing to try to learn in a late-night tired situation, it is better to go to sleep and consolidate the day's learning up to that point. This is why, in part, global educational research shows that academic outcomes are no better in countries that undertake lots of homework when compared with countries with lesser homework, because futile learning is more likely in countries with more homework. So, more is not necessarily better in regards to nighttime learning.

A lot of recent media attention has been given to global education data that shows that Australian school students are slipping down international rankings in terms of their learning outcomes. It is perhaps not coincidental that kids are also sleeping less. Governments and educators are scratching their heads as to why Australia's well-funded and innovative education system is failing its students. Maybe our leaders should be looking not at the system and the teachers but at the kids to explain these failures. We know that even the best teachers, with the best educational resources, are unable to achieve good outcomes in tired kids. Tired kids do not engage in classroom learning.

Recent research by the Grattan Institute showed that 40 per cent of students were unproductive in the classroom. Although a few of these were rowdy and disruptive, the vast majority were found to be passively and silently disengaged in the classroom. These kids were tuning out, largely because they were sleep deprived. They are often not noticed by teachers because they are quiet rather than rowdy, and were thus well described in this study as 'classroom ghosts'.

SO, LET'S GET PRACTICAL

As you can see, the reasons behind teen tiredness are multiple. However, it is easiest to think of tired teens in three distinct categories.

1. **Those who simply do not get enough sleep.** These are 'won't sleepers'. They choose late school-night bedtimes and are sleepy because they don't get enough school-night sleep. This group form the majority of sleep-deprived teenagers. They don't necessarily know they are tired because most of their peers are also tired, so they think this is all normal. This group can usually be fixed by the home-based, parent-driven treatments outlined below, whereas those teens in group two or three are more likely to need further treatment from a sleep professional.

2. **Those with a late body clock.** These are 'can't sleepers'. Even with the best intentions and good sleep habits, these kids cannot get to sleep at a reasonable bedtime for their age. As previously described, they are wide eyed and alert late at night and hopelessly tired and cranky with sleep inertia first thing in the mornings.

3. **Those with psychological issues that prevent them getting to sleep on time.** These are, like late body clockers, 'can't sleepers' rather than 'won't sleepers'. An example would be a teenager who worries at bedtime. The worry prevents sleep and the trouble getting to sleep results in more worry and anxiety, and so it spirals.

This all seems pretty simple; however, some of the teenagers I see have combinations of the above categories, with several different factors at play.

So, now I will outline the strategies you can undertake as a parent to improve sleep. In most teenagers, these will be sufficient, but in a minority, professional help will be needed. I will guide you through this process. Hopefully you will rediscover your smart, happy offspring through these solutions.

IDEAL WORLD SLEEP SOLUTIONS

If I had the power and magical cleverness to do it, this is what I would do.

First, I would lengthen our current twenty-four-hour day by three or four hours. We could all enjoy, say, a twenty-seven-hour day. This would allow busy teenagers to comfortably fit in all their daily activities and still have time to get their quota of sleep.

Second, I would delay high school starting times by about two hours for part of the year, and by three hours during daylight saving time. School finishing times would be delayed also, so total teaching time would be unchanged. This would allow high school students to sleep in, and be fresher and more alert during class time. It would especially help the 15 per cent of teens who have a late body clock. In fact, many US states have legislated late high school starting times, resulting in startling improvements in academic outcomes.

Third, I would limit homework to a level that would fit well with sleep requirements. A healthy balance between homework expectations and sleep need is an important way of avoiding late-night learning impairment.

But in our non-ideal, real world, consider the practical strategies that follow.

THE REAL WORLD SOLUTION PATHWAY FOR PARENTS

Step 1: Have a chat about the power of a good sleep routine

Sit down and have a chat with your tired teenager about sleep. Sleep is a low-priority activity and is poorly valued by most teenagers. Therefore, just having a chat, in itself, can help create the opportunity for an increased amount of sleep time. Don't do this late at night when everyone is tired and emotional. Be careful not to be too prescriptive or dogmatic. Often the initial step in improving sleep is to provide insight regarding the benefits of good sleep. Mention the emotional, learning and even sporting benefits of good sleep. Many teenagers are not that interested in sleep as such, but some become interested when they learn, for example, that sporting ability improves with optimal sleep. In fact, many professional sporting teams now employ sleep coaches in order to gain competitive advantages for their athletes. Ask what they think about their current sleep patterns and whether they think their sleep issues are impairing their moods. The aim of this chat is to establish if your son or daughter has a degree of insight regarding sleep, or whether they think it is all a non-issue.

Additionally, this chat may spark motivation to make positive changes. Increasing sleep time of course means either reducing some awake activities and/or improving organisational skills and efficiencies related to these activities, so that they can be completed more quickly. Sometimes a written after-school and evening timetable is helpful. Prospective planning is helpful in avoiding all-nighters just before a big homework project is due. Remember also that tired kids are more likely to procrastinate, and therefore they tend to delay homework and study until late at night.

The bottom-line aim here is to forge an agreement on a sensible, regular, weeknight bedtime. In an ideal world, the best bedtime is that which achieves nine hours' sleep. This is typically a very hard sell, particularly to those at or beyond mid-teenagerhood (fifteen years and older), so in practice I tend to broker some sort of compromise, say, eight hours' sleep. An achievable sleep time, rather than an ideal world sleep time, is usually more palatable to tired teenagers.

Be aware also that many teenagers tend to normalise their abnormal sleep patterns. Research shows also that they are likely to underestimate their tiredness and overestimate the amount of weeknight sleep. In this context, do not assume that because your teen is in their bedroom, they are asleep.

Because sleep deprivation gets progressively worse across adolescence, and given that older, more independent teenagers are less receptive to a sleep chat, I strongly encourage parents of tweens and young teenagers (ten to fourteen years old) not to procrastinate about this. Earlier-age chats are better, easier and more likely to be successful in achieving a reasonable and regular bedtime.

Step 2: Establish a pre-sleep routine

Suggest a couple of routine relaxing activities in the thirty minutes before bedtime. Going to bed immediately after undertaking brain-alerting activities, such as studying or gaming, means that the brain is not in the mood for sleep, and so thoughts race through the brain after lights out. Sleep is then hard to achieve and this may induce further worry and anxiety, resulting in more wakefulness and so on.

The best pre-bedtime activity is a hot, deep bath thirty to forty minutes before lights out. After the bath, one's core body temperature reduces, and this is sleep inducing. Other helpful pre-bed activities include reading (not from a backlit device, though); listening to music (a chilled music playlist is best), and a small snack and drink (make it the same each night). If these activities are undertaken in the same order and at the same time each night, they set up what we call 'sleep onset cues' after a few weeks of practice, i.e. the pre-bed activities tell the brain that sleep is coming soon, so the brain gradually drifts into sleep mode. This is all a bit like Pavlov and his dogs. So at lights out, the brain is relaxed and sleepy, rather than racing with unhelpful thoughts.

A simple pre-bed routine also separates alerting activities from sleep. Initially, pre-bed routines can be viewed as boring and a waste of time, but often, after three to four weeks, teenagers begin to enjoy them, particularly when getting to sleep becomes easier. Remember that sleep improvement is not instant, as the brain takes a few weeks to learn these positive sleep associations.

Step 3: Retrain the brain

This is a pretty easy and straightforward step. It simply is that bedtime and lights out occur at the same time. This means avoiding undertaking any activities in or on the bed that are not related to sleep. This step is aimed at reducing 'conditioned arousal' (this term is explained in detail in the 'Digital Heroin' section, earlier in this chapter). Like many aspects of improving sleep, this may take some time as it involves reconditioning the brain to change from thinking about the bed as a place of wakeful activities to thinking of it as a place of sleep. So be patient, and expect a gradual, rather than instant, improvement.

Step 4: Avoid having digital devices in the bedroom

The best way to address this is to have a talk about nighttime electronic screen use. This is not likely to be a popular topic of conversation! However, it is a chat that needs to be had (unless your teenager is one of those extremely rare species that doesn't use electronic screens at night). Electronic screen behaviour is very hard to change, as these devices are great fun, extremely addictive and they are the key means by which teenagers stay socially connected outside of school hours. The potential FOMO (fear of missing out) created by nighttime screen limitation is a powerful force. So, selling 'dream time' as a replacement of 'screen-time' ain't easy. Pretty much all teenagers will need your help in changing their nighttime screen habits, or, put another way, you need to act as a screen media mentor. At the same time, ensure that you are a good digital role model, and do not constantly check your own device for updates.

The ideal way to manage this step is by discussion and verbal agreement, sometimes called a 'digital contract'. I will explain below how screens can be limited by force, and although this choice should be part of the discussion, it is better for everyone if this step is undertaken by cooperative agreement.

You have read earlier in the chapter about the many ways screens can sabotage sleep. In order to limit these effects, devices should not be used in the hour before lights out, nor subsequently during the night. Ideally, devices should be turned off and placed on their charger pre-bed. To avoid the strong temptation to use the device at night, the device should charge in a location away from the bedroom. This is part of what we call 'sleep hygiene', which means creating a bedroom environment that is conducive to good sleep. Having your teen's smartphone or other device(s) living away from the bedroom overnight also lessens the likelihood of so-called 'infomania' developing. Infomania is the excited expectation of a return text or email, and when this occurs late at night it is a powerful disturber of sleep.

Many parents feel totally disempowered in regards to teen screen management. They do not wish to create conflict by confronting their teenager over this. When you get responses like 'you are ruining my life', 'my friends will never speak to me again', 'I hate you so much' and so on, remember that such responses are common during initial discussions, because the fear of missing out on nocturnal electronic connectivity through screen-time limitation is a strong force. Your teen will learn that their friends still do talk to them each morning, even following a late-night screen lockdown. Remember that your ultimate aim is not to be your son's or daughter's best friend, but rather to bring them up in the best possible way you can. Optimising their moods, happiness and education through good sleep health is a great investment, despite the difficulties you may encounter along the way.

If your attempts at mutually agreed screen limitation are resisted, and if this issue becomes an ongoing battle that you are not ultimately going to win, you should seriously consider fighting your teen's overuse of their electronic gadgetry, with a screen-limiting electronic gadget of your own. Such screen-limitation devices place you in control and help your teen overcome their FOMO, their nocturnal electronic addictions and the other factors that conspire to prevent them voluntarily reducing screen exposure at night.

There are a number of online platforms and software programs that help with screen management in young people. These allow you to lock out screens overnight or, more preferably, you can negotiate a voluntary digital agreement, whereby screens will not be used beyond an agreed time on school nights. In this case, should your teen use their device outside agreed times, thus breaking this agreement, you will be immediately electronically alerted, and can intervene. Again, the 'voluntary' method is better than the 'enforcement' method.

Family Zone is an excellent screen management platform that has been developed by Australian parents.

You may notice that I haven't mentioned drugs or sleeping tablets as treatments. This is because drugs, at best, help for a day or two, and at worst don't help at all. Also, most sleep drugs actually impair sleep quality. I guess if drugs did work, the treatment section of this chapter would be very short!

SO WHAT NOW?

We know that at least eight in every ten tired teenagers will respond positively to the four-step parent sleep solution that I have outlined above. This is despite the fact that few teenagers will embrace all the strategies completely. There will be various levels of engagement and motivation. Adherence to these strategies will wax and wane. Pressure and stress can occur acutely, and compromise sleep even as sleep is improving. Try these treatments for at least three to four weeks, and try to be patient and supportive without pushing too hard.

As sleep slowly improves, you will see better moods, increased energy levels, especially first thing in the mornings, and sleep-ins will lessen in duration. When this occurs you can assume, but won't necessarily witness first hand, improved short-term memory, better engagement in the classroom and improved learning efficiencies. At this stage, if possible, obtaining feedback from class teachers is helpful in reinforcing good sleep outcomes, and therefore continuing the above strategies in the long term. This builds resilient sleep, which is not then compromised when the inevitable next stress comes along.

WHEN THIS ALL BLOWS UP IN YOUR FACE – WHAT THEN?

If you have one of the 20 per cent of teenagers whose sleep does not improve, or whose recalcitrance means they totally refuse to partake in any of these strategies, don't despair, help is at hand.

Failure of parent-driven treatments suggest that a teen may have a quite late body clock, and/or there may be significant psychological factors present that prevent the above treatments from being fully effective. In this situation a specialist sleep doctor or sleep psychologist may be able to step in and assist in or take over sleep treatment, either online or via face-to-face consultation.

FACE-TO-FACE SLEEP CLINIC

One of the big barriers to addressing this common problem is the fact that there are very few sleep clinics that specialise in helping adolescents with their unique sleep needs. Although paediatric sleep clinics have been established in all state capital cities in Australia, usually within children's hospitals, most assess and treat sleep problems in babies and young children only. None is specifically focused on adolescent sleep issues.

To address this problem, I helped establish Australia's first adolescent sleep clinic at The Woolcock Institute, Sydney University, in 2014. The key people in our team are adolescent sleep physicians like myself, and adolescent sleep psychologists. At the time of writing this chapter you might be surprised to find that there are only three clinics like this in Australia. Ours is in Sydney and there is another in Melbourne and another in Adelaide. While there are sleep clinics around the world dealing with different sleep problems, the treatments they offer to patients may vary considerably. At The Woolcock Institute, after a booking is made (www.sleepshack.com.au) treatment would proceed along the following lines.

Prior to your visit we send you some sleep diaries to fill in each morning, and these give us a picture of your teen's sleep pattern over several weeks. We ask lots of questions about school, extracurricular activities, stresses, moods, daytime sleepiness, academic performance, sleep issues in other family members, lifestyle, bedroom environment and, of course, electronic screens. From all of this we work out which factors are contributing to sleep deprivation. We then formulate a written treatment program, which we outline in detail. With each component of treatment we forge a verbal contract with your teen, asking their agreement to follow our advice. Sometimes we need to compromise on one or two components of treatment in order to obtain a verbal contract. Throughout the consultation we assess insight and motivational factors, and improve these if needed.

Treatment will include the components outlined in the parent solution pathway above, as well as extra body clock and psychological treatments that are tailored to your son's or daughter's needs. We may use morning sunlight exposure to reduce the sedative effects of high melatonin levels, and this then helps 'reset' a late body clock. Funnily enough, treatments are more likely to be undertaken when delivered by a health professional than when delivered by a parent. The treatments are usually undertaken for six weeks, with ongoing mapping of the sleep pattern on sleep diaries. Phone support is available if there are any speed humps along the way. A follow-up visit then assesses the response to treatment and fine tunes any remaining issues. Teens with a late body clock are prescribed a relatively late bedtime in initial treatment, and they then have a further four weeks of treatment to reset their bedtime to an earlier and appropriate time. This is called 'bedtime fading'.

From this point onwards, most families can continue to apply the treatment strategies in a self-managed fashion. Even when sleep is optimised it is important to continue to prioritise sleep and regulate sleep patterns. This creates resilient sleep, which protects the mental and physical health of teenagers when the inevitable next stress rears its ugly head.

For information on a sleep clinic in the UK, visit your GP or clinician with your son or daughter to ask about referral to a specialist clinic or hospital department that provides help for those with sleep problems.

COME ON IN TO SLEEPSHACK

If you live in Sydney, Melbourne or Adelaide, help for tired teens is readily available, but what about those adolescents who need help elsewhere? This is why we developed the world's first and only personalised online sleep diagnostic and treatment programme for teens and tweens. It's called SleepShack (www.sleepshack.com. au) and it's designed for young people from ten to eighteen years of age.

I encourage you to have a look at it. There is a short introductory video on the home page that explains how SleepShack works and the sleep issues that we assess and treat. Essentially, SleepShack replicates in the online world what we do at the sleep clinic. Families are electronically rather than physically connected to us. Dr Amanda Gamble, adolescent sleep psychologist, and I personally assess your teen's sleep patterns, and we then formulate and prescribe tailor-made treatments for your son or daughter.

SleepShack is not only a solution for those who live far away, it's also valuable because it allows you to get help immediately. Long clinic waits were resulting in many teenagers catapulting into crises because of worsening sleep problems, and SleepShack totally overcomes wait times. Assessment and treatment is undertaken online within a forty-eight-hour period, following a period of three weeks where you and your teen compile electronic sleep diaries online. We know that the longer teenagers go without sleep treatment, the more difficult they are to treat, so trying to nip these problems in the bud by avoiding clinic waits is very important.

The majority of teenagers prefer online sleep treatment, both because they are generally attracted to screens and the internet, and also because many are uncomfortable in a clinic setting with a sleep doctor and their parents hovering over them. Some feel, in this situation, as if they are what we term 'therapeutic prisoners' and they are being trapped and forced into a situation that compromises their autonomy. If this sounds like your son or daughter, then SleepShack, rather than sleep clinic, may be the way to go.

Although SleepShack is primarily a diagnostic and treatment platform, it is also an educational tool, aimed at further helping parents understand sleep science and health. There are lots of free educational resources, as well as a Facebook forum, on the website.

Beyond this, if you have further questions, or are unsure how to proceed with your tired teenager, you can email me via SleepShack for advice and direction.

The educational arm of SleepShack is free, as is any email advice from my team and me. To help us cover the costs of running this online service, SleepShack's formal sleep assessment and treatment programme costs A$140. The programme is of six weeks' duration for most teenagers; however, those with a late body clock undergo an extra four weeks of treatment of bedtime resetting.

PREVENTION IS BETTER THAN CURE – SLEEP HEALTH EDUCATION FOR SCHOOLS

Adolescent sleep health should, of course, be taught in all schools. Providing students with sleep insight is the first step in motivating them to more highly prioritise sleep and undertake good sleep habits. The Sleep Connection, unlike most school-based sleep education programmes, is able to identify students with sleep problems and direct families towards solutions.

Author biography

Dr Chris Seton is a paediatric and adolescent sleep physician in Sydney. Chris assesses and treats all types of sleep problems in babies, children and adolescents.

Chris helped establish Australia's first Paediatric Sleep Investigation Unit at the Children's Hospital, Camperdown, in 1990, and has worked as a Staff Specialist in Sleep Medicine and Respiratory Support, at what is now The Children's Hospital Westmead, since that time.

In 2015, Chris developed SleepShack, the world's only online sleep diagnostic and treatment programme for sleep deprived teens and pre-teens.

www.sleepshack.com.au

See also:

Chapter 3: Understanding the Teenage Brain

Chapter 5: Healthy Habits for a Digital Life

Chapter 6: Online Time Management

Chapter 7: Problematic Internet Use and How to Manage It

Chapter 8: Computer Game Addiction and Mental Wellbeing

Chapter 14: Advice for Parents: Be a Mentor, Not a Friend

Recommended websites:

NHS: www.nhs.uk/livewell/childrenssleep

US National Sleep Foundation: www.sleepfoundation.org

UK Sleep Council: sleepcouncil.org.uk

Online sleep diagnostic and treatment platform: www.sleepshack.com.au

The Woolcock Institute of Medical Research – Adolescent Sleep Clinic and Adolescent
    Sleep Seminars in Sydney: www.woolcock.org.au

Further reading:

Carskadon, M, Raffray, T, Van Reen, E & Toarok, L, 2011, 'Circadian Rhythm Disorders',
    Sleep in Childhood Neurological Disorders, Demos Medical Publishing, New York,
    pp 219–234.

Manocha, R (Ed), 2017, *Growing Happy, Healthy Young Minds: Generation Next*, Hachette
    Australia, Sydney.

Mindell, J & Owens J, 2010, *A Clinical Guide to Pediatric Sleep: Diagnosis and Management of
    Sleep Problems*, Lippincott Williams & Wilkins, Philadelphia.

We also recommend the very popular companion volume **GROWING HAPPY, HEALTHY YOUNG MINDS** – resilience, bullying, depression, anxiety, body image and many more important issues.

 For more online resources visit:
generationnext.com.au/handbook

2. EMOTIONS AND RELATIONSHIPS SHAPE THE BRAINS OF CHILDREN

Dr Michael Nagel

Humans are social beings. We thrive when relationships are positive, and when they are not we can face myriad physical and psychological challenges. This is true of all people regardless of age but arguably more so during childhood, when the brain is busy maturing and evolving through the interplay of nature and nurture. As such, understanding the links between emotional and social development and relationships is integral to anyone who works with children or who is interested in child development and welfare.

INTRODUCTION

The emotional development that occurs throughout childhood is often taken for granted by most adults. This could be due to the fact that such development is so much a part of our daily lives and so invisible to the naked eye. We can track signs of physical development without much difficulty and readily observe advances in many aspects of language and cognitive development. But it could be argued that we rarely think about how emotional abilities are rapidly evolving and instead are puzzled, or exhausted, when a child's emotions become openly displayed in the most public of places and when least expected or desired. To that end it is imperative to note from the outset that emotional development and associated aspects of social development may be the most important aspects of child development because they help to establish the foundation on which every other cognitive and psychological skill can flourish. Simply stated, emotions and relationships matter and this becomes very evident when one explores this through the lens of neuroscience.

As noted above, the emotional development of a child is linked to social development and relationships and is perhaps the most important foundation for all other types of development. Disregarding social context limits any understanding of emotional development because emotions are often generated in the context of relationships with others and are often managed with the help of other people. Considerable volumes of research tell us that regular social interaction is critical to all measures of healthy child development leading to adulthood. Indeed, all measures of healthy development depend on the quality and reliability of a child's relationships with the important people in his or her life, both within and outside the family. Numerous studies have even identified that the development of a child's brain architecture depends on the establishment of these relationships. We also have mountains of evidence telling us that emotional development is an important consideration with regards to academic achievement and school success.

Given the importance of a child's emotions, relationships and social interactions and their links to a variety of measures of success in school and later life, this chapter explores emotional and social development through the early stages of childhood leading to adolescence.

We know that the first few years in the life of a child are perhaps the most critical for all aspects of development and that the relationships that surround a child have a profound impact on that child's immediate and long-term mental health. In order to fully understand these important components of development, a good starting point can be found by looking at some important structures and systems of the human brain. From there we can then look at how emotional development can be positively influenced and, equally important, how it can be negatively compromised.

EMOTIONS, FEELINGS AND THE BRAIN

Whenever researchers discuss the brain they generally identify three major areas: the brainstem, limbic system and cerebral cortex. In terms of understanding emotional development, it is the limbic system that is of most interest; however, a brief look at each region not only helps to frame this chapter but serves as a reminder that each of these areas is intimately connected with and influences one another.

At the base of the brain, connecting it to the spine, is the brainstem. This important region is primarily involved with reflexes and autonomic functions including our fight-or-flight reflex as well as many of our inner drives, including hunger and sleep. While you are reading the words on this page you may start to feel hungry but you are likely unaware that it is your brainstem that is not only triggering your desire for food but also monitoring your heart rate, circulation and breathing. It should come as no surprise that significant trauma to the neck can present many problems or even be fatal.

The region of the brain that likely pops into people's thoughts when considering structures of the brain is the cerebrum, which is comprised of two hemispheres. This area of the brain sits relatively high above the brainstem and is usually identified as the region of the brain where thoughtful, organised thinking occurs. The four lobes of the cerebrum are what separate us from all other species on the planet and damage to any part of any of the lobes in either hemisphere can create myriad difficulties in terms of how we engage with the world around us. For example, a stroke in the left hemisphere can result in impaired and often irreversible difficulties in putting our thoughts together and articulating these through speaking.

In terms of emotional development, regions of the cerebrum, and in particular the prefrontal lobes, assist in regulating our emotions and such regulation, under normal circumstances, improves with age as all areas of the brain mature. It is worth acknowledging the importance of the prefrontal lobes here. This region of the brain, which does not fully mature until the third decade of life, works to inhibit impulses, guide decision-making, encourage long-term planning, mediate emotions and delay gratification. Because the emotional part of the brain, or limbic system, matures much sooner than the prefrontal lobes, children often have difficulties regulating their emotions and display degrees of emotional immaturity that generally fade with age.

The limbic system, as noted above, is the emotional epicentre of the brain. Nestled in the middle of the brain and between the brainstem and cerebrum, structures in the limbic system are not only responsible for our emotions but also play a part in motivation and various aspects of memory. Interestingly, there appears to be a greater number of neural connections running from the limbic system to the higher-order thinking regions of the brain than there are going in the other direction, suggesting that emotions can literally drive our behaviour and actions. Remember also that the limbic system matures sooner than the higher-order thinking regions of the cerebrum.

Overall brain development and maturation occurs from lower regions to higher regions and roughly from the bottom up to the front and from the inside out. Such a developmental trajectory is an important evolutionary principle in that our most instinctive and primal reactions to threats occur through the interplay of structures within the limbic system and brainstem. Consider, for example, what would happen if you were standing waist deep in the ocean and noticed the large dorsal fin of a great white shark approaching you. If the higher-order regions of the brain matured before the limbic system and brainstem, you would likely marvel at the magnificent beast moving freely through the water towards you before realising it might be a good idea to make your way to the shore as fast as possible. Because of how the brain matures, however, your limbic system may invoke memories of shark attacks witnessed on the news or in movies and your fight-or-flight response would initiate immediate action to ensure your survival. On more familiar terms, the maturation timeline of the brain is one of the reasons why infants can react immediately to any form of environmental stimuli, such as crying due to an unexpected loud noise, while older children and adults temper such actions with some measure of thoughtful analysis, such as seeking out the cause of the noise.

The differences between how infants and adults might react to particular events not only remind us of how regions of the brain work in concert to process environmental stimuli, but also illustrate that emotions are not solely isolated to the limbic system. For example, while it is certainly the case that some structures within the limbic system are responsible for generating emotions, it is the cerebrum where feelings of anger, sadness and anxiety, among others, are experienced. In other words, the limbic systems acts as an emotional relay station for passing on information to the higher-order thinking areas of the brain where it can be translated into feelings, moods, motivation or social awareness. This is an important consideration in that emotional and cognitive development are linked at a neurological level and this development impacts on all aspects of behaviour, thinking and learning. Equally important is recognising that while the terms 'emotions' and 'feelings' are often used synonymously, they are, in fact, not the same thing. In order to help illustrate the difference, consider the following scenario.

You are walking down a neighbourhood street when suddenly, and unexpectedly, a large dog barks loudly and lunges at the fence that stands between you and its gaping teeth. All of your senses come alive as you capture a vast array of stimuli via structures in your limbic system, which work with other regions of the brain to trigger an emotional response such as surprise, fear or anxiousness. In other words, emotions activate particular neurological circuits that prioritise our experiences into things we should pay attention to or simply ignore, while feelings are the subjective psychological labels that emerge as a result of such activation. Emotions precede feelings; they are physical and instinctual and can be measured by looking at blood flow, brain activity, body language and micro-facial expressions. Feelings, on the other hand, are the mental representations and subjective reactions that are influenced by personal experiences, memories and beliefs. While we all may understand the feeling of being afraid, it is important to remember that fear, and indeed all feelings, is the by-product of each unique brain perceiving and assigning some meaning to an emotion; one person's fear of heights is another's adrenaline rush.

It is sometimes difficult to remember the differences between emotions and feelings but perhaps it is easiest to think of emotions as mental states that can be associated with a wide variety of feelings, thoughts and behaviours. Fear, for example, may give you the sensation of your hair standing up on the back of your neck while sadness can impede you from doing anything productive at work. Arriving at those types of emotional states as well as others is the product of myriad processes between the limbic system and other regions of the brain that rely on physical sensations, attention, memory, perceptions, self-reflection and reasoning. Simply stated, almost everything we do begins or is linked to our emotions and, as such, the importance of the interplay between emotional and social development cannot be understated.

LINKS BETWEEN EMOTIONAL AND SOCIAL DEVELOPMENT

Experiences in the real world matter. For example, as our prefrontal lobes mature we get better at controlling our impulses, but our experiences of controlling our impulses also assist in the development of the prefrontal lobes and such real-life experiences literally shape our brain. The dynamic developmental interplay needed for all aspects of healthy neural development, behaviour and learning is a social process requiring cascades of interactions between individuals and the environment and real-life experiences. We learn to make better decisions and become better planners by making not-so-good decisions and then correcting our behaviour. Such decisions, corrections and, indeed, all aspects of behaviour are not made in a social vacuum but instead rely on continuous feedback from others and, as such, our emotional and social development are inextricably linked.

The links between emotional and social development should be self-evident. Children are born into a world in which they are very dependent on adults, and as they grow, social interactions become increasingly mutual. Mutuality encourages cooperation and an adult's response to a child's emotions not only helps to shape important qualities, such as empathy, but also shapes future social interactions. It is likely that most adults are unaware of the tremendous impact they have on a child's emotional and social development, let alone the impact they are having on a developing brain. When an adult consoles a crying infant or child they are literally shaping that child's brain and this is a prime example of how nature and nurture work together. Our social and cultural life is shaped by our biology and vice versa, and this is evident in the very earliest stages of a child's life.

In terms of overall development, the first six months of a child's life are dominated by emotional and social development. For the infant, this is about survival, in that they need food and security, and early infant behaviour looks to meet those needs via the limbic system. When hungry, a baby cries, then smiles when fed and perhaps laughs when content. These early emotions and feelings shape a child's learned behaviour through the responses it receives. When an infant smiles or laughs and sees an adult smiling back, the child's understanding of social interactions is strengthened from the feedback it receives. Over the first twelve months, expressions of fear, shame and shyness emerge first and then are followed by contempt and an expanding emotional repertoire each successive year.

The developing range of expressions noted above mirrors changes in the maturing brain. After six months of age, significant changes and growth in the neural architecture of the brain provide for greater connectivity between the emotional and rational parts of the brain, and by two years of age these regions are communicating with greater efficiency and expediency. As a result, children's emotional responses become increasingly evident in body language and facial mannerisms, and as language emerges and develops, feelings can then be expressed orally. This maturational journey relies on interactions with other individuals and, as such, emotional and social development are interconnected. This is evident in toddlers who, through social interaction and relationships, 'begin' to demonstrate an awareness that other people may have different emotions to their own, which helps to facilitate a very important quality known as empathy.

Empathy is a critical aspect of emotional and social development. Our capacity for empathy allows us to sense the feelings of another person. Infants have limited capacity for empathy and true empathetic behaviour emerges roughly around two years of age as the higher-order thinking regions of the brain mature. It is around this time when children discover that their sense of self is distinct from other people, and as their capacity for empathy improves, they come to understand a wider range of emotions and become more adept at assessing other people's emotions. Importantly, as children mature physically and become more mobile and independent, their experiences also increase in variety and this diversity in experience also shapes the emotional and social brain. The increasing independence of children helps to develop other important aspects of emotional and social development including attachment, temperament and emotional regulation.

Many experts in the fields of psychology and child development would suggest that attachment is perhaps one of the most important aspects of a child's emotional development. Simply stated, attachment refers to a child's emotional bonding with another person or the creation of an enduring emotional tie between two people. Attachment and bonding with an adult is a child's first and principle source of security and provides many other important emotional attributes and social skills. Attachment and bonding are not just emotional necessities but are influenced by powerful neurotransmitters and chemicals in the brain. Perhaps the most prominent of these is oxytocin.

Oxytocin is present in both males and females but females have much higher levels of this important chemical. Oxytocin has been referred to as the 'love' or 'bonding' hormone, due to its links to various behaviours including sexual and maternal behaviours along with trust and attachment. In terms of relationships, numerous studies have demonstrated that positive relationships heighten oxytocin levels while diminishing stress hormones and even physical contact itself elevates oxytocin. Infants and children who find comfort in the arms of their parents or a loving caregiver are not only being soothed but are also experiencing an important social interaction that positively impacts on brain development and overall wellbeing. As children grow and mature, attachment need not always be physical but through visual or audible contact or what can be referred to as 'abstract' attachment. However, the first five years of a child's life are particularly important in terms of creating environments and social contexts that foster relationships that positively affect attachment and healthy development through social contact. Such contexts also assist in shaping a child's temperament.

Temperament is something that many parents and those who work with children may find challenging. Temperament basically refers to a person's emotional and/or social style and the individual differences people demonstrate with regards to emotion, attention, arousal and reactivity to various situations. This is particularly evident in new or novel situations and while the terms 'temperament' and 'personality' are often used interchangeably, they are not the same thing. Temperament is one component of personality and the exact nature of a person's temperament lacks clear consensus among researchers. However, there is general agreement that temperament is biologically based and influenced over time by genes, environment and experience. Again, nature and nurture work together to shape this important aspect of our emotional self.

One of the most interesting and yet confounding aspects of temperament is the differences that can exist between siblings. Most parents, excluding those with identical twins, will have some stories about how one child may be easygoing, for example, while another might present very difficult behaviour when both are experiencing similar scenarios. This is perhaps one of the reasons why temperament is often described as being a biological or genetic disposition, and there is some evidence to suggest the existence of neurological contributors to temperament, particularly in relation to dopamine and serotonin.

Dopamine and serotonin are neurotransmitters or the chemical messengers in the brain that facilitate communication between neurons through synapses. Elevated levels of serotonin have been linked to improved impulse control and reduced aggression, while low serotonin activity has been associated with poor impulse control, risky behaviour and aggression. Dopamine, on the other hand, plays a role in the brain's motivation and reward systems and influences sensation-seeking behaviours. High levels of dopamine activity in certain regions of the brain provide a sense of pleasure and enjoyment which in turn influences intrinsic motivation and a desire to repeat any experience associated with such feelings. After reading this, some might assume that helping a child control their impulses and aggression might simply be a matter of regulating these neurotransmitters in some way. Unfortunately, the brain is far more complex than the descriptions provided above.

Earlier it was noted how the various regions of the brain, while somewhat distinct in purpose, work together. Numerous studies have demonstrated that temperament, emotional regulation and behaviour do not reside solely in the limbic system but, rather, are the products of complex activity between the emotional and higher-order thinking regions of the brain. For example, one study looking at aspects of temperament in four-year-old children during play sessions found that children who had been identified as 'aggressive extroverts' and 'fearful introverts' showed greater neural activity in the right prefrontal cortex than 'non-aggressive extroverts' and non-fearful shy children. In fact, the non-aggressive extroverts and non-fearful shy children had relatively stronger activity in the left prefrontal cortex during play group. It is noteworthy that the researchers concluded that those children who were less aggressive and shy may have been employing the language regions found in the left hemisphere in association with other cognitive processes more effectively and, as such, demonstrated overall positive play behaviour. Equally noteworthy, however, is that such studies should not be taken to suggest that a child's behaviour is fixed in the brain as a constant throughout life but, rather, that some children may require different forms of guidance and assistance when it comes to coping with their individual emotions and temperament. This is also true in terms of another important component of emotional development alluded to above and known as emotional regulation.

The term 'emotional regulation' is an umbrella covering a number of important capacities, but it is probably easiest to think of emotional regulation as an individual's ability to manage emotional stimulation effectively and use this purposefully to regulate thinking, learning and behaviour. For children, the development of emotional regulation is a process that generally improves with age and increasingly allows for greater control of behaviours that may assist in the achievement of goals or, conversely, diminish success. Emotional regulation is a mix of emotional, physiological, behavioural and cognitive processes that allow individuals to adjust to experiences. For an infant, this can be as simple as turning away from unpleasant stimuli while young children might talk to themselves or use 'private speech' to solve problems, and an adult might take a deep breath and refrain from saying anything or walk away from something they find equally unpleasant.

Like many of the components of emotions and emotional development discussed above, emotional regulation involves a complex array of structures and processes in the brain, generally improves with age, and is a product of both nature and nurture. At the risk of appearing repetitive, experiences (nurture) matter and, as such, relationships and strategies for positive relationships and emotional development are critical considerations for any individual raising or working with children.

RELATIONSHIPS AND STRATEGIES FOR SUPPORTING THE DEVELOPING EMOTIONAL BRAIN

The information provided in the sections above was not only set out to inform but also to strongly present the case that environments and experiences have an exceptionally strong influence on emotional development and, indeed, all aspects of development and brain architecture. Within the scientific literature there is now little, if any, argument that development is shaped for better or worse by relational and social contexts. Moreover, it is now generally accepted that it is the dynamic interaction of nature and nurture that facilitates changes in children's brain growth, function and capacities. Environments and experiences mediate the potential with which children are born and the strength and quality of relationships between children and the adults around them are fundamental to the positive and effective development of a child's emotional wellbeing and overall neurology.

For example, a lack of positive relationships, inadequate supervision of and involvement with children have all been strongly associated with increased risk of behavioural and emotional problems. In extreme cases where neglect associated with a low level of various sensory inputs such as touch, speech and social interaction occurs, the likelihood of underdevelopment of the brain is almost absolute. Experiences matter; unlike the complexities associated with the brain, fostering positive experiences is actually, if you will pardon the pun, child's play.

Children need to be loved and supported. In the very early stages of life this means ensuring they are attended to when in an apparent state of distress and not ignoring crying as some form of training or character-building exercise. When children are in a state of distress, it is important for adults to remain calm in order to maintain a positive relationship. Like adults, children often experience stress when situations are new, novel or unfamiliar. That is one reason why routines are so very important and why creating a predictable world for children facilitates healthy emotional development. It is okay to just say no to a child, but that response must remain constant for similar situations. Giving a child a biscuit just prior to dinner one evening and then forbidding it another evening sends mixed messages to that child and is not helpful in terms of developing emotional regulation. Structure and routines are important.

Emotional development also involves learning and developing new skills though a wide range of experiences. New and novel activities therefore need to be supported by warm and responsive relationships. This requires adults to be emotionally and physically available at the nexus of providing environments that are safe and secure. On a more practical level, parents, caregivers and all those who work with children can facilitate healthy emotional and social development through the following.

SPENDING QUALITY TIME WITH CHILDREN AND ENGAGING THEM IN CONVERSATION

Modelling positive and effective emotions and social skills: Decades of research has laid a pretty solid framework, noting that 'children see, children do'. If anger is displayed by an adult when frustrated, a child may learn to do likewise. It is also advantageous to describe and label emotions and link those emotions to events and behaviours when possible.

Being predictable: Tell children what is happening in the moment and in the future.

Being aware of a child's emotions and emotional signals: All brains, and indeed all children, are unique and will react in different ways to different situations. Children will have preferences for how they might engage with the world around them and these need to be understood, supported or, when necessary, altered. This in turn requires adults to understand the meaning of a child's behaviour and not entirely focus on the outcome. It is natural to focus on the outcome of an angry outburst, for example, but understanding the meaning of the anger is very important. Some children will act up in anger due to fear while others may do so out of frustration, boredom, anxiousness or myriad other feelings.

Having fun: Sing, dance, play, tell and read stories and seek as many ways as possible to have fun. Having fun not only builds relationships and supports emotional development, but also releases powerful chemicals and engages the brain's neurochemistry in a positive fashion, diminishes stress and anxiety and boosts the immune system.

The ideas and strategies above are not an exhaustive list but represent a few of the very simple things that can be done to facilitate and enhance emotional and social development. It is, however, critical to stress that healthy emotional and social development depends a great deal on the quality of a child's relationships with the important people in his or her life, both inside and outside of the immediate family. As noted, many studies have found that the quality and stability of a child's human relationships lay the foundation for a wide range of later developmental outcomes that really matter. Concurrently, neuroscience supports generations of instinctive habits related to child rearing and relationships and provides a compelling scientific argument for the types of nurturing that occur when adults proactively engage in positive relationships with children. In simpler and more eloquent terms, and using the words of the esteemed development psychologist Urie Bronfenbrenner: a child requires progressively more complex joint activity with one or more adults who have an irrational emotional relationship with the child . . . somebody's got to be crazy about that kid. That's number one. First, last and always.

Relationships matter for children's emotional development, and the more warm, positive, loving and numerous, the better!

Author biography

Dr Michael Nagel is an Associate Professor at the University of the Sunshine Coast, where he teaches and researches in the areas of cognition, human development, behaviour and learning. He is the author of ten books on child development and learning used by teachers and parents in over twenty countries. Dr Nagel has delivered over three hundred workshops and seminars for parents and teachers nationally and internationally. Nominated as Australian Lecturer of the Year each year since 2010, Dr Nagel is a member of the prestigious International Neuropsychological Society, is the Queensland Director of the Australian Council on Children and the Media, and is a feature writer for *Jigsaw* and the *Child* series of magazines, which collectively offers parenting advice to more than one million Australian readers.

www.michaelnagel.com.au

See also:
Chapter 3: Understanding the Teenage Brain

Recommended websites:
Mumsnet: www.mumsnet.com
Family Lives: www.familylives.org.uk/advice
Virtual Lab School: www.virtuallabschool.org/preschool/social-emotional/lesson-4
Zero to Three: www.zerotothree.org

Further reading:

Aamodt, S & Wang, S, 2011, *Welcome to Your Child's Brain: How the Mind Grows From Conception to College*, Bloomsbury, New York.

Bell, MA & Wolfe, CD, 2004, 'Emotion and cognition: An intricately bound developmental process', *Child Development* 75(2), pp 366–370.

Brazelton, TB & Greenspan, SI, 2000, *The Irreducible Needs of Children: What Every Child Must Have to Grow, Learn and Flourish*, Perseus Publishing, Cambridge, Massachusetts.

Crugnola, CR, Tambelli, R, Spinelli, M, Gazzotti, S, Caprin, C & Albizzati, A, 2011, 'Attachment patterns and emotion regulation strategies in the second year', *Infant Behavior & Development* 34(1), pp 136–151.

Damasio, A, 2004, 'Emotions and feelings: A neurobiological perspective', in Manstead, ASR, Frijda, N & Fischer, A (Eds), *Feelings and Emotions: The Amsterdam Symposium (Studies in Emotion and Social Interaction)*, Cambridge University Press, Cambridge, pp 49–57.

Diamond, M & Hopson, J, 1999, *Magic Trees of the Mind: How to Nurture Your Child's Intelligence, Creativity, and Healthy Emotions from Birth Through Adolescence*, Penguin Putnam Inc, New York.

Dowling, M, 2014, *Young Children's Personal, Social and Emotional Development* (4th edition), Sage Publications, London.

Eisenberg, N, Valiente, C & Eggum, ND, 2010, 'Self-regulation and school readiness', *Early Education & Development* 21(5), pp 681–698.

Faull, J & McLean-Oliver, J, 2010, *Amazing Minds: The Science of Nurturing Your Child's Developing Mind with Games, Activities and More*, Berkley Books, New York.

Fox, SE, Levitt, P and Nelson, CA, 2010, 'How the timing and quality of early experiences influence the development of brain architecture', *Child Development* 81(1), pp 28–40.

Goleman, D, 1995, *Emotional Intelligence: Why it Can Matter More Than IQ*, Bantam Books, New York.

Goleman, D, 2006, *Social Intelligence: The New Science of Human Relationships*, Random House, London.

Hershkowitz, N & Hershkowitz, EC, 2004, *A Good Start in Life: Understanding Your Child's Brain and Behaviour from Birth to Age 6*, Dana Press, New York.

Kochanska, G, Coy, KC & Murra, KT, 2001, 'The development of self-regulation in the first four years of life', *Child Development* 72(4), pp 1091–1111.

Manocha, R (Ed), 2017, *Growing Happy, Healthy Young Minds: Generation Next*, Hachette Australia, Sydney.

Nagel, MC, 2012, *In the Beginning: The Brain, Early Development and Learning*, Australian Council for Educational Research (ACER), Camberwell.

Nagel, MC, 2012, *Nurturing a Healthy Mind: Doing What Matters Most for Your Child's Developing Brain*, Exisle Publishing, Newcastle.

Nagel, MC, & Scholes, L 2016, *Understanding Development and Learning: Implications for Teaching*, Oxford University Press, Melbourne.

National Scientific Council on the Developing Child, 2004, *Young Children Develop in an Environment of Relationships* (Working Paper No. 1), Centre on the Developing Child, Harvard University, Cambridge, p 1.

Raver, CC, 2002, 'Emotions matter: Making the case for the role of young children's emotional development for early school readiness', *Social Policy Report* 16(3), pp 3–18.

Shonkoff, JP & Phillips, DA (Eds), 2000, *From Neurons to Neighborhoods: The Science of Early Childhood Development*, National Academy Press, Washington.

We also recommend the very popular companion volume **GROWING HAPPY, HEALTHY YOUNG MINDS** – resilience, bullying, depression, anxiety, body image and many more important issues.

For more online resources visit:
generationnext.com.au/handbook

3. UNDERSTANDING THE TEENAGE BRAIN

Dr Michael Nagel

Until recently, very little was known about brain development during the teenage years. Advances in research and technology have now provided us with very important insights into the developing teenage brain, which in turn should help us to better understand and engage with young people.

INTRODUCTION

Our understanding of brain development has grown exponentially over the last couple of decades. Neuroscientific research has merged boundaries with many other fields and, as such, the science surrounding the brain and mind is now available to parents and all those who work with and engage young minds every day. In other words, we are gaining far greater access to, and understanding of, the developing brain, and there is indeed much attention to be given to the teenage brain. However, in order to better understand the teenage brain and provide a foundation for understanding some of the behaviours associated with being a teenager, a brief introduction to the brain's structures and how they develop is necessary.

THE DEVELOPING BRAIN

The human brain is an amazingly complex, still poorly understood organ. Consisting of various layers and structures, the brain possesses hundreds of billions of cells that bathe one another in chemical messengers that influence moment-to-moment changes of the mind, behaviour and experience. Its complexity is so unmatched by anything in nature that the brain has been described as the most unimaginable thing imaginable, and although we have learned a great deal, most neuroscientists would likely agree that we probably only know about 1 per cent of what we would like to know. What we do know, however, is that the brain starts out as a small collection of cells that becomes a complex super-highway of electrochemical impulses that shape who we are and what we do.

Chronologically speaking, the brain begins to form about seventeen days after conception. This marks the beginning of an amazing journey of neural development where neurons will generate and migrate to different regions of the brain. Neurons are a type of brain cell that resemble bulbs, with sprouting roots called 'dendrites' and a tail-like structure known as the 'axon'. The dendrites of neurons act like antennae and receive information from other neurons and/or from environmental stimulation. As you read these words right now, your brain is gathering information that passes through your eye to your occipital lobes where it is interpreted and dispersed to other areas of the brain. An important, and sometimes difficult, thing to remember is that seeing isn't happening in your eyes. Nor does hearing take place in your ears or smelling happen in your nose. Your sensory organs take in information, which is translated into electrochemical signals and passed between neurons while your brain decides what to do with the information. This passing of information between neurons occurs across a small gap between axon terminals and dendrites, which is commonly referred to as a 'synapse' and facilitated with the assistance of 'neurotransmitters' (chemical messengers). Everything that you experience is the product of an electrochemical dance that is choreographed for future attention or deemed unimportant and forgotten.

The process of passing information noted above is how the brain 'learns'. When axons send signals that are received by dendrites via a synapse, learning takes place; and the more that these types of connections are made, the faster and more efficiently the signals move and the more permanent they become. An important aspect of this communication between neurons is that if synapses are used repeatedly, over time they will become 'hardwired' pathways and part of the brain's permanent circuitry. Conversely, if they are not used repeatedly or often enough, they are usually eliminated and much of this occurs during the teenage years. This 'hard-wiring' of pathways appears to be a use-it-or-lose-it process whereby nurture helps to shape nature. In other words, experience plays a pivotal role in 'wiring' the brain. This is perhaps one of the greatest examples of how nature and nurture work together with the end result being the overall development of the mind. Moreover, all human behaviour can be traced to the communication among neurons whereby every thought and experience you have, every emotion you feel, every moment you make and all of your awareness of the world around you is possible because neurons talk to each other. This neural chatter is rampant in the first few years of life and by age three, a child will have more connections in its brain than the paediatrician it visits when unwell. In essence, the brain overcompensates by producing more connections than are needed and then it gets rid of many of those connections during the teenage years. We will revisit that later but at this point it is also significant to note all of this early neural activity leading to a mature brain relies on some important chemicals and for a number of functions to occur over time. The brain does not fully mature until we are in our third decade of life and, as such, full neurodevelopment is actually more marathon than sprint. During this marathon, the teenage years see significant changes to the brain and also the potential for significant behavioural manifestations. There may be some very good reasons why teenagers will do things that leave adults bewildered and those reasons can be found in the changing structures and functions within the teenage brain.

STRUCTURES OF THE BRAIN

The structures of the brain and the maturation of those structures offer important insights into the world of teenagers. The number of structures at play inside anyone's head at any one time are vast in scope and detail and therefore it is prudent to limit this part of the discussion to a broader and perhaps more general perspective of those things going on inside the head of a teenager. In adopting this position, we can start by looking at three regions of prominence within the brain: the brainstem, the limbic system and the cerebrum. It is significant to note that isolating these areas is primarily for descriptive purposes, given that they are intimately connected and work in concert with one another.

The brainstem or region closest to the spine is responsible for functions not under conscious control and where survival responses such as fight or flight are activated. The limbic system or central part of the brain harbours and processes our emotions and memories. Finally, the cerebrum, which contains the occipital, temporal, parietal and frontal lobes, has been recognised as the region where processing environmental stimuli, thinking and consciousness exist. Within the cerebrum, the frontal lobes are integral components of who we are and what we do. In the context of understanding the teenage brain, some very important and relatively new insights have emerged regarding these areas and brain function.

First, there was a time when some believed that many of our cognitive capabilities were mature and readily available on or about the time puberty kicked in. We now know that this is simply a whimsical notion and that the teenage brain undergoes a massive remodelling of many areas that affect everything from logical and responsible thinking to impulse control to sensation seeking and the controlling of one's emotions. Full brain maturation extends beyond the teenage years but there is a lot of work going on between the ears of teenagers. In terms of maturation we know that the survival mechanisms of the brain along with the limbic system or emotional hub of the brain are mature long before the analytical and logical processes of the prefrontal lobes come fully online. This means that teenagers are hot-wired for emotion but often lack the brakes to slow down those emotions when they speed down life's highway of experimentation and experience.

We also know that during the teenage years the brain travels down a pathway of deconstruction whereby it discards unused synaptic connections or prunes away those connections developed in the first three to four years of life as it works towards becoming more efficient. Interestingly, this restructuring occurs in concert with an increase in myelin, or the white matter of the brain. All of these changes are significant and amid all of this restructuring, pruning and growth in myelin, it is important to remember that the brain seems to mature roughly from the bottom up and around to the front, and in different areas and at a different rate for males and females. These changes can have a profound impact on various mechanisms of the mind and on teenage emotions and thought processes, or the lack thereof. The implications of this incredible neural transformation are evident in teenage behaviour and, quite simply, in how teenagers engage in and deal with the world around them. A more detailed look at the changes noted provides us with a great deal of food for thought when it comes to working with and engaging teenage minds. The production of myelin offers a good starting point for such exploration.

MYELIN AND SYNAPTIC PRUNING – THE MATURING BRAIN

Myelin is the white matter of the brain and is actually a fatty material that grows like a sheath around the axons of neurons and acts as an insulator and conductor. Because it acts as an insulator, myelin aids in synaptic communication. Simply stated, more 'myelinated' axons mean a faster and more efficient brain with the end result being that certain activities are easier to learn when regions of the brain are sufficiently myelinated or when our brains become 'fatter'. This is very evident in the early years of a child's life when it is clear that many of a child's capacities do not 'come online' until regions of the brain have received significant myelin growth. For example, vision and motor coordination are very limited at birth because the neural networks responsible for sight and movement aren't working fast enough due to the lack of myelinated axons. Importantly, the last regions of the brain to myelinate completely are the frontal lobes and in particular the prefrontal lobes. This is the region of the brain that considers what is a reasonable response to an adult, what are the implications of getting a piercing and myriad other teenage dilemmas.

This process of myelin development noted above is referred to as myelination or myelinisation and is a lengthy journey lasting well into the twenties and resulting in the tripling of the size and weight of the brain. Interestingly, while the teenage brain is expanding its volume of myelin, it is also decreasing its total volume of connections through a process noted earlier as pruning or, more accurately, synaptic pruning.

Synaptic pruning is a vital process with regards to overall brain development. Remember that in the first few years of life, a child's neural connections will come to outnumber those of an adult. On or about the time pubescence begins, and most notably through the teenage years, the brain starts to discard or prune those synaptic regions that are seldom used. This allows the brain to refine itself, become more specialised and more efficient, and process stimulation and information faster. The greatest influence on the connections that the brain maintains and what it decides to discard is found in an individual's own life experiences and environment. Synaptic pruning is an extremely important process of development where the saying 'use it or lose it' attains great implications for teenagers in that the brain is actually being remodelled or reconstructed. Therefore, the experiences that teenagers have – or don't have for that matter – not only impact on teenage emotions, thought processes, learning and behaviour but quite literally shape their brains.

Another important aspect related to the pruning of synapses is that, like the production of myelin, the last regions of the brain to be pruned are the prefrontal lobes, or the brain's 'chief executive officer'. As teenagers engage with the world around them, myelination and pruning are part of a natural developmental stage that can impose on, and give rise to, specific behaviours. Before looking at some of those specific behaviours there is one further aspect of teenage brain development worthy of consideration, namely the influence of certain neurotransmitters.

NEUROTRANSMITTERS AND THE BRAIN

As I mentioned at the beginning of this chapter, neurotransmitters are the chemical messengers released during the communication of information from one neuron to another via synaptic transmissions. The brain produces probably at least fifty, and maybe as many as one hundred, different chemicals that it uses to communicate. During the teenage years some of the important neurotransmitters in our brain seem to have a mind of their own. Three of those that are most pertinent to this discussion on teenagers are melatonin, serotonin and dopamine.

Melatonin is a neurotransmitter that forms part of the system that regulates the sleep–wake cycle associated with our circadian rhythms. This important chemical is produced in the centre of the brain by the pineal gland and when the sun goes down and darkness grows, melatonin levels increase and we feel sleepy. It appears, however, that once puberty kicks in, the release of melatonin declines and seems to be pushed back a couple of hours. Many parents can tell stories of how sleep patterns changed in their children once the teenage years took a foothold on life and their kids would go to sleep later. And while it is true that social events, homework, sports, television, social media and evening jobs might impact on a teenager's sleep, there is now ample evidence showing us that internal biological processes also influence adolescent sleep.

While melatonin levels appear to change and impact on teenage sleep patterns, serotonin levels also appear to vary during the teenage years. Serotonin is an important chemical for helping us to feel calm and relaxed. It can have an impact on mood fluctuations, anxiety, impulse control and levels of arousal, and low levels of serotonin have been associated with depression, sleep disorders and a variety of behavioural disorders. Some of the latest research available also suggests that serotonin plays a powerful role in moral judgement and decision-making, and influences social behaviour. During the teenage years, levels of serotonin can temporarily decline and teenage girls are especially susceptible to lower levels of serotonin given that this neurotransmitter is influenced by oestrogen during the menstrual cycle. High levels of oestrogen enhance levels of serotonin, oxytocin and dopamine, while low levels see corresponding decreases in those chemicals. The potential for low-to-high fluctuations of serotonin during the teenage years has led a number of researchers to speculate that serotonin is complicit in increased impulsivity and greater risks of depression during adolescence.

While serotonin can impact on moods and aspects of behaviour, dopamine is another powerful neurotransmitter that can influence how we feel and act, and it appears to fluctuate markedly during the teenage years. In itself, dopamine is often referred to as the brain's 'pleasure' neurotransmitter, given it plays a role in novelty and reward-seeking behaviours, and feelings of wellbeing and motivation. New experiences, especially those associated with some element of risk, thrill or degree of danger, can elevate dopamine and produce feelings of intense pleasure. So influential is dopamine that low levels have been associated with a range of challenges from difficulties maintaining attention on a task to Parkinson's disease, while exceedingly high levels are evident in those who suffer from schizophrenia, Tourette's syndrome and obsessive-compulsive disorder. It should be apparent that levels of this neurotransmitter can have a profound impact on a person.

During the teenage years, dopamine levels are at their highest and then begin to decline as adulthood approaches, and this can impact on behaviour, given how dopamine engages the brain's reward systems. So strong is the influence of dopamine in teenagers that neurodevelopmental studies have identified that there seems to be a dopamine 'power play' between the higher-order thinking regions and the more primal emotive systems, resulting in the immature prefrontal cortex of teenagers giving way to the powerful emotions associated with impulsivity and risk-taking. Importantly, while it appears that all teenagers will take part in some measure of risky behaviour, there are also individual differences in the chemicals and systems noted above, suggesting that some teenagers will engage in far riskier behaviours than others and this can also be impacted on by the brain's reward systems.

Without going into the fine neuroscientific details of how the brain senses, interprets and mediates rewards, both human and animal studies tell us that the reward systems of the brain undergoes massive changes during the teenage years, resulting in greater sensation-seeking, reward-seeking and risk-taking behaviours. This change may account for links between teenage risk-taking behaviours and increased mortalities, health-compromising behaviours and harmful outcomes during this time of life. Moreover, changes in behaviour associated with risk-taking, impulsivity and mood swings in teenagers are compounded by all of the other developmental changes noted earlier, and it seems that the teenage brain is primed to do things that might make a six-year-old child cringe in disbelief. It is these types of behaviours and approaches to working with teenagers that are explored next.

UNDERSTANDING AND WORKING WITH TEENAGERS

Understanding teenagers?! Many generations have tried but we can view teenage behaviours differently and develop a better understanding of teenagers if we continually remind ourselves that the teenage brain is a work in progress. From the outset, then, it is important to remind ourselves that teenagers, regardless of physical appearance and size, are not smaller versions of adults. The brain is changing during the teenage years and it is awash with emotions amid a stage of restructuring and, at times, the potential absence of logical reasoning. Emotions can be both positive and negative in terms of teenage behaviour and, as such, behaviour should be seen as a biological symptom as well as a result of social circumstance. Teenagers may do some beguiling things, but this is part of a normal stage of identity formation. From that perspective, *it is important to ensure that boundaries and guidelines are clear, concise and unambiguous. It is also important to foster lines of open communication and carefully temper any teenage need for independence with the experience of an adult* – in this sense mentoring programmes and positive relationships with the adults around them are important considerations when working with, and raising, teenagers.

A further consideration lies in recognising that *the teenage brain is primed for sensation-seeking and risk-taking activities.* These types of activities will vary according to gender, experience and exposure to a variety of environmental stimuli. Sensation seeking may also occur in the guise of experimentation and *teenagers are particularly susceptible to chemical addictions including to nicotine, alcohol and other drugs.* Whenever possible, *creating opportunities for teenagers to take risks in a positive and pro-social way may assist in providing an environment for them to extend themselves and avoid harmful alternatives.* The key to all of this lies in providing supportive environments that allow teenagers to take risks on various levels and in various contexts. Once again, however, firm boundaries and structures are needed. *Many teenagers take risks through extracurricular activities such as sport and music but it is important to find alternatives for those who don't.* One relatively easy way of accommodating this would be to *develop 'rites of passage' activities that not only allow for the facilitation of pre-arranged elements of risk but also offer opportunities for individuals to recognise and affirm their transition into adulthood.* Teachers, counsellors and parents alike can do this in various contexts and with a variety of positive outcomes.

In understanding that teenagers will engage in risk-taking and sensation seeking, it is also important to remember that *teenagers may not always understand the implications and consequences of their choices and decisions and, as such, talking to and supporting teenagers is important.* However, *it is also important for adults to listen, listen and listen some more and, in doing so, also remember that they were once teenagers as well.* Every generation seems to think the current younger generation is problematic but it turns out that that is not the case and simply a matter of misplaced opinion. Neurologically speaking, current generations of teenagers aren't any different from previous generations and while they live in different times and contexts, they still share a need to be heard with those of us who grew up some years ago. Empathy goes a long way when working with teenagers. Furthermore, there is a common tendency to demonise teenagers in the media and it is not uncommon to see headlines such as 'teens run wild' in newspapers. *Always remember that for every teenager who does something that makes the news in a negative fashion, there are thousands who don't and we should celebrate the teenage years regardless of how many challenges they present.* Showering young people with positives and striving to ensure positive environments go a long way towards enhancing brain maturation. Cognitive energy channelled in this manner will go much further than trying to find a solution to an arguably unanswerable question such as 'What could they be thinking?'

Along with being empathetic when needed, *it is also important to model the types of behaviours you expect and to encourage teenagers towards self-regulation. Teenagers do value their peers but we also know that the most significant person in a teenager's life is typically an adult role model,* usually a parent but often a teacher, coach or other adult. Teenage brains are particularly susceptible to emulating the wrong role models and social media can provide far too many of those. Adults need to model the types of behaviours that they want the teenagers around them to emulate, which also helps to build self-regulation in the teenage brain. *A teenager presented with appropriate models for dealing with anger, frustration or other emotions will increasingly become aware of their own behaviour, understand the importance of controlling it when necessary, and display positive approaches to dealing with life's highs and lows.*

Finally, avoid rushing teenagers into maturity or 'growing up'. There is nothing that any adult can do to hurry the natural developmental timelines of the brain. The discussion above has offered broad guidelines towards understanding and working with teenagers but each brain, and each teen, is different. Take hope from any examples of maturation you see and be sure to acknowledge those things that appear to be the actions of a maturing mind. It is equally important to remember that while our understanding of the brain has improved over the years, there are some time-honoured concepts that remain true. *Teenagers respond well to adults who value and love them and they listen to and trust those adults who care about them, avoid judging them and invest time in, and with, them.* The teenage brain is a work in progress and it can be guided to grow emotionally, socially and intellectually in a positive and healthy manner. It just needs time, attention, encouragement, guidance, love and the voices of experience from those who grew through similar times of change, experimentation and self-discovery. In the end, understanding the teenage brain is not just about understanding the young people around us, but in understanding the teenage brain, we are also offered a mechanism for remembering who we once were so that we can now provide the support needed for healthy development. In short, we don't have to just accept the neurodevelopmental changes outlined in this chapter, we can actually shape and change them.

Author biography

Dr Michael Nagel is an Associate Professor at the University of the Sunshine Coast, where he teaches and researches in the areas of cognition, human development, behaviour and learning. He is the author of ten books on child development and learning used by teachers and parents in over twenty countries. Dr Nagel has delivered over three hundred workshops and seminars for parents and teachers nationally and internationally. Nominated as Australian Lecturer of the Year each year since 2010, Dr Nagel is a member of the prestigious International Neuropsychological Society, is the Queensland Director of the Australian Council on Children and the Media, and is a feature writer for *Jigsaw* and the *Child* series of magazines, which collectively offers parenting advice to more than one million Australian readers.

www.michaelnagel.com.au

See also:
Chapter 2: Emotions and Relationships Shape the Brains of Children

Recommended websites:
Mumsnet: www.mumsnet.com/teenagers
Relate: www.relate.org.uk/relationship-help/help-family-life-and-parenting/parenting-
    teenagers

Further reading:
Blakemore, SJ, 2007, 'The social brain of a teenager', *Psychologist*, vol. 20, no. 10, pp 600–602.
Carew, TJ & Magsamen, SH, 2010, 'Neuroscience and education: An ideal partnership for producing evidence-based solutions to guide 21st-century learning', *Neuron*, vol. 67, no. 5, pp 685–688.

Carskadon, MA, 2002, *Adolescent sleep patterns: Biological, social, and psychological influences*, Cambridge University Press, Cambridge.

Casey, BJ, 2013, 'The teenage brain: An overview', *Current Directions in Psychological Science*, vol. 22, no. 2, pp 80–81.

Chassin, L, Hussong, A & Beltran, I, 2009, 'Adolescent substance use', in Lerner, RM & Steinberg, L (Eds.), *Handbook of adolescent psychology: Volume 1: Individual bases of adolescent development* (3rd ed), John Wiley & Sons. Inc, Hoboken, pp 723–763.

Dahl, RE, 2003, 'Beyond raging hormones: The tinderbox in the teenage brain', *Cerebrum*, vol. 5, no. 3, pp 7–22.

Feinstein, SG, 2009, *Secrets of the Teenage Brain: Research-based Strategies for Reaching and Teaching Today's Adolescents* (2nd ed), Corwin, Thousand Oaks.

Giedd, J, 2010, 'The teen brain: Primed to learn, primed to take risks' in Gordan, D (Ed), *Cerebrum: Emerging ideas in brain science*, Dana Press, New York, pp 62–70.

Howard, PJ, 2006, *The Owner's Manual for the Brain: Everyday Applications from Mind-brain Research* (3rd ed), Bard Press, Austin.

Manocha, R (Ed), 2017, *Growing Happy, Healthy Young Minds: Generation Next*, Hachette Australia, Sydney.

Medina, J, 2008, Brain Rules: 12 Principles for Surviving and Thriving at Work, Home and School, Pear Press, Seattle, Washington.

Nagel, MC, 2009, 'Mind the mind: Understanding the links between stress, emotional well-being and learning in educational contexts', *The International Journal of Learning*, vol. 16, no. 2, pp 33–42.

Nagel, MC, 2014, *In the Middle: The Adolescent Brain, Behaviour and Learning*, Australian Council of Educational Research, Melbourne.

Nagel, MC, 2012, *Nurturing a Healthy Mind: Doing what Matters Most for your Child's Developing Brain*, Exisle Publishing, Newcastle.

Nagel, MC & Scholes, L, 2016, *Understanding Development and Learning: Implications for Teaching*, Oxford University Press, Melbourne.

Ponton, LE, 1997, *The Romance of Risk: Why Teenagers do the Things they Do*, Basic Books, New York.

Sousa, D, 2009, *How the Brain Influences Behaviour*, Corwin Press Inc, Thousand Oaks.

Spear, LP, 2010, *The Behavioral Neuroscience of Adolescence*, W.W. Norton & Company, Inc., New York.

Strauch, B, 2003, *The Primal Teen: What the New Discoveries about the Teenage Brain tell us about Our Kids*, Doubleday, New York.

Walsh, D, 2004, *Why do They Act that Way? A Survival Guide to the Adolescent Brain for You and Your Teen*, Free Press, New York.

KIDS IN CYBERSPACE

4. ONLINE GROOMING AND CYBER PREDATORS

Brett Lee

This chapter outlines the strategies online child sex offenders use to lure their intended victims. It then details simple steps parents and families can take to reduce the risks in their home to virtually zero.

INTRODUCTION

Learning offender strategies and the types of vulnerabilities they prey on helps police detectives pick up the trail of child sex offenders. It requires studying profiles of typical offenders and their victims. As well as pretending to be a child online, a detective learns about predators by infiltrating groups and becoming a part of their online community. They study predators' methodology, interact in their communities, gain their trust and identify individual threats and potential victims.

What becomes obvious using this approach is that predators cannot be identified by their outward appearance. There is no profile photo of them under the description of a 'typical' child sex offender. Rather, they reveal themselves and their inward desires by the behaviours they engage in online and, in the case of the more dangerous, later in person. Someone who is scruffy looking and socially awkward in person might be totally trustworthy around children. Conversely, a quiet, neatly dressed man who heads off to an office job every day might harbour dark secrets that not even those closest to him are aware of. No particular physical-world stereotype exists that will help parents identify an online predator or child sex offender in their neighbourhood.

One of the first online sex offenders I arrested could well have been 'the guy next door'. He was a typical, conservative, clean-cut office worker who lived on his own. As often heard when apprehending similar types of defendants, he had been married once, but the marriage had not worked out.

Another offender I arrested was young, solidly built and well dressed. He was your 'average Joe'. Disturbingly, he had been studying at university to be a teacher. During investigations, detectives found online messaging between him and fellow predators, who jested, 'How can you be a teacher?' To which he responded, 'Oh, I would never do it to my own students; that would just be sick.'

And the appearance of one of the most aggressive online predators I ever encountered came as a total shock when detectives moved in to arrest him – he was seriously disfigured and got around in a wheelchair.

TYPES OF OFFENDERS

Some online child sex offenders confine their offences to gathering and distributing illegal materials over the internet, while others further the process and try to meet their victims in person. They include adults and in some cases children who – naively or with intent – create, possess, post or distribute child exploitation materials online. Regardless of their motives, their actions are criminal and punishable by law.

Online predators are usually males, although they may be pretending to be females. They come from a range of different backgrounds. They could be married or single; educated or uneducated; in high-flying jobs or unemployed; straight or gay; well spoken or gruff; physically able or disabled; in their twenties, thirties, forties, fifties or sixties. The oldest offender I encountered was in his late sixties. While I came across adult females online who could have been a direct threat to children, I never had the opportunity to establish their identities. However, women in the US have been found guilty and jailed for such crimes. Sometimes women are accomplices to male criminals. They know abuse is occurring but do nothing about it or, worse still, are coerced to take part in the crime.

Predators in the physical world often turn out to be a family member or trusted family friend. While the source of the online threat is far more varied and can even come from the other side of the world, it can still come from within a family. Complaints are made to police by parents concerned with comments or materials posted to their children by a family member or friend. They have felt their family or friends have displayed concerning behaviours on the internet.

Among the most dangerous online offenders are those who seek to meet their victims in person. They include those who are prepared to commit physical offences against children if given the opportunity and those seeking to commit offences against children specifically.

Opportunists are offenders who, while not looking to commit an online offence specifically against a child, are motivated by sexual drive and control and will offend if an opportunity arises. They may seize on an opening to groom a child for sexual purposes or expose a child to indecent material. They may be prepared, if given an opportunity, to view, post, gather and distribute child exploitation materials or to physically offend against a child.

Predators are offenders who intentionally set out to commit online offences against a child. These offences range from committing psychological harm – by grooming children, exposing them to indecent materials and coercing them to collaborate in indecent acts – to physical harm – by meeting them in person to commit offences.

A predator is more likely to offend because children are their sexual preference. Their motivation is higher, and they are prepared to take more risks. However, an opportunist is equally dangerous because of the effect they can have on their victim. Their methods and negative actions generally evolve as the offences take place and include everything the predator is prepared to do.

WHO PREDATORS TARGET

A predator may prefer to target a child of a certain age, gender, physical build, hair colour, nationality or geographical location. Predators can be very different in their focus. Some target eight- or nine-year-olds, while others think that this age group is too young or too old. Others pursue only girls or boys, while some do not care who they prey on. One of Australia's worst offenders, Dennis Ferguson, who died in December 2012, stalked and offended against babies, either boys or girls. Ferguson saw eight- or nine-year-old children as too old. Ferguson's attitude of 'I do not care; it just has to be a child' made him a very dangerous individual. It is not necessary to describe every offender's persuasion, only to say that online child sex offenders try to achieve the same sinister results online as they do in person when preying on the vulnerable and innocent.

While boys and girls are both targets of child sex offenders, girls are at greater risk because far more predators target girls.

In the physical world, to be close to children, offenders join sports clubs, drive school buses and become teachers. Sadly, society's awareness of their presence casts suspicion on most people who serve in these pastimes and occupations. Online, the big difference is that an offender can strike from anywhere in the world within seconds.

Other predators visit dating sites to look at a woman's profile and whether she has children. Chillingly, the first aspect of her profile the predator will check is whether she has children. How many? Are they boys or girls? What ages are they? If the predator's approach is 'successful', they can be invited into that family's home. Dating sites attract a lot of predators. The strategy is: 'I know that the children's mother is single and looking for someone. I know that if the relationship works, I can get into that home.'

WHAT ONLINE OFFENDERS SAY

While many predators possess common mindsets and predispositions, they can be very different in how they target children. Some come across as social networkers with wholesome everyday intentions to befriend a child and become a part of their life. Then they use subtle messages to try to obtain what they want. Other offenders are particularly aggressive and fast-moving. They are direct from the outset and communicate something like this to potential victims:

'Where are you sitting?'

'Can your mum see you?'

'Where are your parents?'

'Is the computer facing the door?'

'Is your door closed?'

'What are you wearing?'

'Have you ever touched yourself? How did you feel?'

It might sound far-fetched for someone to say this in the first ten minutes of engaging with a child on the internet; however, that is exactly what more aggressive predators do.

A normal child will most likely respond just as they would in the physical world, with something like: 'Go away; you are disgusting,' or, 'That is ridiculous'.

Then the predator will probably move on. Because so many people use technology, they can have multiple conversations in seconds until they come across a person who responds in a way they are encouraged by. Then the grooming process commences. Online investigators are exposed to these types of conversations a lot:

'I want you to touch yourself.'

'I want you to get a pen and insert it in yourself.'

'When you go to school, I want you to kiss your friend.'

When offenders use the internet to communicate these types of sinister activities, it desensitises the victim so that they become less and less shocked by the comments and materials being supplied to them. A child can tend to think that they are dealing with two-dimensional data, all the while not suspecting that they are being groomed for abuse.

Pretending to be a child online, detectives encounter every ploy imaginable from predators daily. 'Have you got a picture of yourself that I can see?' is a classic line from these people as they seek to find out as much personal information as possible.

When they establish contact initially, predators want personal information so they can make their victim real in their minds. It heightens their sexual experience to believe they are 'doing it' online with a child. They are creating a picture, a profile of their victim. This is the first basic step predators take to groom a potential victim.

CREATING FALSE IDENTITIES

The threat can come from anywhere because the internet enables predators to create false identities. What a person sees on the screen is very often not reality; it is just what has been put on the screen. A child may think they are communicating with a thirteen-year-old girl or fourteen-year-old boy, but the person on the other end may be a fifty-year-old. The child only sees what is on the screen. Thus, when educating a child about safe internet usage, it is important to remind them that what is seen is often not reality; it is just what has been put on the screen.

Child sex offenders pretend to be the perfect internet friend, the person they want a vulnerable child to think they are. In a child's mind, they also become the person that child wants them to be. There is a strong psychological effect, with the child wanting and believing them to be real. They can become more real, important and special to the child than anyone in the physical world. Adults fall for similar ploys too. The stalker is creating a false persona in line with what the victim wants them to be. That is part of being groomed online.

THE FIVE STAGES A PREDATOR FOLLOWS

Even a well-taught child is not fully equipped to take all the necessary safeguards against strangers. No child can deal with every issue or situation in the adult world. It is not about how intelligent, well balanced, mature or IT savvy they are; they simply do not possess the level of life skills or instincts adults possess. Adults look at the world through different eyes. Predators use techniques designed to break through the defences of even the best-trained children and, unfortunately, the nature of technology provides the perfect environment for them to achieve this.

I advocate that proactive parenting is the first line of defence in protecting children from predators. By the time law enforcers become involved, damage has already been done to a child's wellbeing. Parents must be vigilant at all times in looking out for their children, both in the physical world and online. Knowing the five basic stages a predator follows will help in this.

Stage One – How they identify a potential victim

Selecting a child might involve viewing their Facebook profile picture: 'That child is about ten, female, blonde ... yep, that's the type of child I would want.'

While some predators are less discriminate, they normally look for someone based on a set of criteria:

- age
- sex
- location
- build
- features (e.g. hair colour).

Most predators require some form of profile when it comes to a victim, however slight, even opportunists. It might be a preference for boys over girls. Those who require no identification profile are the most dangerous. It broadens their threat level if they just want access to any child.

Stage Two – How they gather information about the child

The predator delves into the child's life, visiting sites where they can be found. They explore what the child looks like in different scenarios through their social network photos. This makes the child more real to them.

Gathering information satisfies two main requirements of the predator. First, it makes the victim real in their minds, heightening their illegal fantasy or activity. Second, it helps them determine whether the child is susceptible to being manipulated.

Information collection can include identifying the child and where they live. These details can be gathered not only from the online activity and communications with the potential victim but also from friends' or contacts' information.

Stage Three – How they identify and begin to fill a need

'Ah, so that's what they are missing – perfect!' They take notice of what the child is talking about online and what is happening in their lives through information provided on the internet.

A young girl might feel she is not as pretty as her friends. Her low self-esteem is evident to the predator, who tunes in to her self-deprecating comments, images and posts. This gives the predator the opportunity they need to get the attention of this person. For example, they could take the opportunity to pose as a teenage boy, telling her she is the most beautiful girl he has ever seen and that she is the answer to all his prayers. The predator's strategy is to fulfil the young person's need.

The gathering of information helps the predator begin conversations that interest the victim. They begin to form an online relationship. They establish trust, credibility and rapport with their targeted victim. The child's natural defences can be lowered because the supposed anonymity of the internet gives them a false sense of security.

Arrested predators often confess to looking for an 'in' or a need in the following types of children:

- Young people who are dissatisfied with themselves and isolated from friends or family.
- Children who oversexualise themselves and readily share personal information with strangers.
- Children who try to portray themselves as being older.
- Children who act differently online than they would for their age in the physical world.

Predators have explained to me these behaviours indicate a need or that the child has low self-esteem. A child might indicate directly or indirectly that they are from a broken family and that there is no father in the home; they might need a father figure. Another child exploring self-harm might need a sympathetic shoulder to lean on. Perhaps a child and their parents are clashing in the home and an adult who finally understands is welcomed. Or a child is unhappy with their physical appearance – this covers many young people during adolescence – and welcomes compliments on how attractive they are.

A predator does not need to be told what a child's need might be. They can identify it by silently observing a child's online activity and behaviour. They watch, wait and prepare to capitalise.

After pinpointing the child's weakness, the predator is perfectly positioned to commit an offence through grooming, threats, blackmail or intimidation. Predators often get aggressive if they discover a target victim talking to someone else on the internet. 'Where have you been?' they press. 'Why have you taken so long to respond?' They become possessive and jealous.

Stage Four – How they desensitise the victim

The child's inhibitions are lowered by the predator showing them photos and videos and talking through inappropriate things online.

'Now play through this, and in just a little bit, we'll watch this' – the victim is enticed.

'You should meet me.'

'We should do sexual things.'

'All your friends are doing it; you may as well do it with me' is a ploy that makes the victim feel left behind and unimportant.

As I engaged with these predators as an online detective, I felt the force of their persuasiveness, and it revolted me to know that they thought they were destroying a child's innocence. Detectives are required to keep the computer running and the video rolling as offenders think they are performing their disgusting acts in front of young children. One of my colleagues used to keep sticky notes on hand and paste one over the explicit parts so he did not have to see it all.

Even after all this time I cannot shake some of the more explicit and disturbing images I witnessed. After viewing the depraved material predators expose a vulnerable young person to, it is inconceivable to fully understand how damaging it would be on a developing child's mind. It would not only desensitise or normalise depraved acts but it could very easily leave a permanent imprint in a child's memory. That is why this material should never be thought of as, 'That's just what children look at.'

Stage Five – How they initiate abuse

The offender explores how far they can go in subjecting the child to further online abuse, all the while capitalising on the illegal groundwork already laid. Increased online abuse often involves seeking increasingly explicit online encounters, and resorting to blackmail if the victim does not continue.

'I have got those photos and video of you from the first time. If you don't meet me and do this again and more, I am going to make sure that your parents, friends and school see those images. You will be humiliated, and get into a lot of trouble.'

The most dangerous predators initiate an interest in meeting face to face in the physical world. They may indicate they want to meet in real life and take naked photographs of the child for money.

Some are prepared to travel from another region to take photos or engage in sexual acts in exchange for monetary and other material rewards: 'I can get to your town, book a room, and you can meet me there.'

As a detective gathering evidence, predators thinking I was a child arranged to meet me in hotels, shopping centres and at railway stations. On one occasion, I arranged to meet the man in a park virtually next door to where the online investigation was being conducted.

After the filth I was exposed to in reaching that point, I took quiet pleasure in the predators' surprise when, at an arranged meet-up with their intended victim, they were confronted not by a helpless child but by a police detective with handcuffs.

FIVE CORE SAFEGUARDS IN THE HOME

If parents take the following steps in safeguarding their children, they will reduce online risks and potential issues to virtually zero.

The internet is a valuable and indispensable part of modern life. Putting the right safeguards in place in the home is not about preventing children from using technology, it is about helping them be a part of that world and making it safer for them.

Never overcomplicate the process. The rewards for following my advice will include less family conflict and avoiding the dangers and consequences other families may have to deal with.

Safeguard 1 – Parents, take charge

You are the one who controls technology and makes the final decisions.

This is not about 'mistrusting' children; it is about acknowledging that they are children, they look at the world through different eyes and may not make the choices required to stay safe. As children grow, parents can let them make choices with less guidance but ensure their choices remain consistent with family requirements. The main decisions parents need to make are:

- When technology is used.
- Where technology is used.
- What programs, apps and sites are allowable.
- Who a child can connect with.

Don't allow technology to take charge. Do not believe that a program or website's popularity, user numbers or profitability give it credibility or suitability.

Safeguard 2 – Use parental controls

Parents have a right to know where their children go and who they communicate with.

Most schools have software or programs designed to monitor online activity. They do this because they have a duty of care for students. Parents should also have systems in place. If parents whose family has been devastated by online issues could turn back time and detect a potential problem early, they tell me that of course they would use monitoring or filtering software to prevent the issue arising in the first place.

There will be those who claim this is 'spying' on children, as though parents are doing something wrong. Am I spying on my teenage daughter because I want to know where she is going with her friends on Friday night and who will be there? Of course not. I need to know this to ensure she is safe. When children become adults, they will not harbour a grudge; they will thank their parents for caring enough to monitor their activity and most likely do the same with their own children.

Parental controls work on a device or account to monitor or control information or activity. A variety of programs are available and some can be downloaded for free. Common functions include:

- Blocking concerning websites.
- Setting time limits and ensuring curfews.
- Recording websites visited.
- Recording conversations in certain programs.
- Limiting the downloading of particular apps.
- Notifying a parent of concerning activity.

If parents start using monitoring or filtering programs early, it will become a part of their child's online world. They will be accustomed to it at home, just as they can expect to encounter it at school and then in the workplace.

Warning – filtering or monitoring software should never be relied on as a total solution or a replacement for broader parental oversight.

Safeguard 3 – Stay current

Parents should increase their knowledge base as needed.

This does not mean staying current with all technology, only technology relevant to the family. Parents of five-year-old children do not necessarily need to know about Facebook yet. Staying current does not require parents to become technology experts. It involves being aware of what children generally do on the internet, and keeping up to date on:

- What devices can connect to the internet.
- When those devices are connected.
- Where kids are going online and what programs and games they are using.
- Who they are connected to.

Parents stay current by talking to their children and other adults, seeking advice or asking questions from teachers and schools, and seeking information online.

Safeguard 4 – Set rules and boundaries

These are not optional.

Parents and children have rules and boundaries in every area of their lives. Rules don't stop them having fun; they protect them from themselves and others. Parents can be confident they are making a difference by putting rules in place. Rules can be changed if it is found they don't suit. As children grow, parents should not be afraid to modify a rule, taking care not to move outside their values, beliefs, morals and ethics. Rules and boundaries provide security, letting children know where they stand.

The rules must be enforced or there is no point having them. They will not be taken as seriously if they can be continually broken or challenged. On the other hand, it is not weakness to allow a few more minutes playing a game.

General rules might include:

- Time limits and curfews.
- An understanding of what language is acceptable.
- Guidelines on where in the home technology can and can't be used.
- What websites, games and apps can be used.
- What to do if something of concern happens or a mistake is made.

Safeguard 5 – Communicate

Create an environment of openness about technology and talk about it with your kids.

This is the most important and effective safeguard against online issues. It is powerful to tell children, 'If you have a problem on the internet, or even if you make a mistake, I want you to talk to me about it and I promise I will help you solve the problem so you can keep having a good time online.'

Healthy communication about technology occurs by seizing the opportunities when they arise, such as:

- Take ten minutes each day during school drop-off or pick-up.
- If you notice an unusual facial reaction after your child looks at a screen, ask what they saw and if everything is okay.
- Have a chat around the dinner table about what's happening online.
- Direct children to and discuss media articles about technology.
- Take other times to chat to children about what is happening online.

Never underestimate the value of face-to-face communication. Research has shown that families who sit around a dinner table at least three times a week and talk are less likely to experience cyberbullying. The child ends up with a real feeling of support. If a child sex offender approaches them online and learns that their parents know about their internet usage, they will not hang around.

As children grow, the way parents communicate with them changes. When they are young, parents 'tell' them; as children move into their teens, the tone changes more to discussing, guiding and suggesting.

Parents should never stop communicating. They should continually talk to their children, other parents, friends, family and schoolteachers.

TAKE-HOME MESSAGES FOR PARENTS

- Keep internet usage out of the bedroom and out in the open.
- 'Friend' your children on Facebook and predators are more likely to leave your child alone and look elsewhere.
- Use privacy settings and predators are more likely to pass over your account.
- Posting photos that depict your child with other family members can deter a potential predator.

TAKE-HOME MESSAGES FOR TEACHERS AND SCHOOL COUNSELLORS/YOUTH WORKERS

- Youth will always rely on your life skills and instincts.
- Quality online behaviours can be instilled.
- Never underestimate the power of the screen.
- You, along with parents, are the only line of defence.
- Technology will change but our protective practices, responsibilities and beliefs stay unchanged.
- Always believe you are making a difference.

Author biography

As a former police officer and undercover internet detective, Brett Lee spent five years online pretending to be a young person to gather evidence against child predators. He frequented chat rooms and messaging programs, and was part of multiple online gaming communities. He spent thousands of hours assuming fictitious identities in social networking sites. Through his undercover work as a 'teenager', Brett arrested eighty-nine adults for their online activity. He subsequently founded training company INESS (Internet Education and Safety Services) and online training resource Internet Safe Education. The father of four now speaks to students, parents and teachers about safe and responsible internet use.

www.internetsafeeducation.com

See also:

Chapter 5: Healthy Habits for a Digital Life
Chapter 6: Online Time Management
Chapter 7: Problematic Internet Use and How to Manage It
Chapter 9: Sexting – Realities and Risks
Chapter 13: Talking to Young People about Online Porn and Sexual Images

Recommended websites:

Think U Know: www.thinkuknow.co.uk
UK Safer Internet Centre: www.safeinternet.org.uk
Child Exploitation and Online Protection UK: www.ceop.police.uk

Further reading:

Lee, B with Morris, D, 2014, *Screen Resolution – A Detective Enters the Predator's Lair Disguised as a Child*, Aurora House, Bowral, and on www.internetsafeeducation.com
Manocha, R (Ed), 2017, *Growing Happy, Healthy Young Minds: Generation Next*, Hachette Australia, Sydney.

 We also recommend the very popular companion volume **GROWING HAPPY, HEALTHY YOUNG MINDS** – resilience, bullying, depression, anxiety, body image and many more important issues.

 For more online resources visit: **generationnext.com.au/handbook**

5. HEALTHY HABITS FOR A DIGITAL LIFE

Dr Kristy Goodwin

This chapter will outline possible risks to kids' health, learning and development if screen-time isn't used in healthy and helpful ways. It will detail practical strategies that parents and educators can implement to mitigate any potential risks associated with technology (because digital abstinence is not a viable solution!).

DIGITALISED CHILDHOODS

Kids today are growing up immersed in a tsunami of screens. They're learning to tap, swipe and pinch often before they've learned to tie their shoelaces, grip a pencil or ride a bike. They're spending more and more time on digital devices and often at increasingly earlier ages too (for example, in the 1970s the average age at which children were introduced to technology was four years and in the twenty-first century it is now four months).

As parents and professionals working with young children, navigating the digital terrain is both confusing and concerning. Australian and international studies have found that kids' screen-time habits are a universal health concern for parents and professionals alike.

Raising kids in a digital world is confronting and overwhelming for many parents and professionals working with children because, unlike most other parenting conundrums faced, they have no frame of reference when it comes to the digital world. Most parents (and teachers and professionals working with families) grew up experiencing analogue childhoods, where they stared at the sky and not at screens. However, now they're raising and working with 'screenagers': children who often spend more time with pixels than with people. They're raising and teaching kids who are experiencing digitalised childhoods and this is affecting their behaviour, learning preferences and physical health and development.

Therefore, it's only logical that many parents, educators and health professionals are worried about how technology and screens are impacting on young children. In particular, fears about the amount of time children spend with screens (and what this time actually displaces in terms of developmental priorities) and potential health risks associated with screen use, as well as a raft of other concerns related to cybersafety are universal digital dilemmas facing parents, educators and health professionals.

TIME ON SCREENS

Kids are spending increasing amounts of time on digital devices. Reports suggest that many young children are spending a significant proportion of their waking hours each day with screens. Some studies have found that 40 per cent of eighteen-month-olds are spending more than two hours with screen media on a daily basis. Other studies have shown that 45 per cent of eight-year-olds and 80 per cent of Australians aged twelve to seventeen use screens more than the recommended limit of two hours per day. It's important to note that not all screen-time is toxic or unhealthy. However, too much screen-time can adversely impact kids' basic developmental or health needs (see later explanation in this chapter).

OPPORTUNITY COST OF SCREEN-TIME

The use of screens isn't necessarily an unhealthy or unhelpful activity. Research confirms that if technology is used intentionally and in developmentally appropriate ways, then there is a host of documented educational and social benefits for children (more so if children are aged over eighteen months of age).

However, excessive amounts of screen-time can derail students' health, learning and development. Put simply, too much screen-time can displace time for key developmental priorities: there's an opportunity cost associated with screen-time. For example, research confirms that excessive amounts of screen-time can erode opportunities to be physically active, engage in play and sleep.

SEVEN DEVELOPMENTAL NEEDS

As outlined in my book *Raising Your Child in a Digital Age*, neuroscience and developmental science research have consistently identified that kids have seven basic, unchanging developmental needs:

* forming relationships and attachments;
* hearing and using language;
* sleeping;
* engaging in play;
* being physically active;
* developing executive function skills (these are higher-order thinking skills and include impulse control, working memory and mental flexibility skills);
* consuming good-quality nutrition.

Too much screen-time, especially in the early years, can displace opportunities for these developmental needs to be met. This problem is amplified in the early years because, (i) young children have limited waking hours, and (ii) a significant amount of brain architecture is being established in the early years (some estimates suggest that 90 per cent of a child's neural pathways are formed in the first five years of life). However, pre-teens and adolescents are not immune from developmental risks associated with inappropriate or excessive amounts of screen-time.

HOW MUCH SCREEN-TIME IS 'SAFE' FOR KIDS?

Most parents and educators want to know if there are safe amounts of screen-time. While we do have screen-time guidelines, as outlined below, it's important to note that these guidelines haven't been empirically tested. They are based predominantly on research that has examined passive use of technology, i.e. watching television and films. The current Australian guidelines consider all screen-time as passive, non-productive time. However, advances in technologies, such as tablets and gaming consoles, have resulted in kids having access to much more engaging types of technology experiences, where children can assume a much more active and interactive role with screens.

The Australian Government's Department of Health released screen-time guidelines in 2014 in Australia's Physical Activity and Sedentary Behaviour Guidelines.

Australia's screen-time guidelines (correct at November 2016):

0–2 years old – no screen-time

2–5 years old – one hour per day

5–12 years old – no more than two hours per day

13–17 years old – should limit electronic media for entertainment to no more than two hours per day and break up long periods of sitting as often as possible.[1]

LIMITATIONS OF CURRENT AUSTRALIAN GUIDELINES

The current Australian screen-time guidelines:

- Are not based on current practices where screens are frequently used both at home and school.
- Are not grounded in current research that examines the impact of more interactive technologies.
- Are considered by many parents, educators and health professionals to be outdated and unrealistic. Studies have

shown that only 26 per cent of Australians aged two to four years met the recommended Australian screen-time guidelines of accumulating no more than one hour per day. Further, only 29 per cent of Australians aged five to seventeen years met the recommended Australian screen-time guidelines of accumulating no more than two hours per day.

- Fail to address *what* children do with screens, as well as other equally important factors such as when, where, how and with whom kids use screens. The screen-time guidelines class all screen-time as equal. However, there are obvious qualitative differences between a child spending thirty minutes creating a digital storybook on a touchscreen device and thirty minutes watching mindless and age-inappropriate content on YouTube.

Children and adolescents definitely need boundaries around how much time they can spend with screens, but it's unrealistic to suggest that parents and professionals working with children and adolescents can prescribe universal screen-time limits simply based on a child's chronological age. Parents and professionals need more comprehensive guidance when it comes to determining healthy screen-time limits.

Pleasingly, in October 2016, the American Academy of Pediatrics (AAP) revised their screen-time recommendations after mounting pressure that the existing recommendations were outdated and would become obsolete because they were unrealistic for many families.

American Academy of Pediatrics screen-time guidelines

0–18 months: No media use at all is recommended for children under eighteen months. The only exception to this recommendation is if families use Skype or FaceTime (video-chat technologies) to stay connected with one another, so long as parental support is included as part of this screen-time activity.

18 months – 2 years old: Parental co-viewing, otherwise referred to as shared media use, is strongly encouraged at this age. Where possible, children should be using and viewing media with an adult and should be using quality, educational media (and limited entertainment at this age). There are some distinctions between educational and entertainment media.

2–5 years old: Limit media use to no more than one hour per day. This is despite studies that show most preschoolers are consuming two hours a day of screen media. Again, parents should be seeking high-quality educational and prosocial media content, and should continue to co-view the media experience with their child.

6 years+: Educators and health professionals must ensure that media use does not supersede essential developmental activities like play, relationships (i.e. time with friends and family), and sleep. Parents are also encouraged to take time away from screens and engage in other (off-screen) activities with their child. The AAP suggested that children really need active media mentors who are alert, aware and involved in their children's online activities.

Parents should also consider establishing tech-free zones and times. The AAP now specifically states no media should be used one hour before bedtime and during meals (screen dinners) and in the car.[2]

HEALTH AND DEVELOPMENT IMPLICATIONS OF SCREEN-TIME

As previously stated, current Australian screen-time guidelines predominantly use time as a single metric to determine if screen-time is healthy and helpful. However, this is a simplistic approach as it disregards other essential considerations when determining if screen-time is healthy or harmful for kids and adolescents. It's essential that parents and professionals consider more than just how much screen-time children accumulate each day. To more comprehensively explore possible health and development implications associated with screen-time, parents, educators and health professionals are encouraged to also consider what, when, where, how and with whom children engage in screen-time.

WHAT ARE KIDS DOING WITH SCREENS?

Content is king. Kids' access to inappropriate content can cause emotional problems (e.g. premature exposure to and 'normalisation' of pornography). Parents and educators also need to consider if a child's screen-time is active or passive. Is screen-time being used predominantly for leisure or learning? Are kids communicating and creating with screens (which is ideal as they're cognitively engaged and assume an active role), or are they passively consuming content?

Parents need to carefully regulate and monitor exactly what content their child is creating or consuming online. This is a mammoth job for many parents, as the technology is constantly evolving and kids' technical skills and knowledge often surpass their parents', making it easy for kids to dupe them.

In recent times, anecdotal reports have revealed that children and adolescents are increasingly using deception and decoy apps. These apps, typically disguised as a calculator app, can be used like a regular calculator app, but once a pin or pattern is input, the app unlocks to reveal a private vault of photos, videos and texts. Users can also set up 'guest' vaults, containing decoy images specifically designed to be used if they suspect a parent or teacher may request to view the contents of the vault. Such apps are highly desirable in the eyes of the average tween or teenager who wants to keep their online activity a secret from their parents and/or educators.

TIPS FOR PARENTS TO SELECT APPROPRIATE CONTENT

Be specific – Parents and teachers need to establish very clear boundaries around what content is appropriate for children to view and/or create. Parents are advised to create folders on touch-screen devices with the apps that are suitable for kids of different ages to use. Parents can also create YouTube playlists of appropriate content and can pre-record TV shows or specify channels that they're happy for children to view.

Keep up to date – Parents and educators need to stay abreast of the newest apps, websites and gadgets that are geared towards young children. The not-for-profit organisation Common Sense Media, the Children's Media Foundation website and the Net Aware website all provide a range of digital tools available to guide parents and professionals trying to navigate the digital world (see resource lists at the end of this chapter).

Use filters and set up parental controls on all devices – Children can accidentally stumble on inappropriate content. Research commissioned by Family Zone found that 92 per cent of parents worry about children accessing pornography, being approached by paedophiles and accessing violent content, yet only 16 per cent have set up parental controls on internet-enabled devices. Sadly, children cannot un-see unsavoury content. Parents need to install web-filtering software and set up parental controls on all children's devices.

WHEN ARE KIDS USING SCREENS?

Parents and educators also need to think carefully about when kids use screens. Research has confirmed that the use of screens before nap or sleep time can cause sleep delays, which can accumulate into a sleep deficit.

Sleep delays

Excessive amounts of time with screens can displace opportunities for sleep. Too much time with digital devices can erode the time that's required for sleep. Many adolescents now report staying up later because they're using technology. Parents of younger children are also anecdotally reporting that children are waking up at earlier times to get their daily dose of digital (often unbeknown to their parents, who are still asleep).

Many adolescents are suffering chronic sleep delays because of their screen habits. Traditionally, the onset of puberty causes changes to adolescents' sleep habits because of changes to their production of melatonin, which is the hormone that regulates the wake–sleep cycle. This hormone is secreted by the pineal gland early in the evening in younger children, but around puberty, melatonin production is delayed until 9–10 p.m., meaning that adolescents are biologically wired to stay up later (they're not just being lazy when they want to sleep in for hours at a time). Basically, if kids' screen-time isn't carefully managed it can reduce the amount of sleep kids accumulate, and sleep is vital for overall physical and emotional wellbeing and health, as well as academic learning.

Digital devices, in particular back-lit devices like mobile phones and tablets, can delay the onset of sleep. Mobile devices emit blue light, which can hamper the body's production of melatonin. Insufficient production of melatonin can cause sleep delays. Over time, kids' sleep delays can accumulate into a sleep deficit. Therefore, screens can adversely impact on the quantity of sleep kids amass. Insufficient and/or poor-quality sleep causes a range of physical health and psychological issues and can cause learning difficulties.

The use of screens before bedtime can also have an arousal effect on the brain. In particular, rapid-fire, fast-paced screen action (like video games and some cartoons) can overstimulate the brain and also cause sleep delays. Parents and educators need to carefully monitor the type of screen content children are engaging in before sleep time.

Poorer sleep quality

The presence of digital devices in bedrooms can affect children's sleep quality. Exposure to violent or scary media is a cause for concern in terms of kids' sleep habits. Violent or inappropriate media content can increase the chances of children having problems falling asleep and/or staying asleep or having nightmares. Many families report frequent night terrors in children after they've watched inappropriate media content (such as a violent video game, scary film or distressing events reported in the media). While many parents and educators are aware of limiting kids' exposure to violent films and/or video games, it's also the prevalence of scary or disturbing images or videos that are featured on TV news programmes and distributed via social media that are a concern. Film trailers and promotions are another source of content that can be distressing for kids to consume. These concerns are amplified with children aged under eight as they're susceptible to experiencing intense fear as a result of viewing disturbing images (because they're psychologically unable to distinguish fiction from reality).

SIMPLE TIPS FOR HEALTHY SLEEP HABITS IN A DIGITAL AGE

Set a bedtime for digital devices – Ideally it would be at least ninety minutes before sleep or nap time.

Do a technology swap – Instead of banning all digital devices before sleep time, swap back-lit mobile devices for television (which doesn't typically emit as much blue light and children tend to sit much further away from televisions than mobile devices).

Be mindful of what content is consumed (or created) on devices before sleep times – Fast-action, rapid-fire input can have an arousal effect on the brain, making it more difficult for children to fall asleep quickly and easily.

Avoid scary content with children, particularly before the age of eight – It is not until approximately eight years of age that children can distinguish between fiction and reality, so scary content can terrify young children.

Implement gradual changes – If your child has developed some unhealthy sleep habits and patterns because of screen-time, gradually reduce the amount of screen-time before bed, instead of attempting to go cold turkey.

WHERE ARE KIDS USING SCREENS?

Families must establish and enforce boundaries around where technology can be used in the house. Schools also need to identify specific places and times where technology can and cannot be used in school grounds.

In addition to affecting the quantity and quality of sleep, there are also mounting concerns that digital devices are also impacting on the quality of children's sleep. Basically, kids' sleep quality is diminished if digital devices are present in bedrooms because they can interfere with children's sleep cycles. A typical sleep cycle takes approximately ninety to one hundred and ten minutes to complete. It involves four stages of non-rapid eye movement (NREM) and one stage of rapid eye movement (REM). However, due to alerts and notifications sounding, kids are now often being woken up between sleep cycles. Research has shown that children as young as nine years of age are checking mobile devices up to ten times in the night. As a direct result, kids aren't accumulating a sufficient number of sleep cycles for the brain to perform the necessary restorative and pruning functions that it's required to undertake while kids sleep. As a result, many primary-school-aged and secondary students report feeling chronically exhausted.

Recommended tech-free zones

- **Bedrooms** – Children can potentially access inappropriate or unsafe content if they're using devices in bedrooms away from parental supervision and can develop unhealthy and disruptive sleep patterns.
- **Meal areas (i.e. dinner table, breakfast bar)** – Mealtimes are critical for conversation and relationships, and screens have also been shown to change young children's eating habits and preferences.
- **Play areas** – Research has consistently shown that background TV can interfere with children's play. Ideally, play areas should be technology free to minimise possible distractions. Background music is the exception, if it's soft and familiar music for the child.
- **Cars** – Short car trips are an ideal way to communicate and informally chat with kids (without them being able to be

distracted, or escape parents' conversation). Digital distraction because of mobile devices is another media habit that we don't want to cultivate in our kids. So parents need to model healthy habits in the hope that their children emulate these habits later in life.

HOW ARE KIDS USING SCREENS?

Parents, educators and health professionals are recognising the possible impact of screens on children's physical health and development. While there's a paucity of published research in this area, anecdotal observations from educators and health professionals indicate that there are significant risks to children's vision, hearing and musculoskeletal development because of the premature introduction of screens and the increasing amounts of time that kids are spending with digital devices. Again, digital abstinence isn't the solution. Instead, families and professionals working directly with kids, or digital natives, must teach kids healthy digital habits.

Vision

Anecdotal reports from ophthalmologists and optometrists indicate that there are increasing numbers of children presenting with myopia, which is near-sightedness, and computer vision syndrome (CVS). Early exposure and increasing time spent with screens may put kids at increased risk of vision ailments. Children's screen habits place their eyes under many stressors at earlier ages and often for increasing periods of time.

The rapid adoption of tablet and mobile devices means that children are spending more time with backlit devices that emit blue light. Blue light is potentially harmful because it can penetrate to the back of the eye. Children's eyes haven't yet developed the protective pigments that enable them to filter out some of the harmful blue light.

Healthy vision tips

20-20-20-20 rule – To reduce eye fatigue it's important that children take frequent breaks when using screens. Every twenty minutes a child uses a screen, parents and educators need to encourage them to take (at least) a twenty-second break away from the screen, blink twenty times (this also helps to lubricate the eyes and prevent CVS) and look at something at least twenty feet away (approximately six metres, which helps to develop depth of vision) and do something physically active for twenty seconds (star jumps, run on the spot, stretch to help the body calibrate and reposition so no unhealthy postures are adopted).

Encourage screen-free breaks outside – These rest periods allow the eyes to reorient the focus on long-distance objects and not short-distance screens, and time in natural light is essential for healthy eye development.

Minimise glare – Glare from light sources reflecting off walls and surfaces and off screens can place greater demands on the eyes and cause eye strain. Minimise external glare by closing blinds, shutters or curtains when using screens. Avoid using digital devices in direct sunlight or directly underneath fluorescent lights.

Teach visual ergonomics – For example, teach children that the centre of a screen should be twelve to twenty-two centimetres below their horizontal line of sight and the ideal distance between eyes and screens is forty to seventy centimetres for children using computers and laptops (slightly closer for smaller screens such as smartphones and tablets).

Adjust display settings – Screen brightness should match, not compete with, the surrounding brightness of the room. Eyes should not have to struggle, squint or strain to read a screen.

Limit screen-time – Excessive amounts of time with screens are likely to have a detrimental impact on children's visual health. Enforce screen-time limits.

Hearing

Anecdotally, audiologists confirm that they're treating increasing numbers of young children and adolescents for tinnitus (ringing in the ears) and noise-induced hearing loss (NIHL), which is a permanent condition. The World Health Organization estimates that 1.1 billion people worldwide could be diagnosed with NIHL because of unsafe use of personal music devices including mp3 players and smartphones, as well as exposure to noisy entertainment venues. Many governments around the world have acknowledged that NIHL is a serious threat to children's hearing and are developing public health awareness campaigns, such as It's a Noisy Planet: Protect Their Hearing.

Symptoms of noise-induced hearing loss include distorted or muffled sound, a consistent feeling of pressure in the ear, difficulties understanding speech and/or ringing sounds in the ear in silence (tinnitus). While NIHL can occur as a result of exposure to one loud noise, it typically occurs because of repeated exposure to loud sounds over time.

One of the biggest concerns related to NIHL is children's consistent use of headphones above safe hearing levels. Research confirms that use of headphones above 75dB can cause permanent hearing loss. However, many parents and educators are shocked to learn that most commercial mp3 players can reach more than 130dB (contingent upon the model of mp3 player and brand of headphones used). It's also known that damage is cumulative, which is a potential concern as younger and younger children are now using headphones.

Healthy hearing tips

Volume control – Set maximum volume levels on devices. Many products do not allow users to set a specific decibel level, but you can set maximum levels based on what sounds suitable. Check with individual manufacturers as to how to do this.

Use noise-cancelling headphones – Children should use ear-muff-type headphones (it's not essential that they're the expensive branded headphones that tweens and adolescents will insist on purchasing) as these cancel some of the background noise, making it easier for children to listen to the music without having competing background noise.

Limit time with headphones – Where possible, limit children's time to less than an hour per day wearing headphones.

Discourage headphone use as a pedestrian – Warn children of the dangers associated with digital distractions.

Musculoskeletal development

Physiotherapists, chiropractors and occupational therapists are also anecdotally reporting increasing numbers of children presenting with musculoskeletal problems. They attribute this increase to the early introduction of screens, the amount of time children are spending with screens and the adoption of unhealthy ergonomics.

Studies have shown that more than thirty minutes of touch-screen-time per day could result in potential neck and back issues in adulthood. 'Tech neck' and 'text claw' are colloquial terms used to describe a common phenomenon, where children and adolescents are presenting with musculoskeletal problems because of excessive time and incorrect posture hunched over digital devices.

Again, banning technology isn't a viable solution. Educators, parents and health professionals need to teach children healthy digital habits and this often requires professional development and upskilling on the adults' behalf.

Tips for healthy musculoskeletal development

Encourage regular breaks (see the 20-20-20-20 rule above) – Regular tech breaks prevent children's muscles from fatiguing and they're less likely to adopt unhealthy postures if they have a break. When children get up and move about, if/when they resume using a device they'll be more likely to adopt ergonomic postures.

Teach children correct ergonomic postures – Teach children and adolescents how to adjust workstations to suit their physical needs. For example, when using laptops and desktop computers their feet should be flat on the ground and their knees and spines should be at a ninety-degree angle too. Use chairs with adjustable heights, tilts and lower-back support (or insert a cushion to provide extra support). With mobile devices like tablets and smartphones, encourage children to lie on their stomachs as this keeps their necks in a neutral position (and as an added bonus they tend to lie on their tummies for shorter periods of time than they do if sitting up, so they'll naturally reposition themselves). Another alternative with touchscreen devices is to use tear-shaped beanbags, as this allows them to bring devices to their eye level while maintaining their posture (just remember to switch the device to airplane mode first before popping it in their lap to reduce any possible risks associated with electromagnetic radiation).

Limit the weight of schoolbags carrying digital devices – Many school-aged children are now carrying tablets and/or laptops in school bags. As a general rule, children shouldn't be expected to carry bags that are more than 10 per cent of their body weight. So it's important that parents and educators monitor the weight of kids' school bags and make adjustments where necessary.

WITH WHOM ARE KIDS USING SCREENS?

Research has consistently shown that co-viewing, or joint-media engagement, can enhance educational outcomes when using most forms of technology. Using technology with someone, either a parent, sibling or peer, ensures that kids get the most out of their screen-time and it can also prevent the 'digital zombie' effect (where children enter the psychological state of flow and become entranced with what's on the screen).

Tips for managing with whom kids use screens

Encourage co-viewing – Where possible, encourage children to use screens with someone else.

Know who they're interacting with online – Parents and educators need to have specific boundaries around who kids are allowed to interact with online. Cybersafety dangers mean that kids are often divulging private or sensitive information to strangers. If they're playing multiplayer games, parents must ensure that they know who are the other gamers involved in the game.

CONCLUSION

In summary, technology will not disappear and it's not a phase that children and adolescents are experiencing. Whether we love it or loathe it as adults, we have to acknowledge that technology is here to stay. Parents, educators and health professionals need to teach children and adolescents healthy, helpful and sustainable technology habits. This will equip them with the necessary skills and habits that will ensure that their health, wellbeing, learning and development won't be compromised by screens. Digital abstinence or fear-mongering about the potential harmful effects associated with screens is not the solution. Instead, we need to share research-based information with parents and professionals to empower them to make informed decisions about how to best use technology with kids.

TAKE-HOME MESSAGES FOR PARENTS

- Establish healthy media habits from a young age.
- Enforce media habits consistently so your child understands and respects your parameters.
- Have ongoing conversations about your child's use of technology, so it's not perceived as toxic or taboo.
- Parental involvement is critical in ensuring your child benefits from technology.
- Role model healthy media habits as an adult.

TAKE-HOME MESSAGES FOR TEACHERS AND SCHOOL COUNSELLORS/YOUTH WORKERS

- Remind students about healthy technology habits.
- Focus on what, when, with whom, where and why kids use screens and not exclusively on how much time they're spending with screens.
- Consider what's the 'value-add' of using screens.

TAKE-HOME MESSAGES FOR HEALTH PROFESSIONALS

- Help families to create a media management plan that addresses what, when, where, with whom and how much time kids spend with media.
- Stress the importance of developing and maintaining healthy media habits from a young age to protect children's vision, hearing and musculoskeletal development.
- Reiterate to parents the critical role they play in modelling healthy media habits.

Author biography

Dr Kristy Goodwin is a leading digital parenting expert (and mum who also has to deal with her kids' techno-tantrums!). She's the author of *Raising Your Child in a Digital World*, a speaker, researcher and media commentator with a gift for translating research into practical and digestible information for parents, educators and health professionals.

www.drkristygoodwin.com

See also:

Recommended websites:

The Children's Media Foundation: www.thechildrensmediafoundation.org

Net Aware: www.net-aware.org.uk

Internet Matters: www.internetmatters.org

UK Safer Internet Centre: www.safeinternet.org.uk

Further reading:

Goodwin, K, 2016, *Raising Your Child in a Digital World*, Finch Books, Sydney.

Manocha, R (Ed), 2017, *Growing Happy, Healthy Young Minds: Generation Next*, Hachette Australia, Sydney.

Steyer, J, 2012, *Talking Back to Facebook*, Scribner, New York.

 We also recommend the very popular companion volume **GROWING HAPPY, HEALTHY YOUNG MINDS** – resilience, bullying, depression, anxiety, body image and many more important issues.

 For more online resources visit:
generationnext.com.au/handbook

6. ONLINE TIME MANAGEMENT

Tena Davies

To help young people manage time online, I recommend taking a balanced and collaborative approach. This involves setting boundaries in collaboration with young people and empowering them with tools to help self-manage their time online.

INTRODUCTION

Globally and across Australia, managing a young person's time online can be problematic for parents, with 55 per cent reporting that they attempt to limit their children's amount of time online or restricting what times children can go online. A further 65 per cent report that they have 'digitally grounded' their teen by taking away their mobile phone or internet access.[1]

In my experience working across independent and government schools in Australia, the most pressing issue for parents regarding their children's cyber use is managing their time online. This is not surprising given how frequently young people use the internet, which is estimated to be more than three times per day for most Australian teens aged fourteen to fifteen. This is due in large part to smartphone ownership. Young people are also online late into the night, with 28 per cent of fourteen- to fifteen-year-olds going online after 10 p.m.[2]

What may be surprising, given how much young people resist having their online time restricted by their parents, is that they feel themselves that wasting time online is a major issue. When I survey secondary-school-aged children, they rate wasting time online instead of doing homework or sleeping as the most pressing issue facing them regarding the internet. In my surveys, more than 85 per cent of students typically state that wasting time online interferes with their ability to sleep and do homework. Students rate social media as the biggest time waster, noting that they spend an average of three-plus hours across social media platforms.

The impact of wasting time online is significant. Students report that it leads to them feeling anxious about looming homework. Parents report that attempting to manage their children's time online is a major source of conflict.[3]

HOW TO MANAGE A YOUNG PERSON'S TIME ONLINE

Managing time online is not a simple matter and it is one that will be different in each household. I recommend that families sit down together and discuss how their cyber use is impacting them both positively and negatively across important life domains: friends, family, the internet, school, and any other important areas such as sport. The solutions should aim to reduce the negative aspects of the internet and appreciate and respect the positives that it brings.

Your role as a parent should ideally be to act as a media mentor by providing your child with tools and guidelines to regulate their use. However, it is also important to 'parent' the internet in the same way that you may parent other areas of your child's life, by putting in reasonable boundaries and moderating consequences if your child is not displaying good self-regulating skills.

When discussing your child's internet use, make sure to keep an open mind. The digital world is an important source of social contact for young people. They use the internet to maintain and extend relationships with their peers. When we were growing up we used to talk on the phone or hang out at the local café. Nowadays, social media is the virtual hangout. Therefore, spending time online represents an important way of connecting with peers but it does need to be managed. The expression 'fire is a good servant and a poor master' also applies to internet use.

A CASE STUDY

Rose and Tom were frustrated with their children's cyber use. It seemed that they were always either on their smartphones or iPads. Claire, aged twelve, went to bed with her iPhone under the guise that she needed it as an alarm in the morning. Carl, sixteen, was about to start GCSEs and seemed to be playing online games more and more frequently. He played online games in his room and often went to bed after midnight.

Rose and Tom had tried a number of things to attempt to manage their children's cyber use. They 'grounded' Claire and Carl frequently but this seemed to make things worse and escalated into screaming fights. They would try to take their children's devices from them but this never lasted long and led to family discord. Rose and Tom tried to reason with their children, explaining why their online use was bad for them. Each had practically begged their children to stop using their devices late at night. Often they put in place consequences such as no media for a week, but this was impossible to enforce.

When they came to my office they were at a loss as to what to do and asked if I could please try to reason with their children. I noticed that they were stuck in a cycle of escalating consequences.

What struck me about this case was that although Rose and Tom were competent parents, they didn't seem to 'parent' their children's cyber use in the way they would other areas of their children's lives. Instead, they pleaded with their children to be more sensible. They swung between being overly permissive with their children's cyber use (playing video games and playing on phones late at night) and being overly authoritarian by putting in place harsh consequences, which invariably led to fighting, and which they didn't stick to anyway.

As a first step, I asked the family to come in for a meeting. I asked the family how spending time online helped them achieve their goals across important areas of their lives including friendships, family, school and health. I also asked how their cyber use was negatively impacting each area of life.

The kids noted that it was useful to use the internet to connect with their peers and do some of their homework. They also noted that they probably spent too much time on social media and that after a certain point it was *not* useful, especially late at night. Claire noted that spending too much time online kept her from exercising, which was important to her. Rose and Tom noted they both spent too much time playing on their own phones and too much time fighting about the internet as a family. I asked each family member to come up with a few guidelines to address the issues.

Claire said she would do all of her homework before catching up with her friends online, but predictably this only lasted one day. Carl said he wouldn't fight with his parents but that lasted less than one day! I find that this is common with young people, who sometimes devise well-intended and idealistic solutions that are difficult to implement.

After their initial attempts, over the course of a few weeks I met up with Rose and Tom as well as the family as a whole. I met with the parents to give them tools to 'parent' their children's cyber use. I also made some suggestions for Carl and Claire to experiment with so that they could learn to self-regulate their cyber use.

In the end, we focused on a few simple things. The first was to ensure that cyber use did not interfere with sleep, academic achievement and important family time. The family agreed as a whole to no screen-time during family mealtimes, which were about thirty minutes' duration. The second was to stop using devices at 10 p.m. and wind down for sleep. The trade-off for this for the kids was that the parents would respect their need to connect with peers and have fun online. The rules would also be relaxed during the school holidays. Finally, and this took more work, the kids agreed to use productivity software to ensure their homework got done three nights a week. Carl, who played multiplayer games, agreed to three no-game nights provided he wasn't nagged about it on other nights. Each child also agreed to undertake one face-to-face activity. Claire started taking a yoga class after school that she also followed on Instagram, and Carl joined the local gym.

With Carl and Claire, I worked through what they thought was a fair consequence for non-compliance. They said that if they didn't hand over their phones at 10 p.m. they had to hand them over an hour earlier the next night. They also said that if their grades slipped they knew they would have to revisit their agreement.

Following are some points for managing cyber use with adolescents:

- **Start by asking them how the internet is both enhancing and hindering their life** in important areas such as friends, family, relationships, and their health and wellbeing. Then see if your solutions can reduce the negatives without significantly compromising the positives. An example would be handing over the phone to parents at 10 p.m. on weeknights during the school term so that they can prepare for sleep. This gives them ample time to socialise before going off the grid. Ensure the solution is sensible, workable and one that can be enforced.
- **Aim for reasonable use:** ask them what they think this is. My experience is that young people usually suggest something idealistic such as using it for one hour after doing their homework. Unfortunately, this is not realistic. However, asking them what they think is a good way of engaging them and getting the ball rolling is. When adolescents suggest an unrealistic amount of screen-time, I help them to work out a more realistic solution together.
- **Aim for incremental change:** If your child has until now stayed online until midnight, saying 'no screen-time after 8 p.m.' may not work. Instead, wind it down one or two hours. Then reassess.

- **Focus on time offline rather than restricting time online:** Think about what times are important to be away from technology. The times I think are important are family mealtimes and an hour or so before bed as this assists with winding down to go to sleep.
- **Have periods where rules are more flexible:** Relax rules on weekends and also school holidays and, if possible, even some weeknights. This makes for fewer fights but it also makes for more compliant kids.
- **Balance time online with offline activities:** A great way to get your child offline is ensure they are engaged in an offline activity such as sport or another hobby. Team sports are particularly good because they are active and teach social skills to interact in a group.
- **Model the behaviour you want to see:** How often do you go to a café and see couples and families playing on their phone rather than connecting with each other? It's very common that we are slaves to our devices. However, it's difficult to enforce rules if we are not ourselves living by them. If you want your child to talk to you during dinner, leave your phone away from the dinner table.
- **Focus on the big issues:** Sleep loss is a common issue for adolescents. They tend to go to bed late and wake up early to go to school. Sleep loss has a number of consequences. In addition to young people being tired, poor sleep leads to difficulty with concentration, memory and their ability to learn. This in turn leads to worse outcomes for their learning.[4]
- **Give small consequences rather than issuing big threats:** Agree with your child two or three consequences for non-compliance. Make sure they are limited to one day. For example, for the rule *no phone after 10 p.m.*, if they give you the phone late, deduct that time from the next day.
- **Have as few rules as possible (within reason):** Aim to have no more than three or so rules about cyber use. The rules

I highly recommend are: no screen-time thirty minutes before bed; no playing violent online games (or at least limiting this significantly on weekdays); and using productivity software to get work done.

- **A little less conversation, a little more action:** One of the unhelpful behaviours many of us engage in (myself included) is spending too much time trying to reason with children. We often start off reasonably and end up lecturing or worse. We might say something like: 'We discussed this yesterday and we agreed that you are not to go to bed with your phone. I'm really disappointed in you, if you keep this up I'll cancel your mobile plan and you won't have a phone at all! I should never have bought you a phone. You are so ungrateful!' Notice how as the 'reasoning' goes on it escalates and also notice how there is no consequence, just a lecture and an often empty threat. A better way to go is to agree a consequence with a child for non-compliance of a rule ahead of time, then enforce the consequence when needed without a lecture. It would look something like this: 'Claire, we discussed this and agreed that you'd give me your phone at 10 p.m. It's 10.15 p.m. and you are still on it. Please give me your phone. As discussed, your consequence is that tomorrow night you need to give me your phone fifteen minutes early.' Then take the phone and walk out. No conversation, just action. Be sure to follow through the next night. The fewer the consequences, the better.
- **Implement a no-screen night:** Whether once a week or once a month, having a technology-free night is a great way to reconnect (pardon the pun) with the family. Be sure that you plan something fun like going for a walk or out for ice-cream, or stay in and play board games. Reflect on how the night went and try to implement on a smaller scale at other times (i.e. the *hour of no power* twice a week).

TIPS FOR ADOLESCENTS

- **Use technology to self-regulate time online.** There are many types of productivity software available to download as apps onto smartphones and laptops. The one I use is called Focus Keeper but there are many other types available. A search on Google/ Google Play/iPhone app store will reveal many options.
- **One thing at a time.** Alternate blocks of work with blocks of socialising. While it would be a good idea to do all your homework before socialising, it may not suit you. If that doesn't suit, spend some time doing only homework and then spend another period of time socialising. Trying to do both means that you won't be able to do either well. You can alternate thirty minutes of work with fifteen minutes of socialising. You'll still get more work done than if you try to multitask.

DON'TS FOR PARENTS

Don't set rules you can't enforce. While it may be tempting to say things like 'Don't get a [insert latest social media craze] account', the reality is that your child is likely to do it anyway. Instead of saying, 'Don't get Snapchat', discuss some conduct rules and ensure they are using their privacy settings appropriately. I'd rather say yes and be involved in setting parameters than say no and have the behaviour go underground where I'd have no influence.

Don't set yourself up for a fight. If you go in frustrated, saying something like 'Why are you still on your phone? You are such a problem!' this makes your young person either tune out or respond in kind. Instead, set up a time to talk when you are both calm.

Don't have too many rules. When rules go on and on, adhering to them becomes difficult. I'd have a limited number of rules and one or two consequences for non-compliance instead.

Don't be digitally clueless. One of the things I hear most when working with young people is that their parents have no idea about their cyber world. The problem with this is that it is very difficult to parent what you don't know. So my advice is to be on whatever your children are using so that you can have meaningful conversations with your child about it. After all, good teaching starts with learning your subject matter.

FREQUENTLY ASKED QUESTIONS

I can't take my child's phone away from them at night because they need it as an alarm to wake them up in the morning.
Getting enough sleep is essential for your child's mental health, wellbeing and ability to learn. Viewing bright visual displays at night increases alertness and does not set them up for sleep.

If they need an alarm, buy them one. The sleep battle is one worth fighting.

I can't get my child offline late at night because they are doing homework. Is there anything I should do?
Chances are your child is doing homework at 11.30 p.m. because they were too busy socialising online earlier in the evening. I'd negotiate with your young person about how they might start homework earlier in the night. For example, by doing thirty minutes of homework as soon as they get home to get things rolling. Then they can alternate work blocks and social blocks. Often once they start they will be less prone to procrastinate throughout the night. Productivity software may also help (Google will reveal many options). It may also be useful to speak to your child's year level coordinator to determine how much homework they have and how much they need the internet for this.

My child plays multiplayer games that go for hours. How can they balance this and their studies?
This is certainly a challenging one. What I'd suggest is that they have alternating game and non-game nights. This way they can enjoy their gaming and also their studies. If they prove that they are unable to balance this in a reasonable way, I would consider banning the games during the week over the school term.

WHEN TO WORRY

I think the biggest red flag is a significant change of behaviour and a child who withdraws from life. For example, if a child who regularly used social media to connect with peers suddenly says she is closing all of her accounts, this may indicate something is wrong. This suggests that they have had an adverse experience, such as bullying. Or a child who previously loved sport now spends most of his time in his room playing a multiplayer game. If you find yourself saying, 'They used to play soccer/love music/spend time with the family', that's a sign that they may be withdrawing from life. Have a calm conversation with your young person or seek professional advice from a registered adolescent psychologist. See British Psychological Society (www.bps.org.uk) to find a trained psychologist in your area.

Author biography

Tena Davies is a Melbourne-based psychologist and cyber expert. She has recently completed a Clinical Psychology Master's degree with a thesis on parenting the internet. She works with young people and families to help support a young person's cyber wellness.
www.tenadavies.com

See also:
Chapter 1: Understanding Teen Sleep and Drowsy Kids
Chapter 3: Understanding the Teenage Brain
Chapter 5: Healthy Habits for a Digital Life
Chapter 7: Problematic Internet Use and How to Manage It
Chapter 8: Computer Game Addiction and Mental Wellbeing
Chapter 14: Advice for Parents: Be a Mentor, Not a Friend

Recommended websites:
Pew Research Center: www.pewinternet.org
US Natinal Sleep Foundation: www.sleepfoundation.org
UK Sleep Council: www.sleepcouncil.org.uk

 For more online resources visit:
generationnext.com.au/handbook

7. PROBLEMATIC INTERNET USE AND HOW TO MANAGE IT

Dr Philip Tam

This chapter will describe practical, useful ways for a concerned family member or parent of a child with suspected internet-related problems to begin to assess the situation. It will also be of assistance to a non-specialist clinician or youth-health worker in the appraisal and formulation of a case of Problematic Internet Use (PIU) in a teenager or a child.

INTRODUCTION

Problematic Internet Use, also commonly dubbed 'internet addiction' or 'video game addiction', first emerged as a novel clinical disorder in the mid-1990s, initially described in North America and then in Europe and East Asia. Over the next two decades, possibly in association with the marked rise and spread of computers and internet-related technologies, there was a major increase in the clinical recognition of the phenomenon, especially in younger people, with specially designed 'internet addiction treatment centres' emerging to treat clients in many countries. There has also been a steady rise in international research interest into the phenomenon, with many thousands of research papers having been published on the broad topic of 'internet psychology' to date and numerous scientific journals dedicated to publishing research in this field.

Successful and effective treatment of a person with suspected PIU is dependent on the clinician accurately and sensitively assessing the young person, taking into account underlying social, personality and mental wellbeing factors, and appreciating his or her internet usage is a complex and ever-changing phenomenon. Practical methods and strategies to assist this assessment process are outlined in this chapter.

ASSESSMENT OF PROBLEMATIC INTERNET USE: GENERAL PRINCIPLES

The first clinical reports of a new and potentially serious disorder emerged in the mid-1990s in North America, led by Professor Kimberly Young and others, and subsequently in other regions, most notably East Asia. In the following two decades there was a major emergence of research interest into this disorder globally, which coincided with it becoming increasingly recognised as a challenging mental health problem in young people, to the extent that it is currently regarded as a significant public-health concern in countries such as China and South Korea. Active debate also continues in clinical and research communities as to whether PIU should be classified as a mental disorder in its own right.

One key observation to emerge in the research around the world is that PIU is very strongly associated with a range of underlying mental health, social, or family-based problems.[1] Indeed, PIU may better be considered as a complex 'end-point behaviour' of a whole range of pre-existing disorders or conditions, rather than as a disorder in its own right, and it is this perspective that will underpin the chapter about assessment and appraisal of a young person presenting with internet or computer-related problems. It is well established that many other addictive behaviours, such as alcoholism or pathological gambling, also arise as a result of underlying issues such as depression, anxiety or personal problems. Thus, it is clear that taking a very thorough, sensitive and holistic assessment is needed to fully appreciate all the complexities in the young person.

An important initial question to be answered is: how do we define what problematic internet use actually is? A useful, practical definition is that PIU is the pervasive, long-term usage by a person of internet, computer and related technologies (ICT), which results in a clinically significant impact in that person's daily functioning or role/expectation, and which persists despite efforts in the person, or in the social circle, to reduce that usage. A key point in this definition is that in order to have the disorder, there needs to be a significant impact on the young person's roles – these would commonly include his or her commitments to school activities and studies, sleeping patterns, having family meals together, and taking regular exercise. Looking at this another way, if the young person is using the computer in a positive, goal-focused and controlled way – even if it is for many hours throughout the day – as long as they maintain those other responsibilities, then they would not have a disorder. It is also clear that PIU, in common with many other mental health problems, follows a spectrum of severity from mild to moderate to severe. This aspect will be explored more fully in a subsequent section.

THE 'SEVEN DEADLY SIGNS': WHAT FAMILIES SHOULD LOOK OUT FOR

How do concerned parents go about determining whether their son or daughter may be developing an internet- or gaming-related problem, and how might they begin to tackle it? A key starting point is that there will probably be early warning signals that indicate a problem may be developing. I call them the 'Seven Deadly Signs' that all parents should be on the lookout for:

1. Playing computer games, or spending time on the web, for longer and longer periods over successive weeks or months.
2. Going online as soon as the person wakes up.
3. Neglecting daily family routines or responsibilities, such as household chores, daily hygiene or homework.

4. Minimising, or overtly lying about, their time spent online when confronted by a family member with concerns about their excessive usage.
5. Getting irritable, angry or even aggressive towards those family members if their ICT usage is blocked or curtailed – such as by confiscating their device or installing time-limiting software.
6. A drop over time in the young person's grades at school, their ability to concentrate in class or on a homework assignment.
7. A noticeable decline in 'real world' activities, such as sports or hobbies, or going and seeing friends for general play.

Of course, every person will differ in the exact characteristics he or she shows, but my clinical experience indicates that whether the person is in primary or high school, if they show four or more of the above signs, and if these persist or worsen over a period of time, then parents should be taking steps to address the situation.

COMMON MYTHS AND MISCONCEPTIONS

For a phenomenon that has only been with us for no more than two decades, a surprising number of false beliefs and myths seem to have arisen around the concept of PIU. Here are some of the most common, with suggestions for concerned families on how to approach them.

'It's a passing phase that my child will grow out of.' While this may have been true in the past, parents must be aware that the world of the internet and computer gaming is essentially limitless and unending: though their child may get bored of one specific game or website, there are always many more to choose from and visit. Furthermore, parents must be aware that websites and especially social networking sites and computer games are intentionally designed to keep users entertained with new information, updates and challenges, to keep them coming back.

'My child will get left out if they don't keep up with technology.'
Again, it is true that younger generations do expect and indeed demand that they are constantly connected and using the latest devices, but parents must resist the temptation to 'keep up with the iPhoneses' and to set limits on sensible, balanced use at an early stage.

'Violent video games won't affect my child negatively.'
There is increasing evidence that, when played to excess, violent video games can affect a person in their 'real life', to extents such as increased risk of anxiety, of anger problems and even aggression. This is especially the case in vulnerable young people, such as those experiencing a mental disorder, low self-esteem or family stresses.

'Giving them my device is a great way to calm them down.'
Particularly relevant to younger children and even toddlers, the phenomenon of using digital devices as a 'pacifier' should be discouraged. It should not be used in place of sensible, old-fashioned support and structure setting by an engaged parent. It risks the child becoming dependent on a device to regulate their emotions and behaviours, rather than learning over time to calm down themselves.

'I can trust my child to be sensible and responsible in their usage.' While learning self-moderation is an important part of healthy development, parents must be aware that all children lack the self-restraint and self-reflection skills that many adults take for granted; many simply will not be able to resist the many temptations that digital devices offer and will use them excessively without realising it.

THE IMPROVE TOOL: AN ASSESSMENT RESOURCE FOR FAMILIES

To assist concerned parents and families in the challenging task of assessing how much of a problem their child may have, I have put together a simple, easy-to-use resource: the IMPROVE tool.

I: Take an Internet Inventory. This refers to the collecting of data on how much time is spent online or on the computer, what activities are being done, and what time of day (or night) this is occurring – a bit like a detailed diary of all usage. This could be done over, for example, a seven-day period so it can capture usage on a school day, as well as the weekend. More details on the Inventory are given below.

M: Monitor over time. For most of us, digital habits come and go: some specific games of choice get replaced by new ones, and visited websites also go in and out of favour. It is thus important to collect accurate data on how these habits change over time in the young person. Redoing the process about three to four months after the initial inventory is recommended, to allow any major habit changes to be fully formed. This may seem like a lot of work, but it is important for any future treatment plan, and to be able to see if the problem is worsening over time.

P: Parenting factors. Family and parenting factors, both positive and negative, have been shown to play a part in the development of PIU. For example, data could be collected on parenting styles seen at home, if there is consistency or inconsistency between parents, or recent tensions or upheavals. Parents may also be able to assess any role in enabling excessive internet use at home, for example, by being online themselves a lot and not setting a good example, or by buying the child the latest devices or games, without an agreement over sensible usage at home.

R: Real-world activities. This refers to the collection of information on the young person's sporting activities and other social interactions and interests (in the offline world). It is very important to consider these in detail, as increasing internet usage can negatively impact on these real-world activities over time. Having an adequate amount of external activities, interests and friendship groups has been shown to be correlated with having a healthy mental wellbeing.

O: Other (mental health) factors. It is well established that having other mental health conditions or disorders can impact on the development of PIU. Though parents may not feel qualified to make a specific clinical diagnosis in their child, noting the possibility of any mental health concerns will be useful.

V: recent Vulnerability factors. As well as mental health conditions noted above, recent stresses and strains in the young person's life may be relevant to PIU development. For example: have they experienced any bullying (both online or offline); have there been major arguments or significant losses, or have there been perceived 'failures' in a school test or sporting endeavour? All these events can affect a person's self-esteem, and predispose them to PIU.

E: External help needed? By this stage in the IMPROVE process, it should be clear if, or by how much, the young person is affected by PIU. A reasonably informed judgement can then be made as to whether external, professional assistance is now indicated, or if the family members themselves feel confident to address and tackle the problem without help.

WHEN SHOULD A PARENT REFER TO A HEALTH PROFESSIONAL?

As mentioned, every young person with a developing or an established problem around technology overuse will have a unique set of presenting features, but there are some simple observations which may indicate that a referral to a mental health professional is now advised. Such professionals include clinical psychologists, child psychiatrists and the school counsellor. As well as the Seven Deadly Signs and the IMPROVE process, these behaviours may include:

- When confronted by a family member, a refusal in the affected young person that they do indeed have an issue needing intervention (i.e. being 'in denial').
- Acting angrily or very defensively when confronted by family.
- The presence of another mental health problem, such as depression, anxiety or low self-esteem.
- A sudden or marked change in the person's personality, social life or other domain.

If the young person does get referred to a specialist, the findings from the IMPROVE tool, as well as any other observations, will be very useful when that specialist makes their assessment and treatment plan.

In my clinical experience, the biggest hurdle in assisting a young person with PIU is his or her marked resistance to accepting professional help. The possible causes of this resistance are many and varied, and indeed such avoidance is commonly seen in other psychological conditions such as depression, eating disorders and anger problems. Below I expand on the topic of how to build and maintain professional rapport and connection in a dedicated section.

ASSESSMENT PRINCIPLES FOR HEALTH PROFESSIONALS

Assessing the young person, the family and their social circle

It is suggested that the initial clinical assessment consist of two, and possibly three, main components. First, all family members, where possible, should be interviewed together. This will allow details on the problem list and the history to be obtained from all members, including the client, to build up an accurate and sophisticated picture of the issues and how they have impacted on the family system. A joint interview is also useful in allowing observation of the family interactions: how they communicate; what tensions or difficulties there might be and between which members; how they each deal with difficulties and challenges – such as the presenting problem, internet use behaviours.

It will also allow a detailed exploration, involving all family members, of areas such as daily routines (sleep, appetite and food intake, household duties) in the client, which could be incorrectly obtained if the therapist relies on the client alone for this history.

Second, individual interview time with the client is important. Children and teenagers are often reluctant to open up fully in front of family members, especially about personal issues, and this should be acknowledged at the outset of assessment. This part of the interview is often where symptoms and signs of any mental illness or personal stress are revealed. It is also a suitable point to obtain details on the client's interests, social groups, activities and sports/exercise participation – what might be termed their 'social capital'. Particular emphasis should be placed on how their ICT use and overuse might have directly impacted on this 'social capital' domain.

Finally, if time allows, interviewing parent(s) without the client can provide useful background information that family members might not have been comfortable in discussing during the whole-family interview. This may include relationship issues, extended-family mental illness concerns, or information on the client's development or their current problematic behaviour patterns. It also provides an opportunity to assess the parenting style or styles that the client is exposed to, and if there are any inconsistencies or tensions between the parenting styles.

The use of structured questionnaires and surveys

Since the initial descriptions of PIU, a wide range of surveys and questionnaires have been developed to assist in the diagnosis and treatment of clinical cases, as well as in facilitating research projects in the domain. Most of these take the form of a relatively brief set of questions or items (between eight and forty or so) that are completed by the client without the need for guidance or assistance from a health professional. While such surveys are useful to act as a screening tool when looking for the presence of a disorder, and very helpful when conducting research studies into how common the problem is in the general population, they should not be used to make a diagnosis or to decide on a treatment plan on their own. Put another way, PIU – especially in younger people – is a highly complex and multi-faceted disorder that will require a holistic, thorough and empathic history-taking process to explore properly. It cannot be reduced to a simple score on a brief questionnaire, some of which only focus on a specific domain of internet usage, for example, online gaming. Another risk in using a questionnaire without an adequate history-taking process is that the clinician could miss important underlying mental health or family factors relevant to the situation.

One area where standardised questionnaires may be useful, however, would be in monitoring progress in treatment: the client could repeat the survey once therapy has been taking place, to see if scores improve and the client is getting better. Most surveys available for clinicians and researchers were developed for use in young adults and teenagers; it is thus recommended that they not be used at all in the assessment and treatment of children under twelve.

Gender and age-related considerations

Two aspects of the client need some specific consideration in the assessment process: the gender of the person being assessed, and their age. Though the general approach and structure of the interview and assessment should not differ markedly whether the client is male or female, there may be some differences in the patterns of computer and internet usage that the therapist should be aware of during the assessment. The most common and prominent difference – as has been shown by international research – is that boys tend to favour online gaming as the most common ICT activity, and girls enjoy social media and networking. However, in recent years there has been something of a convergence in the differences in activity, with an increasing number of girls enjoying fantasy and action games, and boys utilising social media at a greater frequency. Another key point is that, in general, boys (and males overall) appear to have higher rates of severe PIU than females, and are thus more likely to present to the clinic. This may be related to the specific characteristics of internet-based gaming, where commitments within a game event can take many hours to complete, especially if played as a team. Some studies have shown that young males have up to double the rate of PIU than a comparable population of females.

The other consideration is the age of the client. Broadly speaking, a primary-school-aged child (corresponding to the ages of five up to twelve) will require a differing approach to that of a teenager in high school. It is likely that, in the former case, more of the emphasis of the assessment goes towards the whole-family segment of the interview as a child may show less insight into his or her behaviour, may be reluctant to fully engage, or may simply not fully recall specific details of the history. With a teenaged client, more focus will be on the individual time, as self-reflective capacity, especially with an older teen, is likely to be better. On occasion, a teenager may present on their own for assessment and may decline any involvement of their parents and family in the process; within the bounds of safety and risk appraisal (for example, risk of suicide or risk of harm to others), this request should be accommodated by the therapist.

Building and maintaining a healthy and positive 'clinical rapport' between the therapist and client can, at times, be challenging, particularly when enquiring about personal aspects in their life, both online and offline. Specific strategies to improve rapport are outlined in a following section.

Taking an 'Internet Inventory'

The taking of a detailed internet, computer and gaming-device usage history in the client – what will be termed here the 'Internet Inventory' – is a very important aspect of the assessment process. Clearly, this is of particular importance in school-aged children, who, more than adults, require the clear framework of a daily timetable to allow them to attend school, sleep healthily, engage in family activities, and so on. It would also be relevant to note which specific activities are undertaken online, e.g. gaming, social networking, online shopping or gambling. This is important as different activities undertaken on the web may require differing treatment approaches – for example, tackling excessive online shopping, compared with computer-games playing. Most of the formal research has been done specifically on computer and internet-based gaming, but there is an increasing appreciation that other forms of internet activities can also show the potential to become addictive, e.g. online shopping, social networking, online gambling, and even obsessively viewing videos or collecting online data and information. There is now research being done to investigate those types of activities, most notably gambling, which of course has already had an extensive 'pre-internet' existence.[2]

It is important to map out in as much detail as possible the landscape of screen-based activity. It is not just the total number of hours spent through the day on ICT that is important, it is when in the day or night this usage takes place – for example, does it encroach on mealtimes, on periods when the child should be asleep, doing homework assignments, or even at school? A simple method of tabulating this activity through the day would be having sections for morning, afternoon, evening and, if relevant, nighttime. Similarly, an Inventory should be taken for school-day usage patterns (in the late afternoon and evening, when back at home), and for patterns at the weekend.

Where possible, all online and console-related activities (across all types of devices) that are engaged in by the young person should be tabulated, including the time spent on each one. Screen-based time that is directly related to schoolwork or school assignments, or to employment requirements, such as résumé preparation or researching jobs, should not be included.

The period over which ICT usage is tabulated should not be too lengthy, and should be decided with the young person and their family during the assessment: a two-week period is suggested, which would include two weekends and a representative number of school days.

The Inventory may be gathered in a number of ways, dependent on the situation within the family and the perceived severity of the behaviours. A self-report diary may be of use in less severe cases but this would require a commitment on the part of the young person to regularly complete it, as well as a level of honesty and openness. Another method of gathering data may be through a diary completed by an external observer, such as a parent or carer. This will likely be the preferred method when assessing a younger child who is still in primary school. This method may also lessen the potential for usage under-reporting or even avoidance; a potential negative aspect with this method is that the external observer could be seen as intrusive, even annoying, to the child. Furthermore, being made aware of being monitored and observed through the day could impact on the very behaviours being examined – for example, time spent on gameplay could be reduced by the subject in order to present as less affected by the internet addiction problem. An objective, and potentially much more accurate and representative, method would involve the installation of a web- and computer-use monitoring software package or app. However, it is recommended that such a software package not be installed covertly, without the subject's knowledge and consent, even at a young age, as this could impact on the trust between the young person and the family and therapist.

ASSOCIATED MENTAL HEALTH DISORDERS AND STRESSES

Both clinical experience and international research findings indicate that the presence of other mental health conditions, such as depression or anxiety, are an important risk factor in the development of PIU: a situation that clinicians call 'co-morbidity'. Numerous studies have sought to investigate the association between PIU and a wide range of other mental disorders, including in the teenage population. The disorders which have been shown to have an association with PIU include depression, anxiety, attention-deficit and hyperactivity disorder, autism spectrum disorder (including Asperger's syndrome) and bipolar affective disorder.[3] It is possible that these disorders arose first, and that they then precipitated or caused the PIU to emerge later. For example, a client with depression or anxiety could be using the internet excessively to make themselves feel better or more empowered, or someone with Asperger's syndrome could find the computer-based or gaming worlds much safer and less threatening than real-life interpersonal contact.

Thus, it is very important that the assessment explores the possibility that one or more of these conditions could be present. This, of course, would have significant treatment implications: any treatment plan, for it to be effective, would need to address the associated mental health condition as well as reduce the problematic internet overuse in itself.

As well as formal mental health disorders being associated with the development of PIU, a range of personal, familial or interpersonal stresses and tensions may be important factors that would need exploring in the assessment. Parenting and family styles or attitudes have already been highlighted above, but a detailed history should also be taken about any recent stresses, personal difficulties, losses or other life events that could have been important in the development of PIU.

POTENTIAL ASSOCIATED MENTAL HEALTH CONDITIONS AND OTHER FACTORS

Depression*

Anxiety*

Bipolar disorder (manic depression)

Attention-deficit/hyperactivity disorder (ADHD)

Autism spectrum disorder and Asperger's syndrome

Low self-esteem and low self-confidence

Being bullied by peers*

Having a substance use or alcohol disorder*

Experiencing family dysfunction, instability or isolation

Obsessive-compulsive disorder

* For more information, see *Growing Happy, Healthy Young Minds*

WARNING SIGNS FOR TEACHERS AND COUNSELLORS

Teachers will often be, after family members and close associates of the young person, among the first to notice the development of PIU. Some of the signs that teachers report noticing may include (but are not limited to):

- A sudden, otherwise unexplained drop in school grades or general performance as internet-related issues begin to take hold.
- Being distracted, unfocused or tired in class.
- Arriving late for school, after having been up through the night due to ICT.

- Actively gaming or accessing the web in the classroom, despite instructions not to.
- Spending all of break or lunchtimes on their computer or device, ignoring school friends, not engaging in general play.
- Not turning up for lessons on time, as the ICT usage is such a distraction at break times and they 'lose track' of the time.
- In extreme cases, the client may drop out of school altogether, such is the hold that the ICT use has on him or her (in more extreme cases, it is almost always internet gaming that is the excessive activity).

CONCLUSION

In summary, the assessment of a young person with suspected or actual ICT-related issues will need to be extensive and comprehensive, and may take longer than an 'ordinary' mental health assessment. There are also many useful and practical steps that families can take in understanding and assessing if, or how much, their child may be affected by such problems, and this will require empathy, good observation skills, and at least a modest amount of time and dedication as outlined above.

If a referral to a health professional is made, the general interviewing techniques and history-taking process will be similar to a 'standard' mental health assessment, but some aspects are specific, notably the diligent taking of the Internet Inventory and the particular aspects of building and maintaining rapport with a client who may be resistant, avoidant or even hostile to any suggestion of behaviour change.

Though this assessment process will be time-consuming and occasionally confronting, it is important that it is done properly, as a good history and assessment will greatly improve the chances for a successful treatment path, which will ultimately benefit the young person and their family.

Author biography

Dr Philip Tam is a Sydney-based child psychiatrist, lecturer and researcher with a longstanding interest in the complex domain of internet and video-gaming related disorders. Trained in Cambridge and London Universities, in 2011 he co-founded the Network for Internet Investigation and Research in Australia, to provide practical information and assistance to families struggling with problem internet use. He sits on the DSM-5 group's International Working Group investigating 'Internet Gaming Disorder'.

www.niira.org.au

See also:

Chapter 1: Understanding Teen Sleep and Drowsy Kids
Chapter 3: Understanding the Teenage Brain
Chapter 5: Healthy Habits for a Digital Life
Chapter 8: Computer Game Addiction and Mental Wellbeing
Chapter 14: Advice for Parents: Be a Mentor, Not a Friend
Chapter 16: Could it be Asperger's?

Further resources:

Family Lives: www.familylives.org.uk
The Healthy Digital Diet podcast: accessible for free through iTunes
Network for Internet Investigation and Research in Australia: www.niira.org.au
Professor Kimberly Young's website: www.netaddiction.com

Further reading:

American Psychological Association, 2013, 'Conditions for further Study: Internet Gaming Disorder', in *Diagnostic and Statistical Manual* (5th edition), Washington, VA, pp 795–798.

Beard KW, 2005, 'Internet addiction: A review of current assessment techniques and potential assessment questions', *Cyberpsychology and Behaviour* 8, pp 7–14.

Berle D & Starcevic V, 2015, 'Are some video games associated with more life interference and psychopathology than others? Comparing massively multiplayer online role-playing games with other forms of video game', *Australian Journal of Biology* 67, pp 105–114.

Grusser SM, Thalemann R & Griffiths MD, 2007, 'Excessive computer game playing: evidence for addiction and aggression?' *Cyberpsychology and Behaviour* 10(2), pp 290–292.

Han DH, Kim SM, Bae SJ, Renshaw P & Anderson J, 2015, 'Brain connectivity and psychiatric co-morbidity with internet gaming disorder', *Addiction Biology*, doi: 10.1111/adb.12347.

Hysing M, Pallesen S, Stormark KM, Jakobsen R, Lundervold AJ & Sivertsen B, 2015, 'Sleep and use of electronic devices in adolescence: results from a large population-based study', *BMJ Open* 2, 2:5(1).

Manocha, R (Ed), 2017, *Growing Happy, Healthy Young Minds: Generation Next*, Hachette Australia, Sydney.

Petry N, Rehbein F, Gentile DA, Lemmens JS, Rumpf H-J, Mossle T, Bischof G, Tao R, Fung DSS, Borges G, Auriacombe M, Gonzales Ibanez A, Tam P & O'Brien C, 2013, 'International Consensus Guidelines for assessing Internet Gaming Disorder using the new DSM-V approach', *Addiction* 109(9), pp 1399–1406.

Tam P & Walter G, 2013, 'Problematic Internet Use in Childhood and Youth: Evolution of a 21st Century Affliction', *Australasian Psychiatry* 21, pp 533–536.

8. COMPUTER GAME ADDICTION AND MENTAL WELLBEING

Dr Huu Kim Le

How can we help our children maintain a healthy balance between the real world and the virtual world in an era that is forever more digitally connected? Not all children will develop an Internet Gaming Disorder, but a better understanding of how online games are designed and the effects of excessive gaming will give you the confidence to put in place the appropriate restrictions to maintain control, rather than lose it.

INTRODUCTION

The majority of teenagers are able to play internet games in a healthy way, and to enjoy games without negatively impacting on their life outside games.

However, many parents report difficulties in restricting their child's use of internet games. Some teenagers continue to play excessively even when time restrictions are placed on them by their parents. They might find it difficult to stop even when they experience negative consequences, or in some cases, children continue to play compulsively even when they no longer enjoy playing.

As a parent, you want to confidently guide your child to develop their potential with real-life achievements, relationships and connection to their environment.

AUSTRALIAN STATISTICS ON TEENAGE INTERNET GAMING PROBLEMS

In 2012, approximately 1200 South Australian secondary school students were surveyed from fifty randomly selected schools. This is one of the earliest studies investigating problem teenage video game use in Australia. The study found that approximately 1.8 per cent of students had 'pathological video gaming' and 11 per cent of students had 'pathological technology use'. The distinguishing clinical features of Pathological Technology Use in this study were withdrawal (when not using), tolerance (needing to use more to get the same effect), lies and secrecy (in order to keep using), and conflict (problems due to excessive use).

In 2014, as part of the Second Australian National Survey on Adolescent Mental Health, 3000 teenagers from 6000 families were surveyed in the largest Australian study on teenage use of the internet and electronic gaming. They found that adolescents with major depressive disorder had a higher prevalence of problem internet or electronic gaming behaviour than adolescents with no identified mental disorder.

Adolescents had to have at least four of the following five indicators of problematic use:

- Went without eating or sleeping.
- Feel bothered when not doing (psychological withdrawal).
- Use when not really interested (tolerance, loss of control, lose interest in hobbies).
- Spend less time than should with family or friends or doing schoolwork.
- Tried unsuccessfully to spend less time gaming (unsuccessful attempts to control gaming).

They also found that approximately 10 per cent of teenagers spend nine hours or more on the internet on weekdays.

Approximately 11 per cent of males aged eleven to fifteen years played electronic games for five to eight hours per day on weekdays.

A CASE STUDY

Gary (not his real name) is a teenager who has an internet gaming disorder.

He is a fifteen-year-old Australian-born male who lives with his mother, Mary, and younger sister, Sarah. He has missed five weeks of school, and has difficulty getting out of bed due to spending all night playing online games on his laptop in his room.

Parenting Point #1: Research has shown that if a child has access to a computer in their room, this increases the risk of internet gaming problems. A reason for this is less supervision and increased covert playing of games.

Gary recently ended up in trouble due to his online gaming. His mother had to call his father, David, for help after Gary threatened her with a kitchen knife. This happened after Gary refused to turn off the computer and go to sleep. Out of frustration, Mary unplugged the wifi modem in the middle of Gary's Counter-Strike online game.

Parenting Point #2: When to shut down a child's computer game is a source of arguments for many families. Children with serious internet gaming problems can become aggressive or violent when restrictions are abruptly placed on them. Try giving your child a five-minute warning to save their game and finish. If they are in the middle of an online game with their friends, find out from them when the game is likely to finish. If they continue to play beyond the warning or start another game, you will need to implement a temporary ban (ideally at a time when they are not playing). Unplug in the middle of a game at your own risk. Children are desensitised to violence through repeated play of violent games. A sudden withdrawal mid-game can produce violence that is uncharacteristic of your child in the heat of the moment. If your child places their or your immediate safety at risk, then you must consider police intervention. Not only do you need to keep your family safe, but this is often the wake-up call your child needs to see how their behaviour is affecting those around them.

Gary's mother and biological father separated five years ago when Gary was ten years old. In the last few years, David has been making attempts to reconnect with his children, with both children now in his care on alternate weekends. However, David often takes late-night weekend shifts as a taxi driver to earn extra money to pay for Gary's school tuition.

Parenting Point #3: In a modern world, parental supervision is hard to come by. When both parents are busy working long hours or parents have separated, families can fall into the trap of using the internet as a supervision substitute.

From a very young age, Gary has always excelled academically. There is an expectation in the family that Gary will study hard, get good grades, go to university and get a good job, such as a doctor or lawyer.

Parenting Point #4: Many children find themselves under pressure from their friends and family to perform academically or socially. When these real-life expectations are too overwhelming or not met, many children seek online achievements or social connections as a substitute.

Last year, in Year Nine, Gary's father bought him a powerful laptop computer for schoolwork (all students are expected to have their own laptop in class).

Parenting Point #5: In Australia, all high school students are expected to have not just their laptop for school but multiple devices. Many teachers and parents assume that children must keep up with the latest technology, otherwise the child will fall behind. This is not true. We must prioritise basic reading, communication and physical skills first. Many countries that do not have a 1:1 child-to-laptop policy consistently outperform Australia in academic rankings. If a child does not have the basic educational skills to start with, they will not benefit from this technology and are more likely to play games than learn.

One day, a classmate introduced Gary to Counter-Strike, an online multiplayer game with a military theme, also known as a first person shooter or FPS. Gary quickly became very skilled at this game, and Counter-Strike is his favourite online game. Gary most enjoys the achievement aspects of the game and status of being the best player on his team.

Parenting Point #6: Different children play games for different reasons. When online games meet their psychological needs, children can become very motivated to keep playing.

Gary is able to play eight hours straight on this game and the longest ever stretch of time was ten hours straight when he was at his father's house, where his gaming is unrestricted and his father is often working all night as a taxi driver. He is currently playing approximately fifty hours a week since he stopped going to school.

Parenting Point #7: Although there is no set diagnostic or safe number of hours of play, just remember forty hours of gaming is like working a full-time job but without earning money for your time and effort.

Within six months of first playing Counter-Strike, Gary's academic performance began to fall. Time that was usually spent doing his homework was now invested in playing the online game and his concentration at school deteriorated after late-night gaming sessions.

Even though Gary failed his Year Nine examinations, he was allowed to progress to Year Ten. However, earlier this year he developed a viral illness and spent a week at home. Since then, he has been been feeling overwhelmed by the pressure to achieve academically and believes he is unable to catch up. He has been relieving his stress and anxiety by playing more online games where he is known as one of the top players.

Parenting Point #8: Online gaming is a very effective way to escape negative emotions such as feelings of depression and anxiety. However, children need a toolbox of strategies so they do not completely avoid their problems through games. A school counsellor might be the first port of call. Failing basic strategies or the need for further assessment, a school counsellor might recommend a GP or clinical psychologist assessment. If there is concern of a more serious mental health disorder, an assessment with a child and adolescent psychiatrist might be appropriate.

Gary admits that he has struggled with anxiety in the last three months, especially at school, where he is worried he will say the wrong thing or get in trouble with his teacher. When he plays games online he is able to get 'in the zone' and forget about the pressures of school.

Parenting Point #9: Games are designed to maximise the feeling of flow, which is often described as the optimal experience or the feeling of being in the zone where a sufficient level of challenge is successfully met by an equal level of skill. Often when a child is in a state of flow, this is an effective distraction from their problems; however, this avoidance can worsen the original problem.

Gary often has heated arguments with his mother about the amount of time he spends playing online games and admits to shouting and at times punching the walls in frustration.

Parenting Point #10: When children play games excessively, they might believe the amount of time spent playing is normal. When they are not able to play they might become irritable and frustrated. If they are playing violent games, they can be desensitised to violence.

After reaching the top of the Counter-Strike leader-board rankings, Gary no longer enjoys the game as much as before. The game isn't as exciting as when he first started playing. Lately, he feels obligated to help his teammates and maintain his status in his team. He has also felt more on edge, since his team have now started to play high-stakes competitive games where they bet using virtual items. It was in the middle of one of these games that his mother, Mary, abruptly disconnected his internet connection, which cost him and his team valuable points and virtual items.

Parenting Point #11: To adults, games may seem frivolous or like they don't have any serious purpose or value. But to the many people who invest a lot of time and effort playing these games, they hold much meaning and value, sometimes even monetary value, which can lead to gambling problems and credit card debt.

UNDERSTANDING INTERNET GAME DESIGN

What exactly is my child doing in these internet games and why are they spending so much time there?

As internet gaming technology has become more sophisticated over time, they are no longer just 'games', they are now 'virtual worlds' or computer simulations with layers of game design that do not end. Imagine your child was able to transport themselves to somewhere exotic without your help, for example, Bali. Here, no one would know who they were or where they came from. Your child could interact with others, earn money and build things, even a reputation of high status. They only need to use their existing skills and any resources they discover.

Imagine, in order to get to this place, your child was not limited by the physical difficulties of transport such as flights, or the need for a passport and there were no difficulties with language. Also, if your child was harmed in any way, they could just 'restart', like magic. Well, this is what it is like for a child entering a new game. They are virtually transported to another place, an exotic, digitally designed world. Here there are no rules and there is freedom to explore as they please, yet this world is very structured so that they know exactly what to do and when to act, and success is predictable. Imagine then, in this exciting world, that your child is powerful, maybe even famous, and all their friends are there too. Why would they ever want to leave?

My child is now spending all their time in this virtual world through their online game. I think they have an Internet Gaming Disorder. What do I do?

The dilemma for many parents is that their child is spending a lot of time and effort in this virtual world and their child has nothing to show for all this time spent online (unless you are one of the minority of highly skilled players sponsored by gaming companies to glamorise the gaming lifestyle to other gamers).

In this case, as a parent you are trying to convince your child to spend more time in the 'real world'. This process is much like physically extracting your child from Bali back to their home environment.

From this point, there are generally two approaches: do-it-yourself (DIY) or seeking professional help. But first I need to ask you this question:

Have you ever seen a local tourism ad in your capital city? Do you ever stop to think why the local tourism board would need to entice or convince locals to spend more time and money here? You would think that a local would be aware of all the fantastic local things to do in their own backyard, right?

Wrong!

Many people are unaware of the fantastic opportunities on their own doorstep, naturally opting to escape to exotic locations. However, if a friend or a travel agent were able to convince them, they still might be open to spend time locally.

On the other hand, there are local people who spend their time talking to friends and family, researching what to do and organise their own DIY local holidays without any professional assistance. Well, this is the position many parents find themselves in when managing their child's internet gaming and balancing this with the real world. Every day, parents attempt to bring their children back from exotic online locations, either through enticing their child or restricting their child's time spent online.

Approach 1: DIY – I have met many families that have told me that their child previously had a serious internet gaming problem. However, the parents, through their own research or experimentation, found a solution and were able to extract their child from their internet game, who often say, 'I got my child back.' They describe this almost as though their child had been physically abducted by their internet game.

However, many families lack the support and resources to do this, and are struggling, often feeling lost and do not know where to start. Sometimes the problem requires professional help either with a clinical psychologist or a child and adolescent psychiatrist.

Approach 2: Seek help from a professional who can act as an 'agent of change' – As I am seeing more families in my office with a child with an Internet Gaming Disorder, I have found it helpful to adapt my clinical role as a child psychiatrist and expand this to include acting as an agent of change. In fact, I will go even further and imagine myself putting on a 'travel agent hat' in addition to my 'psychiatrist hat'. That is, I imagine myself as a 'travel agent for the real world'.

By doing this, it reminds me that in addition to treating a serious mental health problem, I also have to persuade a young person that the real world is far better than the virtual world.

This is an extremely difficult task that takes time and, if not done carefully, risks losing engagement with the young person. By shifting my perspective, I enhance the process of working with the child, understanding what is motivating them and negotiating how to return to the real world safely. This is the easiest way that I can explain this process (please note that this analogy is not meant to trivialise the complex connection between internet games, mental health and family relationships).

Once in my office, I use my knowledge of treating mental illness in young people, family dynamics and internet gaming psychology to help a family through this process. This might involve education, talking therapy and, in some cases, medication. A good clinician will attempt to understand the child's predicament, their strengths and weaknesses, and exactly what is so good about this exotic location that they would rather spend all their time there than in the real world.

To promote change, I will often talk to the young person in their own language, developing a working relationship so I can create a plan that suits their needs, often with a detailed itinerary of activities to get them through their management plan safely and give them the best chances of success. Many children relapse, so that is why it is important to work with a clinician with a genuine interest in this area or a subspeciality in Internet Gaming Disorder as your child will want to work with someone who is non-judgemental and compassionate about their problem.

RED FLAGS (WHEN TO SUSPECT YOUR CHILD HAS A PROBLEM)

- My child has stopped going to school.
- My child will not join the family for family outings.
- My child has stolen money from my credit card to buy online gaming credits.
- My child does not have a normal sleeping pattern.
- My child no longer eats meals with our family or skips meals to play internet games.
- My child's academic performance has deteriorated.
- My child has become violent towards me when restrictions are placed on their gaming.
- There have been more arguments in the family over screen-time.
- My child has lied or hidden from me the true amount of time spent playing internet games.
- My child seems depressed, anxious and has difficulty managing their emotions or dealing with their problems.
- My child has given up core extracurricular activities, such as sports and outdoor activities, that they previously enjoyed in order to spend more time gaming.
- My child only has online friends and finds it difficult to spend time with children their own age face to face.

In many countries, internet gaming technology is widely accessible in our homes, schools and public places. However, parents and teachers are ill-equipped to prevent, let alone treat, problem internet gaming.

Increasing your family's awareness of the effect of internet games on your child's development will give you the tools you need to confidently place restrictions on your child's time playing on internet games.

Author biography

Dr Huu Kim Le is an Australian child and adolescent psychiatrist, based in Adelaide, South Australia. He grew up playing computer games and was always fascinated by digital worlds. A chance meeting with a patient who shared their mental illness with their online avatar inspired Dr Le to specialise in psychiatry and follow the growing research on Internet Gaming Disorder (IGD) in children and adolescents.

In 2015, Dr Le conducted an investigation at the Institute of Mental Health in Singapore on IGD in children and adolescents. He has travelled internationally to collaborate with researchers in South Korea, Japan, India and Canada.

www.cgiclinic.com

See also:

Chapter 1: Understanding Teen Sleep and Drowsy Kids
Chapter 3: Understanding the Teenage Brain
Chapter 5: Healthy Habits for a Digital Life
Chapter 7: Problematic Internet Use and How to Manage It
Chapter 14: Advice for Parents: Be a Mentor, Not a Friend
Chapter 16: Could it be Asperger's?

Further resources:

CGI Clinic – This is my free web resource and Facebook page for parents, teachers and clinicians to aid internet awareness for you and your family: www.cgiclinic.com
Network for Internet Investigation and Research Australia – An Australian website linking professionals, clinicians and researchers in this growing field: www.niira.org.au
Common Sense Media – An online resource which is useful for parents to make informed decisions before purchasing a game for their child: www.commonsensemedia.org
'The Spell of Digital Immersion' – My TEDx Talk delivered in Adelaide in 2015: www.tedxadelaide.com.au/video/1816

Further reading:

American Psychiatric Association, 2013, *Diagnostic and statistical manual of mental disorders (DSM-5®)*. American Psychiatric Pub.

Gentile, DA, Choo, H, Liau, A, Sim, T, Li, D, Fung, D, & Khoo, A, 2011, 'Pathological video game use among youths: a two-year longitudinal study', *Pediatrics*, peds-2010.

King, DL, Delfabbro, PH, Zwaans, T, & Kaptsis, D, 2013, 'Clinical features and axis I comorbidity of Australian adolescent pathological Internet and video game users', *Australian and New Zealand Journal of Psychiatry*, 47(11), pp 1058–1067.

Lawrence, D, Johnson, S, Hafekost, J, Boterhoven, De Haan K, Sawyer, M, Ainley, J, Zubrick, SR, 2015, *The Mental Health of Children and Adolescents. Report on the Second Australian Child and Adolescent Survey of Mental Health and Wellbeing*, Department of Health, Canberra.

Manocha, R (Ed), 2017, *Growing Happy, Healthy Young Minds: Generation Next*, Hachette Australia, Sydney.

9. SEXTING – REALITIES AND RISKS

Jeremy Blackman & Lesley Podesta

This chapter aims to provide readers with a deeper understanding of youth sexting and the risks involved, as well as suggest strategies for how to connect with, educate, guide and support young people on these issues.

INTRODUCTION

'The invention of new machinery, devices, and processes is continually bringing up new questions of law, puzzling judges, lawyers, and laymen . . . The doors may be barred and a rejected suitor kept out, but how is the telephone to be guarded?'

Telephony Magazine, 1905

Emerging technologies disrupt social norms. This has been the case for a long time. The telephone – not smartphone – was the original game-changer, way back at the turn of the twentieth century. It made parents worried that legions of young female telephone operators were suddenly able to organise rendezvous with potential suitors without anyone knowing.

Social technologies can be challenging, even confronting, to many of us. But new social tools are often welcomed by younger generations, especially when they are afforded greater freedoms by them. With lives increasingly scheduled and structured, in a physical world that is shrinking, is it any wonder that teens are always looking for a place of their own?

The rise of social media platforms and messaging apps, like Instagram and Snapchat, has given teens the tools to communicate with each other in a variety of ways. Digital communication platforms in the twenty-first century are instant, accessible, cheap (or free), visual, interactive and, notionally at least, private.

'Sexting', a term coined and used by adults, is widely perceived to be a negative and dangerous online behaviour practised exclusively by youth. It has been popular to condemn such 'risky' youth practices, or as Associate Professor Kath Albury from the University of New South Wales notes, 'to dismiss them as evidence of young people's "ignorance", "low self-esteem", "addiction" and/or "narcissism".' However, by openly condemning these practices, we prevent young people from feeling comfortable enough to tell us what they are doing and why they are doing it, thus reducing our ability to assist them when they do need help.

Like many youth behaviours that involve exploration, discovery and risk-taking, there are certainly dangers involved. Serious concerns and consequences include: betrayals of trust; damage to reputation; defamation; breaking the law; blackmail; extortion; links to the world of pornography; and even sexual predation and grooming.

Regardless of our own feelings and opinions about youth sexual practices, we do need to understand the phenomenon of 'sexting' fully if we are to better support the young people in our care. Recent research has shown it is a complex social issue that needs to be understood by adults if the risks are to be mitigated, if the education and support of young people is to be relevant and effective, and if parents are to maintain trust and communication with their children.

WHAT IS 'SEXTING'?

'Sexting', combining the words 'sex' and 'texting', is widely understood to be the sending of provocative or sexual photos, messages or videos using a mobile phone or website.

Young people use their own colloquialisms to describe their practices, such as the generic terms 'selfies' and 'naked selfies', but also more descriptive terms like: 'n00dz', 'dirty pics', 'banana pics', 'sexy texts' and, of course, 'tit pics' and 'dick pics'. However, due to widespread media attention, the formal term 'sexting' is now widely understood by younger generations, if not used by them.

In recent focus groups with young people run by the University of New South Wales, the term 'sexting' was viewed as inherently negative and even sinister, in contrast to the more neutral terminology of 'pictures' or 'pics'.

WHY YOUNG PEOPLE SEXT

As observed in the 2015 study conducted by the Australian Institute of Criminology (AIC): 'While the definition of sexting is broad and can incorporate everything from mutually consensual exchanges of images to coercive and exploitative behaviours, the vast majority of young people who engage in the sending and receiving of explicit images do so voluntarily.'

There are four main motivations for youth sexting. Young people send sexts:

- To people they want to 'hook up' with.
- To show intimacy and trust with someone they are in a relationship with.
- To gain approval, praise and/or acceptance.
- To experiment with sexuality and identity.

THE PROBLEM OF CONSENT

Some argue that youth sexting might be only voluntary in a certain sense, and that peer pressure will generally override common sense and self-protection.

However, we often give young people too little credit. In an American study in 2008, two-thirds of teenage girls said sexting was 'fun and flirtatious' and made them 'feel sexy'. For others, sexting was seen as a form of initiation into the sexual culture. There were similar findings in the 2015 Australian AIC study. Other researchers have found that young girls see sexting as a way they can control how much a boy sees, under what conditions and at what time.

Despite developing strategies to protect themselves and curate their social lives, young people can be tricked into sending naked images – by peers, random strangers and, certainly, online predators.

There is also a significant grey area in consensual relations between young people and the exchange of images and videos. Peer pressure can effectively coerce young people into (reluctantly) creating and sharing personal content. Even one such moment of 'giving in' can have serious consequences, including further requests for material – and increasingly under the threat of betrayal, such as 'outing' or public shaming.

Study after study has shown the youths most at risk online are often the same youths most at risk offline. Age, maturity, experience, education, peer pressure, parental trust and coercion are all factors that impact effective decision-making.

THE DANGERS OF SEXTING

Even though sexting is a fairly common practice in youth communities, the consequences can be dire. There can be emotional, social and reputational, legal and even physical consequences.

Unfortunately for our younger generations, a single act can have devastating effects, thanks to the ruthless sharing capability of digital technologies and the criminal activity of online dealers in explicit images.

Here are four dangers of sexting that parents and teachers should be aware of:

- The recipient saves the images and shows/distributes them to others in their peer group.
- The young person is tricked or coerced into sharing an explicit image.

- The images end up on porn aggregation sites or are used as 'revenge porn'.
- The sexting behaviour leads to criminal charges.

'Revenge porn' is commonly defined as revealing or sexually explicit images or videos of a person posted on the internet, typically by a former (sexual) partner, without the consent of the subject and in order to cause them distress or embarrassment.

PREVALENCE AND INCIDENCE OF YOUTH SEXTING

Whether we personally agree with it or not, sexting is best understood as part of the modern range of behaviours some young people will engage in as an aspect of their sexuality. Placing youth sexting within the context of their broader sexual behaviour is vital, as sexting is primarily an issue of sex education, integrated with digital citizenship and literacy.

It is important to keep in mind that sexting, like sex, is not practised by all young people.

A significant proportion of young people abstain from any form of sexual activity – physical or virtual – and many of them are proud to publicly say so. And some experts have argued that sexting can enable young people to flirt without the need for physical contact and being exposed to the associated risks of STDs and pregnancy. Again, despite one's own feelings about the practice, it is important to accept that sexting is happening and that it is a complex issue that is best addressed with trust, respect, openness and honesty.

In 2013, La Trobe University interviewed more than 2000 sixteen- to eighteen-year-old students across Australia as part of its National Survey of Australian Secondary Students and Sexual Health. The results showed 25 per cent of Year Ten students, a third of Year Eleven students and 50 per cent of Year Twelve students reported having had sex.

Of those who were sexually active:

- 84 per cent said they had received a sexually explicit text; and
- 72 per cent said they had sent one.

Half of this group said they had sent a nude or explicit photo of themselves and 70 per cent reported receiving one.

Lead researcher Professor Anne Mitchell said that for young people, sexting was just part of their sexual relationship.

The 2015 Australian AIC study of sixteen- to eighteen-year-olds found 50 per cent of them reported having sent a sexual picture or video of themselves to someone else. Of thirteen- to fifteen-year-olds, 38 per cent had sent a sexual picture or video, although they were more likely to receive than send an image. Young people commonly reported engaging in the practice as a consensual and enjoyable part of their intimate relationships.

THE TECHNOLOGY YOUNG PEOPLE USE TO SEND IMAGES

The platforms young people use change rapidly. Common sites and apps used at the time of writing this chapter are: Instagram, Snapchat, Kik, Skype, FaceTime, Tinder and Tumblr.

For the majority of parents (and many teachers), keeping up with the technologies is overwhelming; most adults do not have the appetite for finding out about the latest social media or gaming fad. But it is important to stay in touch.

Rather than parents and teachers thinking they have to know each and every app, game and social networking platform that's out there, it is a good approach to become familiar with the functionality the main platforms have. That way, adults can understand what they can do and what the risks might be. They will also be able to have conversations with children and their friends about the types of technology they are using and why.

Here is a simple way to think about the main social media platforms and what they specialise in. Keep in mind that technology is becoming more and more integrated, meaning platforms can do more and more. Most, if not all, apps are multimedia: text, image, video and internet-enabled. Even the humble SMS is trialling 'disappearing' messages.

Type of platform	Example platforms	Key functionality
1. Messaging apps	Snapchat Kik WhatsApp	'Disappearing' messages One-to-one ('private') Image filters
2. Social networking services	Facebook Instagram YouTube	Multimedia Group chat Public profile and networking
3. Games/gaming worlds	League of Legends Call of Duty	Entertainment Peer collaboration
4. Secret/hidden apps	Ky-Calc	Private
5. Dating apps	Tinder Bumble	Meeting new people Location-based markers

The minimum age for using any social media platform is thirteen; some are restricted to older age groups.

It also helps to think about the main motivations for young people using different types of technology. Above all else, they are influenced by their social world. If a parent takes away all technology from their teenager, this is almost equivalent to solitary confinement.

While boundaries and consequences are a common aspect of good parenting and teaching, they are better determined when you understand a little about why the behaviour is occurring.

The top five reasons young people use technology platforms:

- Social.
- The 'yo-yo craze' effect (it's popular because it is).
- Free to use.
- Accessible (mobile, quick/simple, fun).
- Adult-free/shielded.

NOTIONS OF PRIVACY AND CHOICE

Young people often place a fundamentally different value on the notion of privacy. They have grown up in an environment where regularly sharing intimate thoughts, images and videos is the norm. The term 'lifestreaming' has been used to describe this very public, moment-to-moment way of life. American academic Alice E Marwick has identified it as being 'always on' in relation to social media: personal information is shared with an audience in your social media network, and that information in turn creates a digital portrait of the person who is sharing it.[1]

Living in such public view is baffling to most people beyond the age of thirty, and it comes with all kinds of new, blurred understandings of privacy. Many teenagers have developed extremely sophisticated strategies for 'hiding in plain sight', and are often not as defenceless as we might think they are.

Others consciously decide to abstain from sharing on social media, or they may 'hide in plain sight', as identified by American researcher danah boyd, who cites the example of a message created by a young person so that it can be read differently according to who is reading it.[2]

Many young people (as well as many adults) make false assumptions about how social media platforms operate and what they do with their data. There is a deeper irony here that young people are striving for autonomy by seeking an adult-free world but, like most of us, are being monitored more than ever.

GENDER AND SEXUALITY BIAS

Discussions on sexting often include a degree of gender and sexuality bias.

When the issue is dramatised, it tends to do the following things:

- Blames the victim for their 'imprudent' behaviour.
- Frames self-respect and self-protection as obligations primarily for girls.
- Portrays sexting as only practised by young people.
- Portrays sexting as only practised by heterosexuals.

Representations of sexting are symbolic of our society's norms and stereotypes. At best, this lazy messaging reinforces misunderstandings of youth behaviour and, at worst, sabotages our efforts to help.

In Dobson and Ringrose's 2015 article on sext education, they observed that many young people are aware that there are differences in how images of girls and boys are valued. Images of girls tend to be commodified, whereas images of boys aren't taken very seriously. They also state that it is seen as shameful for girls to 'publicly visualise their bodies in a way that marks them with sexual activity or desire'.

This gender double standard can result in girls' sexual activities being stigmatised, disbelieved and/or kept secret. If their behaviour is made public, it can be judged harshly and even punished. Girls who have had their images stolen or sold are often shamed and humiliated.

We need to dismantle these stereotypes to help young people understand how they are being positioned so they can make informed choices.

CULTURE OF SEX AND PORNOGRAPHY

Adding to the pressures of gender stereotypes and bias is the current climate of hypersexuality, amplified sexual desire, and the normalisation of, and easy access to, most forms of pornography. Pornography is influencing almost every aspect of pop culture that young people are engaged with. Bente Skau's thesis 'Who has seen what, when?' found that the average age of first exposure to pornography was twelve years old.

With the value now attributed to sexual desire and its link to self-esteem and even success and fame, many young people might find it difficult to relate to messages of self-respect, caution, prudence or abstinence.

SEXTING AND THE LAW

While It's legal to have sex in the UK from the age of sixteen, it is illegal and a serious criminal offence to take, hold or share 'indecent' photos of anyone under the age of eighteen. The maximum penalty is ten years in prison.

The Association of Chief Police Officers of England, Wales and Northern Ireland (ACPO) have stated that young people engaging in sexting shouldn't face prosecution as first time offenders, but the situation will be investigated to ensure that the young people involved are not at risk. Repeat offenders and more extreme cases are reviewed differently.

From February 2015, 'revenge porn' became a criminal offence in England and Wales. This makes it an offence to share private sexual photographs or films without the consent of the people in them and if the intention is to cause them distress. This includes social networks and sending pictures via text. If convicted, you can face a maximum of two years in prison. (BBC Advice factfile)

WHAT YOUNG PEOPLE FEAR MOST

Despite all of this, research has shown the thing young people fear most is that adults will find out something has gone wrong. That is why knowing what to do to help in the event of an incident is crucially important, so your teenager is more likely to come to you earlier.

Young people have also explained they are often more concerned about being tagged to unidentifiable photos that are not of them.

ENGAGING WITH YOUNG PEOPLE – GENERAL ADVICE FOR PARENTS AND TEACHERS

There is no question that the issue of sex (and 'sext') education is divisive. Many are of the opinion that even acknowledging the behaviour is to condone it.

The vast proportion of our work at the Alannah & Madeline

Foundation is in prevention – from cybersafety to bullying to general wellbeing. Similarly, on the issue of sexting, we advocate for an education-based approach that helps to raise smart, safe and responsible young people.

In seeking an effective approach to prevention, we believe that open communication and strong relationships between adult carers and young people is vital. While strong leadership and messaging from adults is an important component to success, there are risks if this is perceived by young people as outright intolerance. Focusing on embarrassment and shame can actually break down ongoing communication and trust. Framing sexual expression only as a risk can worsen anxieties or feelings of shame that young people may experience in relation to their sexuality.

Also, talking about sexting as solely the responsibility of girls to protect themselves places them in a very difficult situation. It removes boys from any ethical responsibility for their actions and makes it impossible to work through the issue as one of shared concern and respectful relationships. Both girls and boys need to develop shared understandings around what behaviour is acceptable and what is not in their peer relationships. If they have a strong grounding in this area – mainly tied to their self-worth – they are more likely to question and resist the unreasonable and potentially dangerous expectations of would-be sexual advances.

Aim to open, and keep open, lines of communication with young people, and remember these issues are not grounded in the technology as much as they are in social and sexual behaviours.

- Start having conversations as early as possible, depending on the maturity of the child.
- Make conversations a regular occurrence.
- Try your best to make conversations non-confrontational, light and brief.
- Be available for and responsive to any incidents that might arise, however small.

WHAT SCHOOLS CAN DO

In many instances, schools are threatening places for students regarding 'sext education', rather than places of friendship and support. Sext education is mostly separated from general sex education, and facilitated in a haphazard way by staff without the appropriate knowledge and experience.

More effective may be education that seeks to prepare young people with a 'sexual ethics' framework, as suggested by Professor Moira Carmody from the University of Western Sydney, who says that with this approach participants can understand the context of their behaviour, and also ascertain when they are exploiting others, or being exploited. Such a framework also helps young people become aware of mutual expectations that can arise in this 'exchange economy'. Schools should be aiming to create and maintain an environment that is supportive and responsive to students' needs, especially in areas like this that are rarely discussed and often seen by adults and young people as taboo.

It needs to be a school-wide approach, driven by the senior leadership team that includes:

- Proactive policies that effectively address student wellbeing and digital citizenship.
- Reporting procedures, regularly communicated to staff and students.
- Regular targeted sessions for staff learning on a range of youth wellbeing and online issues.
- A focus on promoting pro-social skills across age groups, including 'sexual ethics'.
- Meaningful involvement of young people in the building of a safe and supportive school.
- School-family-community partnerships.

WHAT SCHOOLS CAN DO IF AN INCIDENT OCCURS

- Respond quickly, with empathy and sensitivity.
- Escalate to the appropriate staff member(s).
- Consult with the student or students involved to gather as much information as possible.

Follow school policy procedures, which should include levels of escalation, including when/if you should:

- Notify the student's parents/carers.
- Include other students that may be involved.
- Involve the police.

Schools are extremely busy places, and a student might approach a teacher at a time that could compromise that staff member's ability to effectively supervise other students and fulfil their duty of care. Wherever possible, schools should have options for handling such situations, such as efficient and accessible ways to communicate with the school administration.

Remember that most students' greatest fear is that an adult will find out about a sexting incident. The moment a student approaches a staff member directly to report such an incident, it needs to take priority.

WHAT PARENTS/CARERS CAN DO IF AN INCIDENT OCCURS

- Don't panic – listen with empathy and compassion.
- Allow your child to talk through the whole issue.
- Determine clear next steps, and work through these with your child. This may include:
  - Making an appointment with the relevant staff member at the school.
  - Involving the police.

Bear in mind that not all sexting issues will be worst-case scenarios. The situation may be limited to one person, such as someone the young person is in a relationship with. If they come to you to discuss such issues – let alone the more serious incidents – this is a good sign they feel they can talk to you and believe you will respond quickly and effectively.

REGULAR CONVERSATIONS BETWEEN PARENTS AND CHILDREN

The longer you avoid having conversations with your child about relationships, sexting and sex, the more awkward they will be. Using hypothetical scenarios can be a good way of discussing things without being too personal. This approach will also enable you to get a regular snapshot of where your child's attitudes lie.

The Alannah & Madeline Foundation has developed an online cybersafety education tool called the eSmart Digital Licence, which poses many such scenarios across eight key topic areas.

A new module in this year's product for thirteen- to fifteen-year-olds focuses on relationships and reputation, and is proving to be a great way for adults to broach topics such as sexting and the responsible use of technology. It presents situations in a way that prompts young people to consider many perspectives and value the rights and feelings of others. It also acknowledges that the social world of young people is complex, requires social and emotional intelligence and/or learned strategies, is often fraught, but that bad things won't last forever and there are people around them to help.

Below are two such scenarios in text form – the actual versions are visual and interactive. Visit the website to try the sample quiz: www.digitallicence.com.au

DIGITAL LICENCE SCENARIO 1

Select all the actions that will help protect your online reputation when using a messaging app.

Answer options (correct options in *italics*)

- *Lock down your privacy settings.*
- *Assume each message you send is permanent.*
- Only use the funniest filters.
- Wear revealing clothes in your profile picture.
- Friend/follow people based on their username.

Feedback:

Messaging apps can be great fun, but only you can protect yourself online.

DIGITAL LICENCE SCENARIO 2

You got dumped by your last girl/boyfriend. You feel wretched and want to embarrass them by posting personal images of them online. This course of action is probably . . . (Select all that apply.)

Answer options (correct options in *italics*)

- *Illegal.*
- *Disrespectful.*
- *Unacceptable.*
- Funny.
- Justified.

Feedback:

Sharing sensitive images without consent is a very serious breach of trust and is most likely illegal.

EDITORS' NOTE

The healthy inhibitions of a young person – and of an older adult for that matter – are often bypassed online by the illusion of privacy, anonymity and control that a computer screen provides.

While dictating behaviours to a child or young person is rarely well received, parenting that encourages making sound choices can head off some very damaging consequences of sexting. These might include:

- Police Investigation.
- Arrest.
- Extreme embarrassment.
- Global humiliation.
- Blackmail (others using the images for their own gain).
- Loss of trust among adults.
- Incurring the disappointment of family members.
- Knowledge that others may have and control the image forever.

Sexually explicit content distributed without considering the consequences can fall into the wrong hands. There are no guarantees that even content shared between friends will remain private. The world-wide web provides the possibility of sharing images with potentially three billion people in a split second via smartphone or another internet-enabled device.

Children and their families who have experienced one or more of these consequences invariably regret the incriminating posts ever being made. The ensuing anguish can have a drastic impact on the individuals involved.

The choice by young people to 'sext' is often ill-considered and based on a range of motives, including:

- Acting on impulse.
- The belief it makes them mature.
- 'Everybody is doing it.'
- 'It's not a big deal' or 'It's funny'.
- 'I wanted to feel accepted.'
- 'I don't know, it's just what you do.'

- In response to receiving unsolicited images.
- Pressure from others (either peer or blackmail).
- The desire for another person to like them.
- A lack of education to counter or manage the above.

Sensitive parenting can educate, guide and help a young person to make sound choices without coercion.

When addressing the issue with your child or teenager, it is important they understand their and others' legal responsibilities. Have them consider personal consequences and how they, close family and friends may be affected. This is not to cause fear, but rather to empower them with the facts with which to decide on their actions.

Authors' biographies

Jeremy Blackman is Senior Advisor, Cybersafety at the Alannah & Madeline Foundation. After many years as a secondary school English and digital literacy teacher, his current work focuses on issues surrounding social media and online behaviour, and ensuring youth perspectives are considered in industry initiatives. Jeremy has written, presented and facilitated discussions on these topics across Australia and internationally. One of his ongoing major projects at the foundation is the design of the educational framework and content for the eSmart Digital Licence – an award-winning, interactive cybersafety resource for teachers, parents and children.

Lesley Podesta is CEO of the Alannah & Madeline Foundation. She came into the not-for-profit sector after undertaking a number of senior roles in the Australian Government, including five years as head of the Office of Aboriginal and Torres Strait Islander Health.

www.amf.org.au

See also:

Recommended websites:

NSPCC: www.nspcc.org.uk/preventing-abuse/keeping-children-safe/sexting

Think U Know: thinkuknow.co.uk

Internet Matters: www.internetmatters.org

Connect Safely – US website with e-safety information for parents and teachers:
www.connectsafely.org

Digital Licence – Online e-safety quiz and resources for teachers, parents and children:
www.digitallicence.com.au

Further reading:

Albury, K, 2016, 'Politics of sexting', revisited in *Negotiating Digital Citizenship: control, contest and culture*, Rowman and Littlefield, London.

Albury, K, Crawford, K & Byron, P, 2013, *Young People and Sexting in Australia: Ethics, Representation and the Law*, The University of New South Wales, Sydney.

boyd, d, 2014, 'It's Complicated – The social lives of networked teens', free PDF download: www.danah.org/books/ItsComplicated.pdf

Lee, M, Crofts, T, McGovern, A & Milivojevic, S, 2015, 'Sexting among young people: Perceptions and practices', Australian Institute of Criminology, free PDF download: www.aic.gov.au/media_library/publications/tandi_pdf/tandi508.pdf

Manocha, R (Ed), 2017, *Growing Happy, Healthy Young Minds: Generation Next*, Hachette Australia, Sydney.

Mitchell, A, Patrick, K, Heywood, W, Blackman, P & Pitts, M, 2014, *'National Survey of Australian Secondary Students and Sexual Health 2013', La Trobe University and the Australian Research Centre in Sex, Health and Society*. Free PDF download: www.redaware.org.au/wp-content/uploads/2014/10/31631-ARCSHS_NSASSSH_FINAL-A-3.pdf

Shields Dobson, A & Ringrose, J, 2015, 'Sext education: pedagogies of sex, gender and shame in the schoolyards', *Tagged and Exposed, Sex Education: Sexuality, Society and Learning*, Taylor & Francis, New York.

 We also recommend the very popular companion volume **GROWING HAPPY, HEALTHY YOUNG MINDS** – resilience, bullying, depression, anxiety, body image and many more important issues.

 For more online resources visit:
generationnext.com.au/handbook

10. CYBERBULLYING, CYBER-HARASSMENT AND REVENGE PORN

Susan McLean

This chapter will provide an overview of cyberbullying and other forms of online abuse: what is and is not cyberbullying, methods of cyberbullying, signs and symptoms, what to do and legal considerations.

INTRODUCTION

'Cyberbullying' as a term was first used by a Canadian school teacher, Bill Belsey, in 2007 to describe bullying behaviour that is conducted in the digital environment. He stated: 'Cyberbullying is a way of delivering covert psychological bullying. It uses information and communication technologies to support deliberate, repeated and hostile behaviour, by an individual or group, that is intended to harm others.'

While there is no definitive or universally accepted definition of cyberbullying, the elements considered important in defining an action as cyberbullying, rather than simply being mean, are that the comment, picture, post, share, etc. is deliberate and repeated. One nasty and/or abusive comment, while totally unacceptable, would not be considered cyberbullying behaviour.

Cyberbullying can be described as any repeated harassment, insults and humiliation that occur through electronic media such as email, mobile phones, social networking sites, instant messaging programs, chat rooms, websites and through the playing of online games. Any online or digital site, app, program or game that allows communication between two or more people can be a vehicle for cyberbullying. Cyberbullying, however, is not one nasty, isolated incident. Cyberbullying usually occurs between people who know each other such as students at a school, as members of a sporting club, someone from your social circle or someone you know of, a friend of a friend. It is very rare that there is no connection between victim and bully.

Cyberbullying is pervasive in nature, incessant, ongoing and can occur 24/7. It is not just confined to schools, as reports of cyberbullying also come from workplaces, sporting clubs and youth groups – anywhere people can form some type of relationship. It is now common in domestic and family violence situations to see the abusive partner using technology to continue to abuse, assault and stalk their victim. It's different from bullying in the real world in that the bully can follow you home and into your house by virtue of technology. It often occurs with the perception of anonymity, i.e. an account in a fake name or a blocked number, but in many cases it is clear who is behind the bullying.

Like any form of bullying, cyberbullying can be psychologically damaging, which is often harder for parents to identify and subsequently act upon. It is far harder to see mental anguish than a bruise on a leg, so be aware of any subtle changes in your child's demeanour or behaviour, and investigate. Cyberbullying is often a very public humiliation, as many others see what is written or posted, and once online, it is almost impossible to remove all traces of it. This is one of the reasons that cyberbullying is particularly hurtful to young people who do not have the maturity and life experiences with which to balance out the behaviour.

Statistics as to the level of cyberbullying among Australian teens varies widely, but roughly it averages out to approximately 30 per cent of all Australian children and teens reporting that they have been the victims of cyberbullying. Statistics released by the Office of the Children's eSafety Commissioner for the twelve-month period to June 2016 show the following:

- Cyberbullied: 8 per cent of kids (eight to thirteen years) and 19 per cent of teens (fourteen to seventeen years).
- Exposed to inappropriate content: 9 per cent of kids and 17 per cent of teens.
- Contacted by strangers online: 5 per cent of kids and 9 per cent of teens.

FORMS OF CYBERBULLYING

Forms of cyberbullying can include (but are not limited to):

- Harassing and threatening messages sent using any form of technology.
- Sending nasty SMS (text message), IMs (instant message such as Facebook Chat or FB Messenger), MMS (picture messages including Snapchat) or repeated prank phone calls.
- Using a person's screen name to pretend to be them (setting up a fake account).
- Using a person's password to access their account and then pretending to be them or using the account to bully others, trying to divert the blame.
- Forwarding others' private emails, messages, pictures or videos without permission (you may think it's funny).
- Posting mean or nasty comments on pictures.
- Sending sexually explicit images ('sexting').
- Intentionally excluding others.

Australia's Office of the Children's eSafety Commissioner's research showed the following breakdown in types of cyberbullying experienced.

Socially excluded	Teens – 43%	Kids – 50%
Called names	Teens – 39%	Kids – 39%
Had lies or rumours spread	Teens – 36%	Kids – 28%
Received threats to their safety	Teens – 19%	Kids – 17%
Impersonation	Teens – 9%	Kids – 12%
Account accessed without consent	Teens – 15%	Kids – 9%
Personal info posted without consent	Teens – 10%	Kids – 6%
Inappropriate or personal pics posted without consent	Teens – 9%	

The figures above should serve as a wake-up call to parents, educators and all those who work with and/or care for children. Online abuse in any form is not only wrong and hurtful, it can have a significant negative mental health impact, which makes this issue a public-health concern. Of the young people surveyed, 42 per cent stated that they were adversely affected after experiencing a negative incident online; 58 per cent felt angry, scared, sad or disempowered; 49 per cent struggled with their self-esteem; and 28 per cent lost friendships and/or felt socially isolated. There are no other behaviours with the potential to cause this level of harm to young people. It is not a fad, phase or part of growing up. It is not part of having tech in our lives. It is wrong, disrespectful, hurtful and in most cases illegal as well.

SIGNS A CHILD MAY BE BEING CYBERBULLIED

It is very hard to identify exactly what may be upsetting a child at first glance. Many of the following listed behaviours can be a result of a range of issues, but in the twenty-first century we must be aware that the issue may be a result of technology as much as a result of a medical illness or other issue. There is no definitive list of signs that would indicate cyberbullying, but below are those known to be most common.

Change in mood and/or behaviour: Investigate any change, however slight, in your child's demeanour. This, of course, could be as a result of a lot of different issues, but if something is bothering your child, you need to try to find out what it is.

Lowering of grades at school: A decrease in your child's academic marks should be investigated. Often children who are being bullied show a distinct change in application to study and a lowering of marks.

Not wanting to go to school/sport, etc.: Not wanting to be at the same place as the bully is normal. Going from having no issues heading out the door to school or sport to not wanting to go is a sure sign that something is not right. This can often manifest itself as random and non-specific ailments that occur primarily just prior to having to leave for school or sport. Things such as headaches, stomach aches, or generally feeling sick may indicate an issue other than a medical illness.

Being extra secretive in online activities: Kids often feel that they should have privacy when online and using a mobile phone. Be alert to secretive behaviours, finding them online under the duvet, in a secluded part of the house.

Distinct change in online behaviours: Take note of changes in your child's online behaviour and investigate. Examples include being jumpy when text messages arrive, not putting their phone down, wanting to be online all the time or the opposite – never wanting to be online.

Upset, angry, teary . . . rebellious when not previously: Of course, most adolescents exhibit these behaviours, some more than others. It is a normal and unavoidable part of growing up when hormones seem to take over and your child changes before your eyes. It is difficult to differentiate between normal adolescent angst and something more sinister, but trust your instincts, and if you are concerned, then investigate to try to get to the bottom of the problem.

Change in friendship groups: Again, this can be no more than the normal change in friends that occurs many times during a child's school days, but if you are concerned, act on your worries and at least speak to your child's teacher. They are often aware of these things way before you as they get to see the class dynamic in action every day.

Spending more time with family instead of friends: While it may seem nice, in that suddenly your child wants to hang out with you more than their friends, adolescence is a time where friends become very important and parents less so. Just be aware that things may not be okay in their world (either on or offline) and be there for them. Ask if they are okay, if something has happened that is bothering them, and if they want to talk. If you are still concerned then enlist the help of your GP, school welfare staff or adolescent psychologist.

WHAT CAN I DO IF MY CHILD IS CYBERBULLIED?

Do not be angry with your child: Remember that they are the victim and it is someone else doing the wrong thing. DO NOT threaten to take technology away from them because of what someone else has done.

Praise them for coming to you: This is a big step as most children are frightened to tell a parent about cyberbullying. Even if you don't really understand, let them know that you will help.

Save and store the content: Keep copies of the emails, chats or text messages, comments or posts. Take a screenshot of the evidence or cut and paste it into a Word document, whatever is easier for you. Don't worry if you don't know how to do this, as most children know how to take screenshots. An easy, non-technical way to get hard copies is to bring the content up on the screen of a mobile phone, place the phone on a copy machine and press copy.

Help your child to block and delete the bully from all contact lists: Most reputable sites allow the user to control who has access to them. Sit together to support your child as they do this. Many children feel mean blocking another person, even if that person has already been mean to them.

Do not respond: It is important not to respond to nasty emails, chats, text or comments – this is what the bully wants, so ignore them. Children will need your help and support to do this as it is natural to want to fight back. If your child responds with a threat or other unsuitable comment, then they may get themselves into trouble as well. Although you might like to weigh in with your thoughts, please don't. An adult abusing a child online regardless of what has occurred previously will get you into trouble.

Use the 'report abuse' button: All reputable social networking sites, chat rooms, online games, etc., have a method by which you can let the site know that a particular person/account is behaving unacceptably or bothering you. Tell them the problems you are having and they are obligated to investigate. Accounts can be deleted and warnings sent when users disobey the rules of the site.

Inform your child's school: It is important that they know what is going on so that they can help and support your child and monitor any issues that may spill into the playground or classroom. If the bully is a fellow student, the school will assist to work through the situation and deal with it as they would with any other bullying behaviours reported to them. If the bully is not from the same school, still ensure that the class teacher is aware so that they can also support your child in the same way as they would when any student has a problem. Schools are legally obligated via their duty of care to assist and investigate all reports of bullying, including cyberbullying, regardless of when it occurred. Do not be fobbed off with a comment such as, 'It happened at night, it has nothing to do with us.'

Have some down time without technology: It is important that your child's life is balanced so making sure that they are not online or spending hours on a mobile phone is important for both their mental and physical health (do not do this as punishment, rather as some peaceful time where they are not being bothered).

If unwanted contact continues: In most cases, cyberbullying is successfully resolved with prompt intervention. If, however, this is not the case, you may consider deleting current accounts and starting a new account/s where your child only gives their details to a small list of trusted friends.

Get a new phone number: As inconvenient as it is, this may be the best option if your child is being harassed via mobile phone. If a number that is not 'caller unknown' is harassing your child, then that number can be blocked via the settings in the phone. There are also programs that can be added to a mobile phone that will allow parents to set restrictions on the phone's use. Check with your mobile phone provider. You must also report the abuse to the phone company, which is obligated to investigate. Phone numbers can be changed at no cost if the request for a new number is as a result of ongoing abuse.

If the bullying is ongoing, report it to police: Most school-based cyberbullying is satisfactorily resolved at school level, but there are always exceptions to the rule. Schools cannot report cyberbullying between individual students so it is up to the victim (and parent) to make the report. A police report should not be in place of a school investigation – rather, in addition, if required. Police should always be informed about cyberbullying when, despite the best efforts of the school, it does not stop, when you have no idea who is behind the abuse (fake accounts/blocked numbers) and when threats have been made to your child's personal safety. You don't have to put up with it. By committing an act of cyberbullying a person may be committing a criminal offence under a number of different UK laws.

WHAT IF MY CHILD IS THE CYBERBULLY?

While it often comes as a shock to be told that your child has been bullying another student online, it is important that parents support schools in their handling of the situation. Don't try to make the situation lesser – accept that the school has the expertise to deal with all parties to bullying behaviour. Schools have policies and programmes to deal with students who bully others. Some use things such as restorative justice or similar programmes to support not only the victim but the bully as well.

As a parent, you have a major role to play to ensure that your child does not become or remain a cyberbully. Be involved and aware of what your child is doing online, where they are going and who they are hanging out with. As hard as it can be, children should be supervised when using technology and this is your role as a parent in the twenty-first century. If you see comments that are unpleasant, hurtful or nasty, speak to your child and explain why they should not behave this way online. Be vigilant and be involved. Parents have the ability to prevent the vast majority of online bullying. Once you are aware that your child has bullied someone else online, you can support your child in these ways:

- Help them understand that their behaviour is unacceptable and possibly criminal. Also discuss why it is not okay to be mean online.
- Acknowledge that they may be feeling awful too – they may be upset that they have done the wrong thing, but let them see there are consequences. Don't bail them out!
- Talk to them about their actions and try to find out why they behaved in this way.
- Ask them to imagine they were the victim. How would they feel?
- Work together to improve the situation (apologise, etc.).
- Work towards preventing further incidents. Set clear rules and boundaries about their online behaviour and your expectations. Be vigilant and be involved.
- Enlist the help of school, welfare staff, your GP or a child psychologist.

CYBERBULLYING QUICK RESPONSE CHECKLIST

- Don't respond.
- Block and delete bully.
- Report to the site.
- Keep a copy.
- Tell school (or relevant place) and seek action.
- If ongoing, inform police.
- Support your child. They have done nothing wrong.

Most importantly, stay calm, take a deep breath and try to be rational. Easier said than done, and all parents feel considerable pain when their children are hurt or upset. It is only normal. Often the parent is more upset than the child and kids are very resilient.

Never directly approach another child and/or their parents about a bullying issue. Make an appointment with the school and take all your supporting documents with you. Let the school deal with it, but ensure that they have processes in place to keep you up to date with what they are doing. Remember, they are the experts in these things and need to be supported in order to resolve these issues quickly and successfully. I have often seen cases where the school has acted superbly and the kids have moved on, but the parents want revenge and continue to make an issue out of the situation. Be guided by your children. If they're happy with the outcome then be happy too. If not, take the matter further. By this I mean higher up at school e.g. the headteacher, local education authority or other relevant body. No one has to put up with bullying or inaction, but please remember to be reasonable.

Author biography

Susan McLean is Australia's leading expert in the area of cybersafety and was a member of Victoria Police for twenty-seven years. She was the first Victoria Police officer appointed to a position involving cybersafety and young people. Susan is the media commentator of choice for print, radio and television both in Australia and internationally for her expert and balanced comments. She works closely with Facebook, Instagram, Twitter and Google and is regularly consulted by these organisations for input into their impact on Australian children. Susan is also the author of *Sexts, Texts and Selfies*, a definitive online safety resource.

www.cybersafetysolutions.com.au

See also:

Further resources:

National Bullying Helpline: www.nationalbullyinghelpline.co.uk

eCrime: www.ecrime-action.co.uk

Bullying UK: www.bullying.co.uk

BulliesOut: bulliesout.com

Anti-Bullying Alliance: www.anti-bullyingalliance.org.uk

Childline: childline.org.uk

Revenge Porn Helpline: www.revengepornhelpline.org.uk

Child Exploitation and Online Protection UK: www.ceop.police.uk

Further reading:

Manocha, R (Ed), 2017, *Growing Happy, Healthy Young Minds: Generation Next*, Hachette
    Australia, Sydney.

McLean, S, 2014, *Sexts, Texts and Selfies – How to keep your child safe in the digital space*,
    Penguin Books, Melbourne.

 We also recommend the very popular companion volume **GROWING HAPPY, HEALTHY YOUNG MINDS** – resilience, bullying, depression, anxiety, body image and many more important issues.

 For more online resources visit: **generationnext.com.au/handbook**

11. THE 'GAMBLIFICATION' OF COMPUTER GAMES

James Driver

With the recent explosion of online and mobile gambling there has been a renewed interest in assessing and understanding youth gambling. One factor that may make gambling increasingly accessible and attractive to young people is the developing crossover between gambling and other forms of media – particularly video gaming.

INTRODUCTION

Studies across Australia have been relatively consistent in showing that, within any given year, around 60 to 70 per cent of young people gamble in some form, and around 3.5 per cent of young people meet criteria for pathological gambling.[1] One factor that may make gambling more accessible and attractive to young people is the developing crossover between gambling and other forms of media. Alongside this trend – which has been called the 'gamblification' of games – non-gambling video games are also becoming more sophisticated in the ways in which they encourage and in some cases manipulate players into spending more money. This chapter outlines ways in which certain types of modern video games put young people at risk for transitioning to gambling, or at risk of financial exploitation through coercive approaches to generating revenue.

UNDERSTANDING THE TERMINOLOGY

There are a few terms that we need to understand before taking a more detailed look at this topic: 'gamblification', 'monetisation', and 'coercive monetisation'. 'Gamblification' is the use of gambling mechanics for non-gambling purposes – in the case of games, the purpose is to engage and retain players, and to get them to spend money on the product. 'Monetisation' is the process of converting an asset into money, in other words, the techniques that are used to sell something. Lastly, 'coercive monetisation' describes techniques used to sell something that are based on tricking or exploiting the purchaser.[2] It's also worth mentioning that when I use the term 'games' within this chapter, I am referring to all forms of video games that are not explicitly gambling games, whether they are played on a computer, console or mobile device.

The techniques used to monetise games and to profit from them range from the benign, such as creating a good product that people will want to buy, to the outright coercive and manipulative, such as threatening players with the loss of progress unless they pay up. Gamblification of games is one form of coercive monetisation, relying as it does on various psychological tricks that cause people to want to play more, spend more and be more reluctant to quit. We'll get on to all of that in a moment, but the important thing to understand for now is that while gamblification of games is one form of coercive monetisation, it's not the only one, and other forms of coercive monetisation can be equally effective at addicting players and causing them financial problems.

This distinction is important because it leads to two separate but related problems: the first is that the gamblification of games can lead to people transitioning to real gambling, with all the associated problems of that industry. The second is that some players will continue to play games and never transition to gambling, but may become addicted and financially exploited by these games because of the coercive monetisation methods used.

WAYS IN WHICH GAMBLIFICATION OCCURS

Let's take a look at some of the ways in which gamblification occurs within popular video games. Understanding these different forms of gamblification can help parents and educators talk more meaningfully with young people about avoiding exploitation and manipulation in games.

> ### GAMBLIFICATION
>
> Gamblification in games can be broadly broken down into the following categories:
> - Traditional gambling games available to players within non-gambling games.
> - Free-to-play/non-cash versions of traditional gambling games.
> - Gambling in parallel to non-gambling games.
> - Gambling mechanics (e.g. variable reward schedules) used within non-gambling games.

TRADITIONAL GAMBLING GAMES WITHIN NON-GAMBLING GAMES

Different games use different tactics to get players to spend money, and some really are free to play with no strings attached. It's important for parents to understand the types of games that young people are playing in order to manage potential risks. For a long time now, many video games that weren't really about gambling have included gambling content. Particularly in open-world or role-playing games, players often have the option of entering virtual casinos or gambling within the game world using in-game currency. Examples of this include many popular series such as Fallout or Grand Theft Auto. Although the gambling within these games doesn't specifically point players towards gambling in the real world, it familiarises them with the mechanics of gambling and makes gambling seem exciting and fun; players have the possibility of 'winning big', and the sounds and music that are part of the game can heighten player arousal. More pertinently, the video game is skill-based and these other games are those of chance, thereby perhaps leading the player to believe that there is some skill required to gamble.[3] The ability to 'save' and 'load' your game may encourage riskier gambling behaviour, and hide the significant costs associated with real-world gambling.

FREE-TO-PLAY GAMBLING GAMES

Free-to-play gambling games are games that in all respects look and operate like real gambling with the exception that no real money is involved – players bet using tokens or credits that cannot be exchanged for real cash. These games are potentially a very strong gateway into gambling with real money, not least because many of these games are produced and operated by the same publishers who also own gambling products. Alongside this, many if not most online gambling services that do offer gambling with real money also offer users the opportunity to play for 'free' – using credits rather than money – creating a powerful incentive to later transition to real gambling. Often the rate at which players win when playing in 'free play' mode is inflated, giving them a false sense of how easy it is to make money from gambling.[4]

A UK study into the gambling behaviours of 8017 young people aged twelve to fifteen found that 8 per cent of them had gambled online, and of those who had, nearly a third of them had previously used the 'free play' versions of these games.[5] Another paper showed that about 26 per cent of players who played social (non-monetary) casino games transitioned to real online gambling over a six-month period.[6] Interestingly, this research also showed that the strongest predictor of whether or not players migrated was if they purchased in-game credits with real money in the social games. This makes a strong argument that we need to look at all forms of coercive monetisation as potential links to later gambling behaviours, regardless of whether or not the game itself simulates gambling.

GAMBLING IN PARALLEL TO NON-GAMBLING GAMES

Increasingly we are seeing non-monetary forms of gambling taking place within video games leading to parallel processes of real-world gambling. The most obvious example of this at the time of writing is the popular game Counter-Strike: Global Offensive. In this game, players play as terrorists or counter-terrorists and run around within a virtual environment trying to shoot each other with a variety of weaponry. As players play the game, they receive 'weapon crates', which they can unlock by purchasing a key from the game store. Each weapon crate contains a random weapon, kind of like a Kinder Surprise egg but with virtual guns – a form of non-monetary gambling since the results are randomised. Some of these virtual guns are extremely rare and highly desired by players, leading to businesses creating websites where players are able to trade these weapons with each other for real money.

This has led to a new phenomenon: websites where players are able to gamble using the virtual weapons they have received in exchange for potentially winning other virtual weapons. Because some of these weapons are worth hundreds or thousands of pounds, this is, in all regards, the same as gambling at an online casino – but using fake weapons as chips rather than a more traditional intermediate currency. Due to the fact that these gambling sites only allow players to gamble using virtual goods – even if they can later exchange these for money – these sites are currently extremely poorly regulated, if at all, and are accessible to players who would not be of age to legally gamble through typical gambling sites.

Younger children are increasingly at risk due to new forms of gambling that are not regulated, and forms of gambling that use game cards that can be purchased from supermarkets or local shops – a credit card is not always required.

Gambling mechanics used within non-gambling games

A lot of games use various mechanics that are commonly found in gambling even when these games have nothing to do with gambling themselves. For example, it's a well-known psychological principle that when you give people (or indeed animals) unpredictable rewards for a behaviour, they are far more likely to repeat the behaviour than if you reward it more consistently. In gambling, this takes the form of payouts and jackpots. In video games, it takes many different forms. One of the most common is that many games reward players for playing the game by giving them items that will help them out in the game. Often these items are randomised – some of them have a trivial effect, while others are extremely powerful, so players never quite know what they are going to get. The result of this is that people will often keep playing in order to experience the 'rush' that comes from getting an extremely powerful item or upgrade. One gamer described this eloquently: 'I had this unbeatable rush of adulation and excitement,' he says. 'For someone who didn't get out much I was on cloud nine. And at that point things changed – I started chasing that high.'[7]

Forms of coercive monetisation

Let's turn now to some of the ways that non-gambling games use coercive monetisation to separate players from their cash. These games may never lead players into real-life gambling, but can be equally destructive through the mechanisms they use to promote compulsive gaming and in-game spending. It's worth noting that with most 'free-to-play' games that rely on microtransactions or in-app purchases to make a profit, nearly 60 per cent of their revenue comes from just 10 per cent of players. This means that these games are reliant on a small number of heavy spenders to make a profit, and the industry is well aware of it.

Understanding the tactics used by these games to exploit players is important for parents and educators, so that they can help young people to understand and avoid these tricks.

COMMON TRICKS

Some of the most common tricks used by these games are:

- Hiding the true cost of purchases.
- Playing on emotion.
- Threatening players with loss.
- Targeted deals and advertising.
- Offering rewards and incentives for play and spending.

Hiding the true cost of purchases

Every game that relies on in-app purchases to make a profit requires players to purchase an intermediate currency in the form of credits, gems, gold coins or some other form or currency. Players then use this currency, rather than cash, to purchase items in the game. This serves a number of purposes:

1. Players are less aware of how much real money they are spending for in-game items.
2. It allows the publisher to offer 'discounted' currency. Ramin Shokrizade, a game economist, states that a user who is able to do basic maths equations – which occur in a part of the brain that develops earlier – might feel they are 'saving more' by buying more. The younger the age of the user, the more likely it is to work.[8]
3. It allows the publisher to offer amounts of intermediate currency that means that the player will always have some 'left over'. A common situation is that you spend ten pounds of real money to get a hundred credits. The in-game item you want costs eighty-five credits, leaving you with fifteen remaining – however, there is nothing that can be purchased for only fifteen credits. This motivates players to purchase more coins in order to avoid 'losing' the leftover credits from their purchase.

Playing on emotion

Many games, particularly those targeted at a younger audience, play on people's emotions in order to motivate them to spend money. In the popular game Panda Pop, a game about rescuing baby pandas from an evil monkey, players are confronted with a picture of crying baby pandas when they fail a level. On-screen text then prompts them, 'Don't abandon the baby pandas', with the option of paying in-game currency (requiring real money) in order to continue. An earlier example was the Facebook game Frontierville, which told players that a deer had been wounded by a coyote and needed their help to survive. In this case, 'help' meant feeding it an in-game item that could be purchased for about two American dollars from the in-game store.

Threatening players with loss

Many games threaten players with losing the progress they have made or items they have acquired if they do not continue to play the game. It's well known that humans are highly motivated by loss avoidance, and these tactics are often effective in causing people to continue gaming beyond what they otherwise would. Many popular games like Clash of Clans, Game of War and Mobile Strike obfuscate the source of this threat by making it appear that it is other players rather than the game itself that can cause you to lose your progress, by allowing other players to 'attack' you when you are not playing and steal your resources. These games then often offer you options – for a price, of course – that enable you to better defend yourself from other players. At times, this can lead to a virtual arms race between players, which in some instances has led to players accruing thousands of pounds of charges in game.

Targeted deals and advertising

Most free-to-play games make heavy use of in-game advertising in order to coerce players into spending. Because the game knows how well players are performing, these advertisements are often shown at times when the game knows the player may be more receptive.

For example, after losing a level a player may be shown a screen to the effect of 'you seem to be having some trouble – this item will help you out'. Alongside this, the games may offer what appear to be incredible discounts of 80 to 90 per cent or more – often for a limited time, which creates pressure in players to spend money immediately. Of course, because the items being offered in games have no intrinsic real-world value, it is possible to offer these kinds of discounts that would not be practical in the real world, but which can have a powerful effect on the minds of players who have not been exposed to this sort of advertising before. Many of these games are also capable of sending advertisements to players' phones even when they are not playing the game, creating additional reminders and incentives to spend money.

Offering incentives and rewards

Most of these games also offer various kinds of rewards that motivate players to continue playing and spending. Often players will be given in-game rewards for playing the game every day, with the rewards increasing in value the more days in a row the player plays. Alongside this, players are often given rewards in-game for spending money, by being given VIP status in-game or other bonuses. Sometimes players will be sent notifications to their phone that they will receive a reward if they log in within the next several hours, incentivising them to play at times that they otherwise might not have done so.

THE EFFECTS OF GAMBLIFICATION AND COERCIVE MONETISATION

This section has outlined some of the different types of gamblification and coercive monetisation that exist within modern video games. The details given here are by no means exhaustive, but it's important for those who are concerned about this issue to understand how these techniques and tactics appear within games. One of the best ways to help young people avoid exploitation through online gaming and gambling is thorough education on the psychological tricks used by manufacturers to get players to spend. When young people are able to identify these tricks and understand their purpose, they are much better placed to avoid being manipulated by them. For example, if a young person can be helped to understand that the crying pandas they see are not real and are not suffering – and, in fact, that the game developer is trying to make them feel bad in order to get them to spend money – they will be more able to resist the effects of this sort of manipulation.

Let's turn now to looking at who might be at risk for exploitation by gamblification in games, how to identify the problem and, importantly, what can be done about it.

Signs and symptoms

How can we tell if someone might have a problem with gambling in games, or might be at risk for transitioning from gaming to gambling? A great deal of research and guidance is available on methods for assessment and treatment of problem gambling, and to a lesser extent on problem gaming. Both gaming and gambling can become a problem for someone before they meet the criteria for pathological/addictive gambling/gaming, so it is important for parents and those working with young people to be alert to symptoms that could indicate that gaming is starting to become a problem.

Common symptoms to be aware of would include:

- Preoccupation with gaming – thinking about, reading about, talking about or watching videos about gaming even when not playing.
- Withdrawal symptoms – becoming anxious, depressed, angry or agitated when gaming is taken away or limited.
- Developing tolerance – wanting to spend increasing lengths of time gaming.
- Losing control – having made unsuccessful attempts to try to manage or reduce their own gaming.
- Loss of interest in other areas of their life, particularly other hobbies, social engagements and friends.

- Continuing to game despite experiencing negative effects of their gaming, for example on their schooling, social life, or financial situation.
- Deception of those around them about how much and when they game. For example, lying about the frequency of gaming, gaming at times they know they won't be detected, such as when parents are out or late at night.
- Using gaming as a way to manage negative moods, or to escape from depression, anxiety or stress.
- Experiencing significant loss due to their gaming, such as failing at school or losing friendships.

If a young person is exhibiting more than four or five of these symptoms, then it is possible that their gaming may be becoming a problem – and if the type of game that they are playing is one that involves gamblified content, or which use coercive monetisation, then it is possible that they may be at risk of financial exploitation as well.

Risk factors

While research shows that a not insubstantial number of young people try gambling at some point, not all of those young people go on to develop problems. If we can identify which young people are most likely to be at risk of transitioning to problem gambling, then we will be better placed to target interventions to the right people and at the right time.

Current research has identified a number of risk factors and protective factors that may indicate that a young person is at greater or lesser risk of developing problem behaviours around gambling or gaming, either as a young person or later in life.

Some of the main risk factors appear to be:

- Early exposure to gambling – Adult problem gamblers report being exposed to gambling at a younger age than non-problem gamblers, and so delaying young people's exposure to gambling for as long as possible likely has a protective effect.

- Gender – Men and boys have around a six-times-higher chance of becoming problem gamblers than women and girls, and are about twice as likely to meet criteria for being considered 'at-risk' gamblers.
- Minority status – Research across many countries has consistently shown that those belonging to racial/ethnic minority groups or belonging to lower socioeconomic groups are more at risk.
- Personality – Young people who demonstrate impulsivity, excitability, who are more inclined to take risks or be sensation seeking or become bored more easily, and who show less self-regulation are more at risk.
- Using gaming or gambling as a coping mechanism – Young people who use gaming or gambling in order to modify their mood, or to manage difficult feelings are more at risk.
- Greater life stressors – Young people who have greater-than-average life stressors are more at risk. This could include current factors such as difficulties in the home environment, stress with peers or academic issues, existing mental health problems as well as historical factors such as a history of trauma and abuse, major losses or deaths, etc.
- Existing mental health or addiction issues – Young people with existing mental health or addiction issues are more at risk.
- Poor interpersonal relationships – Young people who lack strong interpersonal relationships, or whose relationships are characterised by conflict, are more at risk. This includes family and peer relationships as well as engagement in the wider community.
- Spending money on in-game purchases – If a young person has a history of spending money for in-game items or boosts, particularly if they have done so frequently or ever borrowed or stolen in order to do so, then they are also more at risk.

While these factors may be potential risks for young people developing problems with gaming or gambling, when the opposite is present this may represent a strong protective factor. For example, a young person who has strong, supportive relationships at home and at school, who has multiple strategies for dealing with stress and anxiety, and who demonstrates a reasonable degree of self-regulation, will be less at risk than someone who lacks these factors.

It is important, then, when considering the possibility that a young person may be at risk of developing problems with gaming or gambling, to look at the wider context of their life. As will be discussed in the next section, part of helping young people involves identifying factors that might create or perpetuate a problem and helping them address these while simultaneously identifying protective factors and supporting them to develop these further. Doing this requires a thorough understanding of the various aspects of a young person's life that may be contributing to the problems they are experiencing.

INTERVENTIONS

While it is crucial to understand how games are structured to promote spending and to familiarise young people with gambling mechanics, and it is important to know what symptoms to look for and how to identify who might be at risk of developing problems, the most important question remains: what can we do about it?

Obviously, early identification and prevention of problems with gaming or gambling is ideal, but at times we also need to have ways of helping young people who may already have developed problems with these issues. Thankfully many of the strategies that can be employed to try to prevent problems developing in the first place are still important and effective once a problem has developed. Ways that parents and educators can support young people to avoid problems with gaming and gambling broadly fall into the following categories:

- Education.
- Modelling.
- Identifying and reducing risk/perpetuating factors.
- Identifying and strengthening protective factors.
- Referring to and connecting with appropriate services.

Education

Educating young people about gaming and gambling is a crucial part of assisting them to make healthy choices for themselves. This education needs to focus not just on the risks and costs potentially associated with gambling and gaming, but also on how to identify the tricks and techniques used by game developers to either motivate them to transition to gambling, or to coerce them into spending more money than they wish to. If parents and educators are well aware of these techniques (as described earlier) themselves, then they will be well placed to help young people understand how these techniques are being employed against them in the game they play. Where possible then, educators and parents can also identify and encourage young people who do want to game to play those games that do not include gamblification or coercive monetisation.

Modelling

It is important for parents to be mindful of what behaviours they are modelling for their children. Since research has indicated that early exposure to gambling is a risk factor for developing later gambling problems, it is important that parents try to limit exposure to this through their own behaviours. Alongside this, modelling appropriate and healthy technology use is important. Young people who start to use technology or gaming for mood-modification — that is, in order to feel better when they are stressed or upset — are more at risk of developing problems. Parents need to be aware of their own coping strategies when they are stressed or unhappy themselves, and avoid modelling strategies that they would not want copied by their children.

Identifying and reducing perpetuating factors

Both parents and educators can play a role in identifying risk or perpetuating factors in young people's lives and helping them to reduce these. As discussed previously, there are a wide range of potential risk factors from personality characteristics through to demographic factors and the wider context of a young person's life. If there are significant risk factors – for example, a young person who is impulsive, socially isolated and has a history of trauma – then it's important to consider ways that these can be managed. Setting and enforcing limits around use, helping young people to develop social skills and build social networks, or providing them support to work through historical issues can all be a part of this process.

Identifying and supporting protective factors

Alongside reducing risk and perpetuating factors, parents and educators can help young people to identify and strengthen existing protective factors. If a young person has strong existing social networks, is involved in other activities or hobbies, or has some capacity for self-regulation and coping, these can all be identified and reinforced through support, encouragement and education/skills training where appropriate.

Referring to and connecting with appropriate services

In cases where a young person might have an existing problem with excessive gaming or gambling, it may be necessary to get additional support from appropriate agencies. There are a number of agencies that can help with issues relating to gambling or gaming, including GamCare and many others. See recommended resource list at end of this chapter.

TAKE-AWAY MESSAGES

- Understand the games that young people are playing, and how those games make money.
- Limit access to games based on 'in-app purchases' or those that simulate gambling.

- Educate young people about the psychological tricks used in modern games.
- Identify and reduce risk factors in young people's lives while supporting them to develop healthy alternatives and effective coping skills.

The worlds of gaming and gambling are rapidly changing and, in some spaces, converging. As developers discover new ways to monetise their products and as the business models of gaming and gambling begin to increasingly overlap, we are faced with a range of emerging public health risks. Since the impulsivity and reduced capacity to accurately assess risk are easily exploited by gaming and gambling businesses, it is perhaps no surprise that it is young people who are disproportionately affected by many of these changes. If we are to understand these emerging risks and be able to help young people to navigate them successfully, then we need to keep up with the rapid rate of change in these industries and understand the nature and appeal of these new forms of gaming and gambling so that we can educate young people about them. When we sufficiently understand the whole context of a young person's life and the mechanisms by which these games exploit players, we will be well placed to help them find alternatives and develop healthy patterns of behaviour.

Author biography

James Driver is a registered psychotherapist and completed his training in Auckland and London. He has worked at a number of addiction-treatment centres and has spent time researching the experiences of people who received treatment for video gaming addiction. He is passionate about improving understanding of the psychological impacts of technology use and helping people to develop healthy habits. James provides training and supervision internationally to mental health clinicians working with these issues and runs a private practice in Christchurch, New Zealand.

www.netaddiction.co.nz

See also:

Chapter 1: Understanding Teen Sleep and Drowsy Kids
Chapter 3: Understanding the Teenage Brain
Chapter 5: Healthy Habits for a Digital Life
Chapter 7: Problematic Internet Use and How to Manage It
Chapter 8: Computer Game Addiction and Mental Wellbeing
Chapter 14: Advice for Parents: Be a Mentor, Not a Friend

Recommended resources:

GamCare Helpline: 0808 8020 133
BigDeal (GamCare's service for young people): 0808 8020 133

Recommended websites:

GamCare: www.gamcare.org.uk
Big Deal: www.bigdeal.org.uk
Be Gamble Aware: begambleaware.org
Gamblers Anonymous: www.gamblersanonymous.org.uk
Games without in-app purchases for older children: www.slant.co/topics/3480/~ios-games-without-in-app-purchases
NHS: www.nhs.uk/Livewell/addiction

Further reading:

Delfabbro, P, Derevensky, JL & Gainsbury, S, 2011, 'Correlates, risk, and protective factors associated with youth gambling', *Health, Medicine and Human Development: Youth Gambling: The Hidden Addiction*.

Manocha, R (Ed), 2017, *Growing Happy, Healthy Young Minds: Generation Next*, Hachette Australia, Sydney.

Monash University, 2011, 'Guideline for screening, assessment and treatment in problem gambling', retrieved from: www.med.monash.edu.au/assets/docs/sphc/pgrtc/guideline/problem-gambling-guidelines-web.pdf

Shaul, B, 2016, Infographic: '"Whales" account for 70% of in-app purchase revenue', retrieved from www.adweek.com/socialtimes/infographic-whales-account-for-70-of-in-app-purchase-revenue/635073.

We also recommend the very popular companion volume **GROWING HAPPY, HEALTHY YOUNG MINDS** – resilience, bullying, depression, anxiety, body image and many more important issues.

For more online resources visit:
generationnext.com.au/handbook

12. VIOLENT VIDEO GAMES AND VIOLENT BEHAVIOUR

Dr Wayne Warburton

Multi-billion-dollar industries such as advertising, Hollywood, television, educational media and training simulators all work on the basic premise that screen-based activities can change the way people think, feel and behave. Research shows that this is also the case for violent video games, which are linked to increased aggression, desensitisation to violence, hostile thoughts and feelings, and decreases in prosocial behaviour and empathy. The secret to managing video game play is aspiring to a healthy media diet: moderation in amount, preferential exposure to helpful content and taking the age of the child into account.

INTRODUCTION

In the latest Common Sense Media Poll of US tweens and teens (2015), thirteen- to eighteen-year-olds spent an average of almost nine hours (8:56) per day with 'entertainment' media, excluding schoolwork and homework, and tweens aged eight to twelve averaged almost six hours (5:55). Average screen use was 6:40 and 4:36 per day respectively. Although television was still the most-used type of entertainment media, video games continue to be very popular. They are played by the majority of children, and the 2015 poll shows that among players, the average time per day spent playing is two hours for tweens and 2:25 for teens. Indeed, around 10 per cent of teens averaged more than four hours of video game play per day. The figures are higher again for boys, as more boys than girls play video games, and boys tend to spend more time playing.

When these figures are compared with other key activities that influence children's thinking and behaviour (for example, kids spend about five hours a day being taught at school and usually much less talking with parents), media use generally, and video game use specifically, are a big influence on many children's lives. For this reason it is important for the modern parent or professional who works with children to understand the potential impacts of media use and video game use.

Although video games have been popular for decades now, in recent years there have been noteworthy increases in average playing hours and changes in content. The advent of tablets and other internet-connected devices, which allow device-based gaming and 24/7 online gaming in any location with internet access, has facilitated a significant rise in the number of hours per day that children play video games, and a decrease in the age of children with access to them. For example, Victoria Rideout found that in 2013, compared to 2011, twice as many US children aged zero to eight used such devices, and time spent on those devices had tripled. The most common activity (63 per cent) was online gaming. In terms of video game content, there have been significant increases in the quality of computer game graphics and programming, in the realism of depicted characters and in the extremity of content.

The thematic content of video games varies widely, but there are many very popular games based around exercise (e.g. dance games, virtual sports), as well as games that facilitate educational outcomes, prosocial behaviour, creativity, cooperation and engagement with moral and social issues. However, a steady staple of the video game industry is in-game violence, with many of the top-selling games consistently having violent content, and sometimes content that is extremely violent. The level of violence and the realism of that violence has steadily increased in recent years, and 'ratings creep' has allowed increasingly violent material to be included into lower ratings categories. Thus, playing of violent video games (VVG) is widespread, even at young ages. Interestingly, there is evidence that for many adolescents, the level of violence in preferred video games rises with the number of hours per week video games are played.

The question this chapter will address is whether this violent video game content has an impact on players.

VIOLENT VIDEO GAMES

When I ask parents whether playing violent video games impacts on children's behaviour, the most common answer I get is that common sense suggests there should be an effect, but that they had heard in the media that this was wrong – that there is little scientific evidence for any negative impacts of playing violent video games or that the scientific community is evenly divided on this issue.

In truth, there is a divide between researchers in this area. However, in contrast to public perceptions, it is not a very even split. The vast majority of scientists who are actively researching this topic accept that there is considerable scientific evidence that playing violent video games can change the way players think, feel and behave, including increases in aggression. In contrast, a small but very vocal group of academics believe that the scientific research linking video game violence to aggressive behaviour is flawed (and that there are, in fact, no negative impacts). This group receives a disproportionate amount of media attention, so their views are widely reported.

Their arguments against the validity of the scientific findings linking video game violence to aggressive behaviour have been carefully analysed by several researchers and, in my opinion, most do not stand up to careful scrutiny. It is no surprise, then, that a number of respected professional bodies have reviewed the research findings and made public statements that there is a causal link between violent media exposure and aggressive behaviour, and/or between playing violent video games and aggressive behaviour. These include the American Medical Association (2000), the American Academy of Child and Adolescent Psychiatry (2000), the American Academy of Pediatrics (2000, 2009), the International Society for Research on Aggression (2012), the Society for the Psychological Study of Social Issues (2014), and the American Psychological Association (2000, 2015).

From my perspective, the argument for a link between playing violent video games and aggressive behaviour is compelling, whether approaching the issue from a common-sense or a scientific perspective. Let's examine this issue from a common-sense viewpoint first.

THE COMMON-SENSE PERSPECTIVE

First, common sense suggests that violent media should influence behaviour in similar ways to other media. Many multi-billion-dollar industries (e.g. advertising, Hollywood, commercial television, educational media, training simulators, etc.) are all built on the premise that screen media (and other media) can affect the way people think, feel and behave. Both scientific research and the marketplace show that such media has a powerful psychological impact across a range of outcomes including knowledge acquisition/ education, voting, developing skills and consumer purchasing. It stretches credibility to believe that violent video games do not have the potential to have a negative impact on the way people think, feel and behave when other forms of media have a profound psychological effect.

Second, every parent and professional who works with children knows that a child's environment influences their psychology and their behaviour. The human brain wires up in response to what we experience every second of every day, and thus the things we experience change what we think, feel and know. Experiences that are frequent or intense lead to changes that are more marked and longer term. There are countless examples: violent homes have an impact on the way children see the world and respond to it; warm relationships with parents and peers are linked with better adjustment and resilience; abusive and chaotic home environments are linked with trauma and a range of mental health issues. If actual and vicarious experiences of violent homes, violent neighbourhoods, violent peers and war zones all affect the way children think, feel and behave, then it seems unlikely that considerable exposure to violent media has no impact at all.

Third, the processes by which all social behaviours (including aggression) are learned and maintained are well understood, and include imitation, observational learning, conditioning, desensitisation and the 'priming' of feelings and concepts in the brain. All of these well-established and highly researched psychological processes predict that exposure to violent media would have some impact on social behaviour.

Thus, based on what we already know about media and psychology and children, common sense leads to one conclusion: a lot of exposure to violent video games should have a psychological impact on the player.

WARNING SIGNS AND INDICATORS (RED FLAGS)

- Becomes aggressive or irritable after playing a video game, a few times or often.
- Becomes angry or aggressive when the parent asks the child to stop playing, a few times or often.
- Talks a lot about violent themes (including game content) between games; has violent fantasies.
- Increasingly aggressive in everyday life.
- Sometimes imitates aggressive content from a video game during non-video-game play.
- Develops an unhealthy fascination for weapons, murder, death.
- Video game content seems to be frightening: nightmares, sleep disturbances, anxiety, fear and/or distress related to video game content.
- A noticeable increase in hostile attitudes, beliefs that aggression is a normal way to resolve conflict, and beliefs that the world is a scary place where others cannot be trusted.

WHAT THE SCIENTIFIC EVIDENCE SUGGESTS

In my view, looking at video game violence from a scientific perspective also points to a clear impact of violent video games on children's psychology. However, before we look at the actual scientific findings, it is important to address why I believe they are trustworthy rather than flawed. Those who disbelieve the research showing a VVG–aggression link suggest there have been problems with the measurement of aggression in the laboratory and a failure to take into account alternative explanations. When the totality of scientific findings are taken into account, these arguments seem less compelling. For any scientific problem, there are strengths and weaknesses for every type of scientific approach. Experiments can prove one thing causes another but the findings may not be relevant to the real world; correlational studies can examine real-world issues but cannot determine whether one factor causes another; studies that examine the impact of a factor on an outcome in the same person over time (longitudinal studies) examine real-world behaviours and can provide inferences of causality, but often do not take into account all the other factors that may also impact outcomes. The key thing to remember is that the strengths of each approach overcome the weaknesses of another, so if a finding occurs across all methodologies, the evidence points to that effect being real. In violent video game research, there have been many studies across a range of scientific research methods, and they converge to find the same outcomes, even when taking into account alternative explanatory factors. For me, this is compelling evidence. Let's have a look at what those outcomes are.

Aggression

There are now many studies showing a link between playing violent video games and aggressive behaviour. Some find causal links between violent video game play and measures of aggression in experimental studies, some find a positive correlation between violent video game play and real-world aggression, and some find that levels of violent game play predict increases in aggressive behaviour over time. The experimental studies test short-term effects. These are short lived (participants tend to show increased aggression for ten to fifteen minutes or so after playing a violent game) and relate only to the mild sorts of aggression that can be ethically tested in a laboratory. Nevertheless, the findings are consistent and clear: playing violent video games increases the likelihood of subsequent aggression.

Across dozens of cross-sectional studies and more than twenty longitudinal studies, a consistent VVG–aggression link is found, suggesting that the short-term effects are also cumulative – those who play more violent video games are also more likely to develop higher levels of aggression over time.

The number of studies examining these effects, as well as impacts on other aggression-related outcomes, is not trivial. Up to 2014 there had been close to 500 tests of these effects across more than 170 000 participants.

Hostile thoughts and feelings

Aggressive behaviour is usually accompanied by internal psychological processes that impel the person towards aggressive actions. Most notably, people might have hostile feelings (such as anger or resentment) or hostile thoughts (for example, attitudes that approve of aggression, the belief that others want to hurt you, or personal scripts for resolving conflict that involve aggression). Experimental studies of short-term effects show that during violent video game play, on average, a player's thoughts and feelings tend to be more hostile than when not playing.

In the long term, there is evidence that heavy consumers of violent media (including video games) tend to develop more hostile ways of thinking. These may include a hostile attributional bias – a tendency to see the world as more violent than it really is, to be less trusting, and to assume hostile motives in others. People with a hostile bias tend to respond to ambiguous events (such as someone accidentally bumping them in a crowded room) as if they are deliberate and provocative, thus increasing the likelihood of aggressive responding.

Desensitisation to violence

There is a substantial and growing body of evidence suggesting that playing violent games causes the player to become desensitised to violence and to the suffering of others, both in the short and the long term. Many of these studies are brain-imaging studies. My favourite study is by Doug Gentile and his colleagues at Iowa State University. They recruited two groups of habitual gamers – one group played a lot of violent games and the other a lot of non-violent games. Both groups played a violent game while in an fMRI (brain imaging) machine. Doug and his group expected the players of non-violent games to have a lot of neural activation in the emotion centres of the brain as they dealt with the feelings associated with hurting others during the game, but expected that the activation levels of habitual players of violent games would flatline, due to desensitisation. What they found surprised them. While the players of non-violent games had the expected spike in the brain's emotion centres, the players of violent games actually suppressed activity in those centres. This suggests that players of violent games may manage the negative emotions linked to hurting others during gameplay by partially turning off the emotion centres in the brain.

Fear

The exemplary work of Joanne Cantor (and others) from the University of Wisconsin-Madison demonstrates that many children find violent media, including the news, frightening. Key things that children find frightening are depictions of dangers, injuries and mutilations, depictions of fearful or endangered people, distortions of natural forms, monsters, frightening supernatural forms and depictions of violent encounters. Unfortunately, all categories are well represented in violent video games. Thus it is not surprising that many children report fear, anxiety, sadness, nightmares, sleep disturbances, stress and trauma symptoms after exposure to violent media, including video games. It is important to note that children under eight tend to be more afraid of the obvious characteristics of a game (e.g. scary-looking creatures), whereas older children are less afraid of things they know aren't real (such as monsters) and more afraid of things they could realistically imagine hurting them, their family or friends (such as a rampaging school shooter).

Empathy and prosocial behaviour

There is now a number of studies showing that playing violent games likely reduces both empathy and prosocial behaviour. This accords with my own experiences talking to parents, who often report the same thing.

WHY WOULD VIOLENT MEDIA INCREASE AGGRESSION?

There are a number of psychological processes that can explain why playing violent games might translate into aggressive behaviour.

Learning aggressive behaviours

There are three key ways in which people acquire behaviour. In associative learning, people link in their mind things that happen together, so that when one of those things happens, the linked thing is also expected to happen. In operant conditioning, people learn to avoid behaviours that have previously been punished or resulted in an adverse outcome, and are more likely to do things that have been rewarded or were pleasurable in the past. In social learning, people imitate the behaviours of others such as their parents, friends or other models, especially models who are attractive, admired, high status, similar or who are rewarded for their behaviour. A vast amount of research shows that aggressive behaviour can be acquired in all three ways.

Because violent games typically involve repetitive violent actions in multiple situations that bring in-game rewards, there is much scope to associate a wide variety of cues with aggression, to find aggression rewarding, and to copy violent role models within the game as well as admired players.

Further, from an educational perspective, Doug and Ron Gentile in 2008 detailed other important ways in which video games are an outstanding medium for learning – they are interactive, exciting, dynamic, repetitive and motivate players to persevere in acquiring and mastering a number of skills. Together, these findings from psychologists and educators suggest that there is much potential for players to learn aggressive behaviour from violent video games. (There is also great potential for learning beneficial behaviours).

Changes in brain activity

There are a number of brain phenomena associated with violent media and violent video games. Research consistently finds that during violent media exposure there is reduced activity in the parts of the brain responsible for higher cognitive tasks such as thinking through consequences and controlling urges. Brain imaging studies also reveal, as noted earlier, desensitisation to violence, and even active suppression of the emotion centres of the brain during violent video game play. Other studies have also found that the right hemisphere of the brain, where negative emotions (such as anger and fear) tend to be processed, is disproportionately activated when watching violent media. Reduced behavioural control, desensitisation to others' suffering and an increase in negative emotions are all factors linked with increases in aggressive behaviour.

Activation in the neural network

Every person's brain is a 'neural network' where every concept and emotion and memory is stored in clusters (nodes) of brain cells. These are highly interconnected, with nodes that are activated together becoming wired together. These links become stronger with more frequent activation. By toddlerhood, people wire together complex knowledge structures that include thoughts, feelings, memories, expectations and action tendencies around specific themes and life experiences. For example, children may have knowledge structures about their bedtime routine or what happens at a children's party. Adults have knowledge structures about a wide range of familiar activities such as shopping in a supermarket, getting the kids ready for school or managing conflict. These knowledge structures are activated automatically in a relevant situation and guide people's behaviour, often outside their conscious awareness. If people's experiences include a lot of exposure to violence and aggression, then they will have a lot of stored concepts and knowledge structures around aggression, and a lot of linked cues that can activate them.

During violent video game play, existing aggressive concepts and knowledge structures are likely to be activated by in-game cues. In addition, when a person plays a violent video game repetitively, they are almost certainly wiring/re-wiring new or existing aggressive knowledge structures, including with multiple cues for aggressive behaviour. Violent video games therefore have the potential to elicit immediate increases in the likelihood of aggression (the sorts of short-term effects seen in laboratory studies) and to produce cumulative effects whereby the person has an increasing number of aggression-related concepts and knowledge structures, and thus an increased likelihood of becoming more aggressive as a person.

HELP! MY SON PLAYS VIOLENT VIDEO GAMES. DOES THAT MEAN HE IS GOING TO BECOME A SCHOOL SHOOTER?

No, no, no!

It is important to emphasise two things here. First, these effects are robust but small. Violent media exposure is never sufficient in its own right to elicit aggression that is anything other than mild. Second, moderate aggression and violence always require there to be a number of other risk factors to occur. That is why all reputable media violence researchers take a risk-factor approach. That is, they believe that violence and more severe aggression only occur when there are a lot of risk factors for aggression that occur together, coupled with a lack of protective factors. Risk factors might include aggressive personality factors, being male, social isolation, being intoxicated, access to weapons, aggressive peers, a violent home and mental instability. Protective factors might include good conflict resolution strategies, a warm and supportive home environment, good communication with parents, an involved and caring community, and peers who are kind. Media violence exposure from this perspective is seen as one of many possible risk factors for aggression, but one of the few that can be managed effectively by parents, professionals and policy makers.

So, if a child plays a lot of violent video games, this may be a risk factor for aggression, but what is most important in determining eventual outcomes is the wider context of that child's life.

MANAGING VIOLENT VIDEO GAME USE

Posture and inactivity

Although the focus of this chapter is on the psychology of violent video game use, it would be remiss of me not to address the physiological issues around heavy gaming. Physiotherapists such as Leon Straker from Curtin University are pioneering research that shows that playing video games (other than active games such as dance games) is an inherently sedentary pastime which involves very little muscle movement. Inactivity is related to a wide range of undesirable health outcomes, and spending long hours hunched near a screen is linked to serious postural problems. In addition, child gamers tend to gain fine motor skills at the expense of gross motor skills. Together the evidence is clear – if children play video games they should not play for extended periods, but rather should have regular breaks and balance out video game play with outdoor exercise that encourages gross motor development.

The importance of active parental involvement

Although many children and teens feel uncomfortable with parents being actively involved in their video gaming, it turns out that when parents make the effort there is a big benefit for children. In one study by Doug Gentile and colleagues, when parents monitored their children's media use more, over time children consumed less media, had a decrease in body mass index, an increase in grades and an increase in sleep. In addition, the children had less exposure to violent media, a decrease in aggressive behaviour and an increase in prosocial behaviour. Clearly active parental monitoring is important!

As well as having an active involvement in their children's video game use, it is also important for parents to be good media-use role models themselves. The Common Sense Media Poll of parents of US tweens and teens (2016) revealed an average personal recreational screen media consumption of close to eight hours (7:43) a day – a level of use hardly conducive to convincing one's children to be moderate in their own screen use and gaming.

A healthy media diet

In modern western society, exposure to media and to video games is part of everyday life. Rather than seek to stop children having access, a more realistic and helpful approach is to work with children and teenagers towards a healthy media diet. Like food, the basic principles are fairly simple: moderation in amount, more of the good stuff and less of the unhealthy stuff, make sure it is appropriate to the person's age.

Although some key organisations are moving away from a numeric indicator of how much recreational media is too much, and focus instead on the healthy management of media use, I think it is helpful to have some sort of number in mind. For me, a healthy level of average daily total screen use is none up to eighteen months, an hour or so for toddlers and pre-schoolers, 1 to 1.5 hours for primary-school-aged children and around two hours for teenagers. How the average is arrived at is less important – children may play more on weekends and less on school days, for example – but letting children decide how they will spend their screen use quota (within limits) is usually a helpful approach.

In terms of content, the basic rule, and one that any child who understands the food pyramid can understand, is that it is healthier to choose more of the good stuff (educational, prosocial, developmentally appropriate media) and less of the unhealthy stuff (violent, frightening or anti-social media, some sexual content, media that vilifies others or is misogynistic). The key is moderation and having parental support when less helpful media is being used.

Clearly, having regard to the child's age is also important.

10 TIPS FOR HEALTHY VIDEO GAME PLAY

1. Aim for your children to have a healthy media diet in the three key areas:
    *   Moderate amount (1–2 hours per day recreational screen use).
    *   Content (more healthy content; less unhelpful content).
    *   Age-appropriateness, especially for children under eight.
2. Keep video games (on any device) out of the bedroom.
3. Aim for more physical activity time than sitting screen-time.
4. When playing video games, have an active break after thirty minutes.
5. Encourage a good, safe playing technique. That is, a technique that:
    *   avoids poor postures;
    *   avoids repetitive movements;
    *   ensures sufficient space for active e-games.
6. Know what games your children are playing and monitor their game use.
7. Set and enforce rules around use.
8. Model appropriate screen use and participation in real-world activities.
9. Have screen-free time before bedtime.
    *   Sleep professionals recommend two hours if possible.
10. Be actively involved in your child's game play.

CONCLUSION

Although there is convincing evidence (in my view) that playing violent video games can have a number of impacts on the player, including increased hostility and aggression, and reduced empathy for the suffering of others, these impacts are generally subtle and can be offset by other factors such as good parenting. The key is to aim for healthy use. Ten tips for healthy gaming are provided as a starting point for parents and professionals who work with children. However, the most important strategies for helping children and teens get the most out of media (while avoiding the pitfalls), are simple: be actively involved and be guided by your common sense.

Author biography

Dr Wayne Warburton is a senior lecturer in developmental psychology and Deputy Director of the Children and Families Research Centre at Macquarie University. Wayne is also a registered psychologist and has a strong research interest in the fields of aggressive behaviour, media psychology and parenting. He has a number of publications in scientific journals and books, primarily on topics around aggressive behaviour and the impact of violent and prosocial media. He is co-author of the International Society for Research on Aggression Statement on Media Violence, the Society for Psychological Study of Social Issues Research Summary on Media Violence, and the world experts' Statement on Violent Video Game Violence in the 'Gruel Amicus Curiae Brief' for the US Supreme Court case of *California vs. Entertainment Merchants*. He is the author of *Growing Up Fast and Furious: Reviewing the Impacts of Violent and Sexualised Media on Children* (with Danya Braunstein).

See also:
Chapter 1: Understanding Teen Sleep and Drowsy Kids
Chapter 3: Understanding the Teenage Brain
Chapter 5: Healthy Habits for a Digital Life
Chapter 7: Problematic Internet Use and How to Manage It
Chapter 8: Computer Game Addiction and Mental Wellbeing
Chapter 14: Advice for Parents: Be a Mentor, Not a Friend

Recommended websites:
The Children's Media Foundation: www.thechildrensmediafoundation.org
Centre on Media and Child Health: www.cmch.tv
Common Sense Media: www.commonsensemedia.org
Distinguished Professor Craig Anderson, world-leading video game violence researcher: www.public.psych.iastate.edu/caa

Further reading:

Anderson, CA, Shibuya, A, Ihori, N, Swing, EL, Bushman, BJ, Sakamoto, A, Rothstein, HR & Saleem, M, 2010, 'Violent video game effects on aggression, empathy, and prosocial behavior in Eastern and Western countries', *Psychological Bulletin* 136, pp 151–173.

Greitemeyer, T & Mugge, DO, 2014, 'Video games do affect social outcomes: A meta-analytic review of the effects of violent and prosocial video game play', *Personality and Social Psychology Bulletin* 40, pp 578–589, DOI: 10.1177/0146167213520459

Manocha, R (Ed), 2017, *Growing Happy, Healthy Young Minds: Generation Next*, Hachette Australia, Sydney

Warburton, WA & Highfield, K, 2016, 'Children and technology in a smart device world' in Grace, R, Hodge, K & McMahon, C (Eds), *Children, Families and Communities: Contexts and consequences* (5th edition), Oxford University Press, Melbourne, pp 195–221.

Warburton, WA & Straker, L, 2015, 'Ten Tips for Healthy Game Play', Australian Council on Children and the Media Fact Sheet, retrieved from: www.childrenandmedia.org.au/assets/files/resources/fact-sheets/parent-strategies/Top-10-tips-for-healthy-game-play.pdf

Warburton, WA, 2014, 'Apples, oranges and the burden of proof: Putting media violence findings in context', *European Psychologist* 19, pp 60–67. DOI: 10.1027/1016-9040/a000166.

Warburton, WA, 2013, 'The science of violent entertainments' in Wild, J (Ed), *Exploiting Childhood*, Jessica Kingsley Publishers, London, pp 65–85.

Warburton, WA & Braunstein, D (Eds), 2012, *Growing Up Fast and Furious: Reviewing the impact of violent and sexualised media on children*, The Federation Press, Sydney.

For more online resources visit:
generationnext.com.au/handbook

13. TALKING TO YOUNG PEOPLE ABOUT ONLINE PORN AND SEXUAL IMAGES

Collett Smart

This chapter provides an overview of pornography as a public health crisis. It also provides practical suggestions for engaging young people in critical thinking about sexual images, and rejecting porn as the norm.

INTRODUCTION

'This is a public health crisis. Like smoking or other public health issues, this will have long-term consequences.'

Dr Joe Tucci, CEO of the
Australian Childhood Foundation, 2016

Pornography is currently labelled 'a public health crisis'. Hundreds of psychologists, academics, sexologists, child advocates and cyber experts are now speaking up about the mind-boggling fact that children are being schooled on sexual practices by hard-core, usually violent, pornography.

Pornography is changing society – and the change is not good.

WHAT DOES THE RESEARCH SAY?

To suitably assist young people to navigate this new reality, parents, schools and communities must first understand what we are facing.

The general consensus is that the nature of contemporary mainstream pornography does not in any way resemble the images today's adults may have been exposed to.

The authors of a 2016 article entitled 'Pornography and the male sexual script' state that pornography is overlooked as a sexual health issue because internet pornography has created a generation gap. Where one generation thinks of pornography as something like a tradesman or delivery boy arriving at a house to find a 'sexually aroused housewife or girl next door', on the internet it has become something else. Most popular and readily accessible pornography contains 'significant amounts of violence, degradation and humiliation of women, are short, and focused almost exclusively on genitalia. Many adults, who are beyond the years of sexual development and exploration and who developed their sexual identities prior to the internet, have not encountered the new sexual scripts internet pornography is inscribing on the sexual identities of younger people.'[1]

A content analysis of the most popular porn found:

- Close to 90 per cent of scenes included acts of physical aggression. The aggressive acts included hair-pulling, gagging, choking and slapping, while only 10 per cent of the scenes contained positive behaviours like kissing, laughing, embracing, etc.
- 48 per cent of scenes contained verbal aggression.
- 94 per cent of those scenes show aggression primarily by males, and overwhelmingly against females.
- 95 per cent of the incidents showing aggression being met with either a neutral or pleasured response by the woman.[2]

Recent research has highlighted the number of critical ways internet pornography is particularly impactful on young people. These include:

- **Ease of access** – Nine- to sixteen-year-olds are more likely to see sexual images online than in other media. Viewing pornography is, for the average young person, as easy as googling or using a hashtag. Video-sharing websites were most frequently mentioned by young people as a source of violent and pornographic content.
- **Increased rates of exposure**, at younger ages, with the age of first exposure being generally lower in boys than in girls.
- **More positive attitudes towards pornography** in boys, from an earlier age, than girls. Boys and men are more likely than girls and women to use pornography for sexual excitement and masturbation. Boys are also more likely to initiate its use, to view it alone and in same-sex groups, and to view more types of images.
- **Adolescents are considered one of the most susceptible audiences** to sexually explicit content. Since they are more frequently exposed to sexually explicit material, their perceptions of the 'social realism' (the extent to which the content of porn is perceived to be similar to real-world sex) and the 'utility' of sexually explicit material increase. I.e. the more porn they see, the more they believe the behaviours and practices in porn to be normal to everyone.

  More than 90 per cent of boys and 60 per cent of girls have seen porn.[3]
- **Young people themselves list porn as their top online concern**, given the remarkable volume and range of sexually explicit online content available, unmonitored and for free. Current popular genres of online pornography are extreme, violent and graphic, and provide novelty and variety (including sex involving multiple partners, double and triple penetrations, bondage, urination and defecation, bestiality, incest, rape or torture porn). A content analysis of the most popular porn found close to 90 per cent of scenes included acts of physical aggression.[4]

- **Children not telling** – Children are often reluctant to report their experiences to parents, due to both embarrassment and for fear of being negatively judged.
- **Distortion of healthy sexual and emotional development** – 'Extensive scientific research reveals that exposure to porn threatens the social, emotional and physical health of individuals, families and communities.'[5]

EFFECTS OF EXPOSURE TO PORNOGRAPHY

A review of research indicates that adolescent exposure to pornography leads to:

- Exaggerated perceptions of sexual activity in society.
- Viewing casual sex, without emotion or responsibility, as the norm.
- Increased sexual risk taking, such as unsafe practices and more sexual partners.
- Encouragement of underage sex.
- The pornographic script, i.e. expectations of what is deemed 'appropriate sex'.
- Diminished trust between intimate couples.
- Belief that abstinence and sexual inactivity are unhealthy.
- Cynicism about love or the need for affection between sexual partners.
- Coercive sexual bullying and forced sex among young people.
- Insecurities about sexual performance and body image.
- Violent and degrading pornography as racist and sexist education, and reinforcing 'the rape myth'.[6]

WHAT CAN WE DO?

We need to be cautious that in addressing this issue, we are not clamping down on children's healthy sexual development. Children and teens are curious about their bodies, their development and sex. Neither sex, nor sexual attraction, are inherently bad. This is part of normal healthy development. We ought to be encouraging young people to be safe, healthy and confident about their bodies and sexual development. The problem is, the sexualised wallpaper of society does not allow for this natural development to occur. With pornography as the number one sex educator, children are forced into an awareness that their bodies and brains are not yet ready for. Young people have questions. They may talk to peers, but their peers are tuning in to the same broken sources as they are. Young people need strong alternative voices to those of 'Pornland'.

THE IMPORTANCE OF RELATIONSHIPS

I believe that relationships are our best defence against the onslaught of porn. It is in relationships that we teach, inspire, connect, fight for a greater good, raise awareness and implore government bodies to act. I also believe we are made for relationships, and research supports that good relationships keep us happier and healthier. Pornography consumption leads to isolation and erodes our human ability for healthy social connections.

If relationships are the key protective factor for both mental and physical health, then adults should invest in modelling healthy relationships to children. Children look to us for authoritative guidance. It is our responsibility to guide them with firm boundaries, high expectations and truckloads of love and acceptance. The purpose of creating scaffolding for our children is not to restrict their every movement or choice, but to build a framework that allows for a wealth of opportunity and development of resilience, while including the necessary protection. This provides a quality of life for them and those around them.

Australian resilience studies indicate that one of the key factors to building resilience in young people is a sense of being connected to adults. And resilient children will be better equipped to push back against porn culture.

I find that schools and parents are still somewhat afraid to address the issue; however, the collective turning of a blind eye is akin to the cultural grooming of children. Young people's exposure to pornography is everybody's concern, everybody's duty of care. Young people need the adults who care about them to help them understand that porn is not reality.

> Parents and schools need to play an active role in monitoring and boundary setting for young people in relation to cybersafety, but this must be done within the context of trusting and respectful relationships.[7]

HOW BEST TO DEVELOP THESE RELATIONSHIPS?

Don't rush it. In our modern age, we want things to be instant (like our coffee), but relationships are hard work and messy. Young people learn values from the adults they spend the most time with, in both the day-to-day joys and the struggles. For children and teens to build healthy relationships requires the adults in their lives to make use of effective communication skills, purposeful discussions and age-appropriate boundaries. We cannot do sex education with just 'the talk'. Today it is about lots of small, frequent conversations with young people. These conversations can only happen if adults continue to build a climate of trust and openness, where young people begin to feel comfortable coming to us for answers, and where no topic is off-limits.

A Canadian study found that 45 per cent of teenagers consider their parents to be their sexuality role model. The findings obviously blew apart the long-accepted stereotype that when it comes to sex, children are mostly influenced by peers and celebrities. The study went on to show that less than one-third were influenced by their friends and only 15 per cent were inspired by celebrities. This landmark survey also revealed that most of the teenagers who looked to their parents lived in families where sexuality was openly discussed and so had a greater awareness of the risks and consequences of STIs.[8]

Children who are well informed and comfortable talking about sexuality with their parents are also the least likely to have intercourse when they are young adolescents. This is contrary to the myth that children will go out and 'experiment' more if they have more information about sex. Teens also describe an increased ability to 'handle pornography satisfactorily' if they had developed positive relationships with others, specifically friends and family. There is a link between good communication between parents and children, with more responsible choices around sexual behaviours and pornography use.

But what if my child doesn't ask?

For those who don't ask, you will need to gauge the appropriate age for discussions, find opportunities to ask questions and then begin with little snippets of information.

A FIVE-STEP GUIDE FOR TALKING TO YOUNG PEOPLE

Stow away your own baggage

Breathe! It is important to be aware of the baggage that we bring into conversations about sexuality with our own children. It's okay to mess up. Just apologise and try again.

Early and often

Be prepared – start talking to children about their bodies as early as language develops. When they ask questions, *listen* and be respectful. Young people need to feel heard, know that their opinions matter and that you aren't just making time to give another lecture.

X-rated versions are already flying around the playground (and the smartphone)

With respect – don't be naive! In my work, I find that most children know more than parents assume. Indeed, if not acknowledged and discussed, the concerns and anxieties of children about images can become too frightening or difficult for them to deal with. Additionally, it may not even occur to them that their information could be inaccurate. No matter what a young person asks, don't make them feel ashamed or dirty – at any age.

Expect each child to be different

Even children in the same family can be very different. Some are very private and like to chat a little bit at a time, while others will chat anytime. Keep your responses age appropriate and in line with your child's level of understanding and emotional maturity. Ask a question to find out how much they know before launching into the topic.

Dimensions of sexuality education

We need to teach children about sex in two parts: the obvious physical details and then the key emotional, psychological and social qualities of sexual relationships.

BROAD AGE GUIDELINES

Toddlers and young children

Obviously, we aren't going to talk about porn to toddlers; however, experts advise that the basic facts about sex and bodies should begin in the early years. Although, don't panic if a child is older and you haven't started yet. It's never too late.

So much of what we teach at this age will be about body safety, 'where babies come from' and the correct terms for genitals. Do not use pet names. This way, if a child is touched inappropriately or sees sexualised media, they can clearly state what has happened. Talk with your child about safe and unsafe feelings.

Parents might make use of opportunities that present themselves at different stages to communicate family values in an obvious manner. As you begin to talk through these issues with your children, you not only equip them with the information they need to make wise choices, but your relationship with them deepens in the process. They learn that they can trust you in the most sensitive areas of life and helps ensure that talking about bodies and development does not become the unspoken taboo.

Using picture books is a fantastic way to introduce new topics, and can be used as a vehicle for asking further questions.

Mid to late primary

You could begin by asking your children how they feel about something you know they have seen or heard. Let them know what you've noticed, e.g. 'I can see you looking worried/upset/interested in . . .' Listen first and then check with them to make sure you've got it correct, by rephrasing what you heard them say: 'So what you mean is . . .'

Pick your times to talk. Driving in the car to sport or kicking a ball outside usually work better than during a favourite computer game.

Between ten and twelve years of age, children need to have discussions about sex and puberty, if they haven't happened already. At this age, it's no longer just about biology and physical development. When talking, start by asking what your child might have heard and what they know about a topic. Ask about colloquial, slang or rude terms their friends might use too (this can bring a bit of humour and realness to the situation).

Make it normal and check in on your child regularly, and don't worry if topics go off track while talking. Most children will remain open if discussions have happened regularly and seem normal in your family. It can be trickier trying to start conversations about sex and porn when other conversations weren't initiated earlier in their lives. Although it is never too late to start talking.

Check your children's everyday TV, movie and gaming diet. Is it age appropriate? Is a child incidentally being exposed to a parent's media choices? Encourage discussions about media.

Although sexuality talks should occur gradually and frequently over the child's lifetime, some parents enjoy taking their tween away for a weekend. This forms a coming of age-type ritual, where chats happen in a neutral setting, over ice-creams or campfires. These aren't meant to be a one-off big talk, rather a starting point for chatting about bigger topics. During lights out, sitting on the edge of the bed or lying next to your child in the dark are also often favoured times for deeper topics. This works especially well for first-time conversations or for children who don't like to make eye contact.

Adolescents

Teens need to feel that at least one adult is trustworthy with big topics. If we want to talk about sex, relationships and pornography, we need to keep working to maintain a relationship with our teens, and to keep their trust. Some teens may need to talk with a safe mentor or youth leader, if they simply won't talk with a parent. Give them permission; in fact, actively encourage them to do so.

Remember that teens can feel deeply yet not know how to express themselves appropriately, especially if they feel disempowered, guilty about something or overwhelmed. Adolescents need opportunities to express themselves and should be encouraged to discuss and debate their thoughts and feelings about problems that affect their world, even if they seem trivial to adults. If it is important to a teen it should be important to you. Debate and discuss popular culture with them, in a way that enables young people to think about their values and make conscious choices about their lives. Use an interest of theirs, a YouTube video or something on the news to spark thoughts about the meanings behind the messages they hear.

Even if you don't agree with an opinion, try to refrain from sounding judgemental of their ideas. You might clearly tell them you do not share their view, but that you are interested in hearing how they came about it. This encourages the development of critical thinking.

Don't be afraid of the pauses and silences.

Remember that it's okay to laugh at yourself or joke around with teens. Not every big topic needs to be done in hushed, serious tones.

Above all, teens need to be told beforehand that even when they eventually mess up (because they will), no matter what they do, no matter what they see, they can talk to you.

Finally, seek professional help if you are concerned about ongoing risky or dangerous behaviour.

Don't always talk in the abstract. It's great to use examples from media, but sometimes kids need you to ask: 'How are you going to make decisions about what you do and don't do sexually?' Sounds terrifying, I know, but this is what college students have said they wanted and needed. You don't have to ask them to tell you where their boundaries are going to be, but ask them to make decisions about that, and to talk with their romantic partners about it. Every single time I've done that, the teenager has come back and told me that they were so glad that they'd had that conversation.

Psychologist Dr Jennifer Shewmaker

WHEN YOU DISCOVER YOUR CHILD HAS SEEN PORN

Just because we talk with our children about the harms of pornography does not mean they will never see it or even seek it out. We've already ascertained that they will see porn – sooner than we feel prepared for – but we are in this fight for the long haul.

When it happens:

- Pause. Don't jump in and blurt out your fears. (If you haven't tackled it well, apologise.)
- Take a walk and think about what you planned to say when it happened.
- Tell them what you found/noticed.
- Ask kindly what happened.
- Expect some initial denial.
- Reassure your child of your love and tell them that you don't think they are dirty and bad.
- Remind them that no matter what they do, you will never stop loving them.
- Remind them they are not alone.
- Talk to your children about wanting to help them and that you will be having more conversations about this issue over time.

- Check whether technology is out of bedrooms, especially at night.
- If not done already, add filtering software on all devices (although *nothing* is completely failsafe!).
- Expect your child to promise that they will *never* look at it again. Many will, even though they don't wish to.
- If you realise viewing has become compulsive, kindly ask if there are steps you might take together to help your child get this under control. Getting them on board with this is very important.
- Help your child notice times that they seek it out (when Mum is still at work? When Dad pops out to drop their sibling at flute?). This gives them more insight and is part of the plan to find healthy alternatives.
- Ensure your child's life is filled with other engaging activities, those that develop self-confidence, self-worth and alleviate boredom.
- Tell them the good news – that their age counts in their favour, because they can develop good habits when put in place early. It's never too late.
- Tell them that it will get easier as you work together.
- Get support from a psychologist, if seeking out porn becomes compulsive for your child.
- For teens already at risk of antisocial behaviour, professionals recommend that parents carefully monitor and severely limit access to pornography on file-sharing networks and elsewhere, for a time.

For schools

It is vital that schools have a plan for talking about pornography with students. Be preventative and empower both parents and students by raising awareness regularly, like you would with alcohol or drug issues. Suggest books, run student seminars, hold parent information evenings, list resources in newsletters. Make it normal to talk about.

Also, be restorative for when pornography use is reported or accessed by students of different ages.

A note to boarding schools: you are the community – the village. In my opinion, many boarding schools are failing this generation of children with their lack of boundaries around technology. Parents place their children in the care of schools as surrogate parents for entire weeks or months at a time. We need to be having serious and urgent conversations about the duty of care to our students in these settings.

TOPIC SUGGESTIONS

Provide young people with questioning and critical thinking strategies to become more media literate.

Encourage everyday empathy

Porn is inherently selfish, so essentially empathy is an antidote to porn. Empathy sees another's humanity.

Question starters for encouraging empathy:

- What is something kind you did today?
- What is one kind thing somebody did for you today?
- Did you notice anyone looking sad today? What do you think was going on for them?

Object to objectification

There is nothing empathetic about treating someone as an object.

Respectful relationships are imperative for teaching children about the value of the whole person at every age. Younger children can learn to recognise objectification through mainstream media, and teens can discuss objectification through porn and sexualised images specifically.

Question starters:

- What is that picture trying to make you think/feel?
- Is that ad trying to change your mind about something?

- What do you think that music video says about the role of women?
- How does that movie lie about real-life relationships? What do you think a real person would feel tomorrow?

Talking to boys

Teach boys that girls are not mysterious or weird. Reinforce that all girls and women have dreams and skills. Teach that hitting or pinching a girl is never a way of telling her he likes her. Teach him how to properly communicate affection – with kind words and gestures.

Indeed, if girls and women are seen as sexual beings through porn, rather than as complicated people with many interests, talents and identities, boys have difficulty relating to them on any other level. This includes working together for higher causes (volunteer work) or enjoying their company as friends.

Talking to girls

Don't focus on appearance and clothing, especially for little ones who should be out playing in something comfortable. Although it's okay to tell your daughters (and sons) they look awesome in the new outfit they have chosen, that should be far outweighed by the times you tell your children how incredible you think their hearts and minds are.

We need to talk to our teen girls about sexualisation too. Many have bought into the pornified lie that their worth is in their bodies, and that all boys want from them is lots of sex. That's simply not true: there are many boys trying to become men of integrity. Teach girls to value so much more than their bodies.

We need to highlight the ability of every teen to exercise self-control, to redirect their thoughts and really look into the person, not simply at the person.

Encourage:

- Not criticising other people's bodies.
- Zero tolerance of rape 'jokes'.

- Opportunities to discuss how popular media portrays women as objects, e.g. Is the person in this image treated . . .
  - Like a tool or an instrument?
  - As something lacking in freedom/autonomy?
  - Without value and integrity?

Porn as a script (a topic for teens)

Young people need to be taught specifically about the lies told by porn.

Discussion ideas:

- Porn does not encourage intimacy.
- Porn sex is not real sex – it is a performance.
- Porn hijacks sexual and emotional wellbeing.
- Porn tells people what they 'should do', 'should want' and 'should enjoy', long before many teens have even had their first kiss.
- A lot of myths and stereotypes are reinforced through porn, e.g. gender roles, race, penis size.
- Pornography is a very poor sex educator.
- Most women do not enjoy the type of sex portrayed in porn – they don't want to be physically and mentally humiliated (even though they appear to be enjoying it in porn).
- Porn treats people as objects to be used.
- Pornography is not how healthy, intimate relationships work.
- Much of porn is humiliating, violent and abusive – not sexy.
- Much of pornography appears to be non-consensual sex and helps fuel the sex trade.
- Porn bodies are not realistic for most men and women.
- Porn sex is not safe.
- The porn industry is a multi-billion-dollar industry and doesn't care about people.
- Sex can be meaningful and better than porn sex.

Boundaries, self-control and consent

If we turn a blind eye to porn we incidentally teach young people that sex is largely based upon seeking '*my* pleasures, *my* desires and *my* appetites' devoid of connection or relationship. If we continue to peddle selfish sex, masquerading as freedom of expression, then we sell our young people short, and are only guaranteed two things:

1. They will have been used.
2. They will use someone else.

If we care for young people, we need to teach them about relationships that exist within the boundaries of mutual intimacy, mutual respect, mutual caring, mutual self-control and mutual commitment.

*   Sex is not easily divorced from emotional attachment.
*   Good sex requires vulnerability. It is about *both* parties working together, which requires being able to actually talk to each other.
*   It requires both parties understanding and being understood.

FOR HEALTH PROFESSIONALS

When pornography access becomes problematic, we need to look at the reason behind the need to engage in certain online activities. Psychologist Jocelyn Brewer asks us to consider what thoughts, motivations and intentions might be present for a young person presenting with problematic internet use.

Some steps to consider with clients:

*   Become familiar with self-defeating habits and recognise the trigger sources. Recognise the routine as it starts, or begins to take over. A journal of triggers may be helpful.
*   Be mindful. Monitor thoughts, feelings and actions. Notice typical thoughts or feelings, or how you start to act. Different states of mind make us more or less susceptible to triggering bad habits.

- Plan for alternatives – think of a better way to handle future situations.
- Enlist the support of a parent, mentor or accountability partner.
- Maintain boundaries with technology use. When and where are the devices stored at home (especially at night)? Is there filtering software installed?

HOPE AND REASSURANCE ARE KEY

I believe it is imperative we reassure young people that many people, the world over, are now working together against the problem of porn. Look for 'good news' stories, activist groups and real life mentors for them to focus on. This helps young people to focus not only on what to avoid, but also their positive goals, their dreams and how they can help make the world a better place.

Young people are looking to us to show them what healthy relationships look like. We must step up to the challenge! If we hope to reverse this trend, we have to join together as communities and be the role models they need.

Author biography

Collett Smart is a consultant psychologist, qualified teacher, lecturer, writer and mum of three. She has spent the last twenty years of her career working in private and public schools, as well as working as a consultant psychologist in private practice and with the media. Collett's knowledge has led to her working with children, teens and their parents around Australia, inner city London and in Africa. She speaks regularly on the impact of pornography on the development of young people and was a speaker at the Pornography and Harms to Children and Young People symposium in 2016.

www.collettsmart.com

See also:

Chapter 1: Understanding Teen Sleep and Drowsy Kids
Chapter 3: Understanding the Teenage Brain
Chapter 5: Healthy Habits for a Digital Life
Chapter 7: Problematic Internet Use and How to Manage It
Chapter 8: Computer Game Addiction and Mental Wellbeing
Chapter 14: Advice for Parents: Be a Mentor, Not a Friend

Recommended organisations and websites:

NSPCC: www.nspcc.org.uk/preventing-abuse/keeping-children-safe/online-porn
Sex and Porn Addiction Help: www.sexaddictionhelp.co.uk
The Mix: www.themix.org.uk/sex-and-relationships/porn
Family Lives: www.familylives.org.uk/advice/teenagers/sex/porn
Collett Smart: www.collettsmart.com
Fight the New Drug: www.fightthenewdrug.org
Go for Greatness: www.goforgreatness.org

Further reading:

Manocha, R (Ed), 2017, *Growing Happy, Healthy Young Minds: Generation Next*, Hachette
    Australia, Sydney.

 We also recommend the very popular companion volume **GROWING HAPPY, HEALTHY YOUNG MINDS** – resilience, bullying, depression, anxiety, body image and many more important issues.

 For more online resources visit:
generationnext.com.au/handbook

14. ADVICE FOR PARENTS: BE A MENTOR, NOT A FRIEND

Tena Davies

In my eleven years working with parents as a psychologist, one of the most common questions asked is which type of parenting is best for their child.

When, as parents, we want to know what the best type of parenting is, we often turn to the internet for answers. This starts early in our children's lives where we google it to find the answer, often gleaning wisdom from the experience of others.

However, the answers on the internet can be confusing. There's attachment parenting, helicopter parenting, tiger mother parenting, positive parenting . . . the list goes on. Given the varied and divergent styles, which is best?

In the psychological research, the most commonly accepted and well-researched parenting styles are: authoritarian, authoritative and permissive,[1] and each is associated with different outcomes in children.[2]

These styles can be categorised depending on their degree of warmth/responsiveness and control/'demandingness' displayed by the parent towards their child. The following is a description of these parenting styles.

AUTHORITARIAN (MY-WAY-OR-THE-HIGHWAY PARENTING)

Authoritarian parents are highly demanding and punitive, and lower on warmth and responsiveness. They value unquestioning discipline rather than democratic give-and-take.[3] Authoritarian parents attempt to shape, control and evaluate the behaviour and attitudes of the child in accordance with a fixed set of standards.

They value obedience as a virtue and favour punitive measures to curb their children's actions or beliefs when they conflict with their standard of acceptable conduct.[4]

Authoritarian parents say things like 'you need to listen to me because I am your father', 'your mother knows best' or 'you have to do what we say because we are your parents'. Authoritarian parents are well meaning but this style of parenting can be associated with negative outcomes, such as decreased academic achievement in adolescents and adults.[5]

As a psychologist, I have noticed that this also leads to a great deal of family conflict, particularly as the child becomes older and seeks greater levels of independence. It also fuels a cycle of punishment and rebellion, where the more the parent puts rules in place, the more the young person rebels.

AUTHORITATIVE (BALANCED PARENTING)

Authoritative parents are both demanding and responsive; they display affection and respond to the needs of their offspring. They discipline their children in a democratic manner, which is characterised as a cooperative give and take rather than coercion. They successfully balance being a mentor or a teacher with enforcing boundaries.

Authoritative parents manage their children's activities and behaviour on a rational case-by-case basis. They do have rules and consequences but these are more democratic and collaborative than those of authoritarian parents.[6]

My experience as a psychologist is that parents who have warm relationships with their children as well as firm boundaries have the most positive relationships with their children. As well, these children tend to be the most well adjusted.

I like to think of authoritative parenting as balanced parenting because it balances guidelines with having warm and connected relationships with young people. Children of balanced parents comply with requests because they know they won't get away with murder and also because they don't want to disappoint their parents.

For my master's thesis I found that children who rated their parents as authoritative were significantly less likely to be addicted to the internet compared to child of permissive or authoritarian parents.

PERMISSIVE (FRIEND PARENTING)

Permissive parents, though they may be warm and responsive, lack control. They tend to be non-traditional and have fewer rules or boundaries compared to authoritarian and authoritative parents. Thus, children of permissive parents are left to self-regulate their behaviour and emotions.

They may allow their children to regulate their own activities as much as possible, and do not wish to insist that their children obey externally defined standards. Permissive parenting can be associated with impulsivity in some adolescents and adults.

It should be noted that while an authoritative parenting style tends to be valued by those living in the English-speaking world, attitudes to parenting styles vary across culture, as do the outcomes. Also, research tells us about the outcomes for groups of people, not individuals. Each parent has to decide for themselves which style is best for each child.

PENDULUM PARENTING

While not technically a parenting style, one pattern of parental involvement I have seen is where parents are inconsistent in their parenting, the most common being parents who are generally permissive but occasionally correct their position during times of stress to being authoritarian and punitive. An example of this is a parent who does not have agreed-upon boundaries about a child's internet use.

The parent may tolerate undesirable behaviour until a crisis hits (the child is bullied) and then punishes the child by removing all of their devices until further notice. This generally lasts a short time and then the pendulum swings again and they resume the permissive stance. This sometimes results in the child decreasing their level of respect for the parent because they know they won't follow through on what they say, and as such they learn that there are few lasting consequences for their actions.

HOW TO BE AN AUTHORITATIVE (BALANCED) PARENT

While there are many different ways to be a balanced parent, the general principles of being both warm and firm but using negotiated boundaries can help guide one's parenting behaviour. Equally important is to take into account the temperament and style of the child. Some children may react very strongly to any sort of rule while others are more compliant. This should be taken into account and accommodated for when putting in place parenting practices.

The following questions may assist you to determine if your parenting is on a balanced track:

- Are you cultivating a warm relationship with your child?
- Do you know your child, their current interests, friends, likes and dislikes?
- Do you spend time together just for fun?
- Are your conversations about enjoying time together rather than addressing behaviour?
- Do you show your child your appreciation of their qualities or take interest in their world even when it is not aligned to your preferences and interests?

If you answered mostly yes, it is likely that you have warm relationships with your children. If you answered mostly no, then it might be worth spending more time and energy fostering a more positive relationship with your child.

- Are your boundaries too firm?
- Do you lecture or threaten your child with punishment for their bad behaviour?
- Do you implement harsh punishments?
- Are the punishments hard to keep?

If you answered mostly yes, then it may be beneficial to think through how to involve your child in setting boundaries.

- Are your boundaries too loose?
- Do you see yourself as hands-off?
- Do you only have half-hearted attempts at discipline?
- Do you have few rules and consequences?

If you answered yes, it may be worth spending more time putting in place a few rules and consequences.

Some guidelines for being an authoritative (balanced) parent

- Give options and choices.
- Ensure the punishment fits the crime.
- Keep it simple and time bound.
- Catch your child being good – it makes the behaviour more likely to occur.
- Spend time doing something fun with your child.

WHAT TO DO IF YOU ARE EMBROILED IN CONFLICT WITH YOUR CHILD

Going through difficult periods with your offspring is very common. It can be easy to lose your way in the relationship. I think the first thing to do is to sit down with your parenting partner or a friend and make a list of all of the issues as they come to mind. Then put everything that bothers you into a priority list from minor to severe. For example, leaving socks on the bathroom floor could be minor and severe could be swearing at you. Then draw a circle around 20 per cent of the items that are worth focusing on and let the 80 per cent go. This will ensure your energy is spent wisely and that you are not souring the relationship by calling out everything that is unacceptable.

I think when doing this you have to also be realistic. If it bothers you that your child has an Instagram account, undertaking a campaign to have them cancel it may be futile. Instead focus on having them remove inappropriate content.

I find that one of the mistakes we sometimes make as parents when embroiled in a difficult relationship with our children is being overly vigilant regarding compliance. As well, we become sensitised to their difficult behaviour and react strongly to even minor transgressions.

I would start with two or three things to address with your child, as focusing on too many rules may feel like an impossible feat for both you and your child and will likely lead to more conflict and less compliance.

Finally, sit down with your child when you are both calm and be frank with them. Start by owning up to your mistakes in handling their behaviour. This could be something like, 'Tom, I know things at home haven't been the best lately. I know I've added to the problem by nit-picking small things and yelling at you when I get frustrated.' At this point don't expect them to own up to their mistakes. The aim is to both model good communication and also to set the scene for a more positive dialogue.

Then move on quickly to the two or three things you need from them. For example, 'Tom, I love you and you are a great kid. I really value and appreciate how you help with your siblings and how when something is important, you can really go for it. And I know we can get along really well. However, there are some things that are getting in the way. What I need from you is to remove the violent and sexual content from your Instagram, to stop using your devices at 10.30 p.m. on weeknights so that you can get some sleep, and to stop swearing at me when you are frustrated. In exchange for this, I'll stop pulling you up on smaller things like leaving your school bag on the floor. And if you hand over your devices at 10.30 p.m., you can have them longer on non-school nights and school holidays. I'll also stop giving you a hard time about going to the skate park with your friends or playing online games at the weekend, as I know you really enjoy doing that.'

One of the most important things to keep in mind is that your child will not appreciate having a boundary set and that they will likely rear up and protest. This is a common adolescent response to having their freedoms/behaviour curtailed. (Did you appreciate it when your parents did this to you?) After all, adolescence is about gaining independence from one's parents. If they become really distressed/angry during the conversation, take a break and come back to it.

Once you get your point across, I would look at engaging them in how to implement the solutions by giving them choices. For example, 'Tom, do you want me to give you a warning that 10.30 p.m. is approaching or do you want me simply to take your phone at 10.30 p.m.? If you want a warning, when would you like this warning to be?'

This type of conversation can take a few goes. Your aim is to model appropriate behaviour by not losing your own cool and to keep coming back to the conversation.

I would also find genuine ways to connect with your child, as having warm relationships with children is central to family harmony and family wellbeing. One way to do this is to engage them through their interests or to find something in common. This could be seeing a film (of their choosing) together, baking, going for a drive. If things are so bad that any contact leads to conflict, start by greeting them and aiming to reduce fights.

On a day-to-day basis, I would also genuinely catch them being good. This may surprise your adolescent but over time will hopefully lead to a better relationship.

A case study

John and Michelle had two children aged twelve and fifteen. As parents, they believed that their children should do as they were told. They expected their children to do well in school and also respect their parents and extended family members.

When the children were young, this worked well. John and Michelle were never the type to have too many rules but they also didn't spend much time negotiating rules. They had positive relationships with their children but as time went on and life got busier, they spent more and more time working rather than spending quality family time. The children themselves were focusing more on their after-school activities and sport, and family time was limited.

John worked long hours and Michelle had gone from working part time while the children were in primary school to working full time when they were in high school. Family dinners were hurried events and didn't always happen.

They came to see me because their daughter, Mara, seemed glued to her smartphone. They had banned the device during the week but they knew she was always sneaking around to get on the phone. Colin was twelve years old and becoming more and more obstinate, refusing to do simple things like clean his room. Neither child seemed to be listening to their parents. The little time they spent as a family was wasted with them arguing about something the children had been doing wrong.

When they arrived at my office, they were fed up with the situation. The children each said that the parents spent all their time picking on them and that there was no point trying to please their parents because nothing was good enough. The parents were tired of pulling their children up on their behaviour.

My first impression of this family was that they were exhausted from fighting all the time and that their good will towards each other had eroded. John and Michelle, while well meaning, had an authoritarian discipline style. The discipline was not always balanced with warmth as they all had been caught up in the business of life and had stopped connecting with one another.

The parents were asked to focus on the top 20 per cent of their children's negative behaviour and to put the rest aside. Michelle and John discussed their issues with their children and negotiated boundaries and consequences.

The next step was bolstering the warm relationships within the family. I started the family session by asking what they would each like to do if they could have one perfect day with the family. Mara said she would go shopping with her mum and then out for ice-cream with the family. Colin said they would go back to the family paintball place they went to last summer. Michelle and John just wanted a day with no major fights.

Following that discussion, the family agreed to do one thing for fun each week. The parents then started catching the children being good throughout the week. While it took time, at the three-month follow-up they were in a better place than when they had started. Michelle noted that the change that made the most significant impact was not nit-picking small things. John found that he was looking for positives in his children's behaviour and also found it helpful to involve them in discussions about rules and consequences rather than expecting them to blindly obey their parents.

FREQUENTLY ASKED QUESTIONS

What do you do when rules cannot be negotiated? For example, for safety reasons?
That is a fair point. In this instance I would make it clear that it is not possible to negotiate on that point. However, I would explain

why that is. For example, it's not okay for you to take illegal drugs because it is illegal, they can have potentially life-threatening effects, can contain harmful substances, affect your brain development, etc.

What if my parenting partner and I parent differently?

It should be no surprise that two parents in a family often have different degrees of a parenting style or different parenting styles altogether. Where approaches are different, they should, where possible, be negotiated between the parents first and then discussed with the children. Where parents are divorced and the relationship with an ex-partner is strained, it is best to focus on what can be done when the children are in your care.

In summary, the way to be a balanced parent is to invest in warm relationships with your children by engaging them, spending time with them, and accepting and taking an interest in who they are. Balance this warmth with firm boundaries but ones that are not excessive and, where appropriate, negotiated with your young person.

Author biography

Tena Davies is a Melbourne-based psychologist and cyber expert. She has recently completed a Clinical Psychology Master's degree with a thesis on parenting the internet. She works with young people and families to help support a young person's cyber wellness. Her approach to working with young people and families is to promote a balanced and practical approach.

www.tenadavies.com

See also:

Chapter 1: Understanding Teen Sleep and Drowsy Kids
Chapter 3: Understanding the Teenage Brain
Chapter 5: Healthy Habits for a Digital Life

Recommended websites:

Mumsnet: www.mumsnet.com/teenagers
Relate: www.relate.org.uk/relationship-help/help-family-life-andparenting/parenting-
    teenagers
Family Lives: www.familylives.org.uk/advice/teenagers
Think U Know: www.thinkuknow.co.uk

Further reading:

Carr-Gregg, M & Shale, E, 2002, *Adolescence: a guide for parents*, Finch Books, Sydney.

Fuller, A, 2002, *Raising Real People: Raising a Resilient Family* (2nd Edition), ACER.

Manocha, R (Ed), 2017, *Growing Happy, Healthy Young Minds: Generation Next*, Hachette Australia, Sydney.

We also recommend the very popular companion volume **GROWING HAPPY, HEALTHY YOUNG MINDS** – resilience, bullying, depression, anxiety, body image and many more important issues.

For more online resources visit:
generationnext.com.au/handbook

15. E-MENTAL HEALTH PROGRAMS AND INTERVENTIONS

Dr Jan Orman

This chapter will help to steer you in the right direction when looking for e-mental health and wellbeing help for young people.

INTRODUCTION

Mental health and wellbeing resources on the internet are known as e-mental health (eMH) resources and fall into three main categories.

The first group is aimed at educating about mental health and wellbeing; the second is designed to promote mental and emotional fitness, and the third is online treatment programs aimed at providing treatment for mild-to-moderate common mental health conditions. Australia is a world leader in developing and researching these resources but, despite the evidence that they are effective (in some studies just as effective as face-to-face therapy), and despite the high levels of psychological distress in the community, these resources remain underutilised.

Parents and carers of children and adolescents, concerned as they are about the potential dangers of the internet, may well baulk at the idea of actually recommending internet-based resources. However, it does look like the internet is not going away anytime soon and there is no question that its use has become a big part of the lives of post-millennial humans.

Children and adolescents searching the internet would do well to have some sage advice about which sites are reliable and evidence based and which sites will do them good rather than harm.

ONLINE RESOURCES FOR MENTAL HEALTH EDUCATION

The division between psychoeducation, as it is called, skills training and online treatment is somewhat arbitrary, as many programs and sites cross over from one category to another.

Adolescents are reasonably well catered for online as far as psychoeducation is concerned. A number of Australian sites have been developed with the needs of adolescents in mind. Of particular note are:

Headspace www.headspace.org.au – A site designed for twelve- to twenty-five-year-olds, which provides lots of mental health information relevant to adolescents including such things as exam anxiety, managing online bullying, coping with body-image issues, dealing with dilemmas around sex and sexuality and more.

e-Headspace www.eheadspace.org.au – Offers a range of services including online and telephone support services and moderated group chat sessions about specific topics. Past group chat sessions are easily accessible allowing users with particular concerns to see what others have said about the issues that are worrying them.

Both Headspace sites provide links to helplines and emergency services.

ReachOut www.au.reachout.com – Provides highly accessible, teenager-friendly information about a healthy lifestyle in areas of particular relevance to that age group. Drop in to the homepage and you'll see that it promises help with 'tough times, sex, friends and drugs' as a starting point. There's plenty of material about personal identity, bullying, harassment, drugs and sex as well as basic mental wellbeing. There are moderated forums to help young people connect with each other for support and a particularly useful guide to apps that may help young people manage their mental health better.

The ReachOut site also includes resources for parents: parents. au.reachout.com, and for professionals working with young people: au.professionals.reachout.com. Information in these parts of the site ranges from how to communicate effectively with teenagers and how to help them manage their use of technology, to tips on working with parents and information about incorporating education about mental health issues into the classroom.

BiteBack www.biteback.org.au – A website developed by a research team at Black Dog Institute in Sydney and based on the principles of positive psychology. It has less of a focus on the things that are wrong than the other sites and more of a focus on the things that are right. It is as much a mental health training program as an information website. It contains information about mental wellbeing as well as games and interactive activities such as a gratitude journal and mindfulness audio tracks. It is ideal for younger adolescents to help them learn to focus on the positive.

MENTAL HEALTH SKILLS ACQUISITION AND RESILIENCE BUILDING

MoodGYM www.moodgym.anu.edu.au – The first Australian-developed online mental health program (and one of the first in the world). Launched in 2001 by the research team at the Australian National University, MoodGYM is a program based on the principles of cognitive behavioural therapy (CBT), originally developed as a mental 'fitness training' program for adolescents (hence the reference to gym in its name). The original research showed that it was very effective in teaching emotional management skills and in raising levels of psychological resilience, especially in boys. Subsequent research has shown that it is also helpful for increasing resilience in adults and effective as a treatment program for both adolescents and adults suffering from mild to moderate stress, anxiety and depression.

Some Australian schools have used MoodGYM as part of their health curriculum for years. I heard a medical student comment recently that while she thought the whole thing was a waste of time when she was made to do the MoodGYM program at school, she realises now that she has survived the stresses of her final school exams and her medical degree using some of the stress-management and self-care skills that she learned from the program.

As parents and carers we do not always have the knowledge to teach the young people in our care the skills they need to survive modern life – and it's not just maths and computer skills! Increasingly, young people need emotional and stress-management skills to navigate the pressures they are under in this new century. Young people and their carers don't need to be mentally unwell or even vulnerable to mental illness to benefit from development of these skills.

Some kids, like Topsy from *Uncle Tom's Cabin* who nobody parented – she 'just growed' – are able to pick things up from those around them (if the people around them have the skills themselves), but others need psychological survival skills to be actively taught. That's where programs such as MoodGYM can be very helpful.

Like many Australian programs, MoodGYM is free to use and entirely confidential. It can be used and discussed in classroom situations (reducing mental health stigma by emphasising the fact that these are skills that everyone needs to flourish) or on a one-to-one basis with a parent or counsellor. Motivated young people, especially those sixteen and over, can even use the program entirely on their own but it is likely that a little guidance will improve their engagement with the program and optimise the gains.

MoodGYM presents its content in a linear lesson-like way and the user works through it from beginning to end. Many people like that, but it doesn't suit everyone.

myCompass www.mycompass.org.au – An online CBT-based program developed by Black Dog Institute which arranges its lessons in independent modules. Once enrolled, the user can complete the modules in any order or just do the one or two they think they need right now and go back for more later if they need to.

While myCompass modules are designed to be used independently, their structure (3 x 10-minute sessions with homework tasks in between) lends itself to adaptation to the classroom environment as well. Like MoodGYM, it is free to use (having been developed with funding from the Australian government), has proven effective in research trials and is completely automated ensuring user privacy.

MyCompass has the added advantage of a smartphone-based symptom-tracking facility that can help the user identify the times and events in their life that affect their mood and their ability to cope. It can show them where and when they might benefit from using the skills they are learning in the modules.

The myCompass website recommends the site for eighteen years and up because the research was done in that age group but a quick review will convince you that most sixteen- to eighteen-year-olds would find the program useful, especially with guidance, and it may suit a mature fourteen- or fifteen-year-old as well.

The Desk www.thedesk.org.au – Another modular program from beyondblue specifically designed to help tertiary-level students with study-specific stressors and lifestyle management. It may also be a helpful resource for students in the latter years of high school.

TREATMENT

MoodGYM and myCompass are not just effective as resilience-building options through mental health skills learning – they are also effective treatment programs for mild to moderate stress, anxiety and depression. Of the available evidence-based Australian online treatment programs, they are the most suitable for use by younger people.

MindSpot Clinic www.mindspot.org.au – MoodGYM and myCompass are both self-help programs. Another option worth considering for older adolescents is guided self-help. This is offered by the MindSpot Clinic at Macquarie University. 'Guided self-help' means that the user is not left to their own devices to work their way through the program but support is provided by one of the psychologists at the Macquarie University clinic. After registration in the program, the user is contacted either by email or telephone by a clinician, and that same person contacts them again after each of the five sessions/lessons in the program to check on their progress and understanding, and help overcome any barriers.

The MindSpot clinic contains a number of different wellbeing programs for various community groups including a program called **Mood Mechanic**, www.mindspot.org.au/mood-mechanic, for young people eighteen and over. There is also a program especially designed for Indigenous users, www.mindspot.org.au/indigenous-wellbeing-course, currently the only one of its kind available in Australia, which is also suitable for older adolescents.

The Mindspot programs are available free of charge to users all over Australia and provide a good alternative to face-to-face therapy for people who are not able or willing to go to see a psychologist, or who are really not unwell enough for face-to-face therapy, but need some help in improving their lives.

The BRAVE Program www.brave4you.psy.uq.edu.au – Anxiety management programs are available for both children eight and over and for young teens. Developed by the University of Queensland, the BRAVE program is designed to help children and younger adolescents understand and manage their anxiety. There are separate programs for eight- to twelve-year-olds and thirteen- to seventeen-year-olds that contain similar information but are presented in age-appropriate ways. The program for the younger age group is designed to be done with a parent or carer helping, while teenagers can manage their program by themselves but would probably benefit more if there was an adult showing an interest.

There is a number of treatment programs for children in the younger age groups that have been developed but are not yet available except in a research environment. Many are still accepting research participants. These include:

Chilled Plus Online www.chilledplus.org.au – A program from the Centre for Emotional Health at Macquarie University for twelve- to seventeen-year-olds who have anxiety and depression.

Cool Kids Online Search for it on www.mq.edu.au – A program to help seven- to twelve-year-olds manage anxiety with the help of their parents or carers.

Cool Little Kids Online www.coollittlekids.org.au – A program for the parents of shy and fearful three- to six-year-olds to help parents improve confidence in this age group.

APPS

The issue of apps is slightly vexed if one is only looking for resources that are evidence based. There are a large number of mental health-focused apps on the market that are simply based on principles that have evidence for their efficacy behind them when used in face-to-face environments, but often no research has been done on the actual apps themselves. Apps are, however, very popular, especially with young people, and can be very useful in helping manage symptoms and increasing engagement in health-promoting activities.

Take the pedometer apps, for example. No research evidence is needed to know that a pedometer can be a useful tool for someone trying to improve their physical and mental health by increasing their activity levels. Having such a tool on your smartphone seems handy and logical. Some research into how widely these apps are utilised and how effective they are in achieving the users' goals would be helpful, but the lack of research is not a barrier to using them. There is no evidence that they are harmful.

The same goes for specific mental health apps. Mindfulness apps are a good example. Mindfulness is a form of meditation which requires learning to be in the present moment without judgement, to notice one's surroundings or internal states and accept them for what they are. We have known for several decades that regular practice of mindfulness (and it does take regular practice for it to be beneficial) has many health benefits, including, on the psychological side, reducing responses to stressful events, reducing anxiety and preventing recurrences of depression. There has been a large number of aids to mindfulness produced over the years, from cassette tapes and CDs of experts leading mindfulness exercises to online programs. Apps are the latest incarnation.

As mentioned earlier, the **ReachOut** site contains a library of app recommendations that may help children, adolescents and adults manage their symptoms. Some are designed specifically for the younger age group. In the toolbox, a filtering questionnaire asks users what their goals are and recommends apps that might be appropriate. Apps worth looking at include the **Worry Time** app, which uses a tried-and-true CBT strategy of isolating worries to a particular time of day to help the user get worry more under control. Also potentially useful is the **Breathe** app, which, as the name suggests, provides breathing-based relaxation exercises suitable for all ages. There's a **Goal Setter** app that lets you set and track goals and apps to support exercise programs, reduced drinking, better nutrition, anxiety management and improved general wellbeing.

To see the sort of creative things that can be done with apps, take a look at an app called **Music Escape**. It comes from Queensland University of Technology. The aim is to use the music on your phone to help manage your emotions. The app takes your personal playlist and allows you to arrange the songs according to how they make you feel. You can then dial up a playlist that, for example, will help you feel calm when you are feeling upset. All these apps are available free of charge from the App Store.

On the parents and professionals section of the ReachOut website, you can find more information about the various apps mentioned on the site and some suggestions about how to use them.

As parents, teachers or carers, it is important that we explore (and even use) these apps before recommending them to young people, just as we would always read a self-help book before recommending it. Occasionally untested apps may make recommendations that are not in line with best practice (like the bipolar app that recommends that the user drink alcohol to help them calm down) so recommend them with caution if you have not heard about them from a reliable source.

It's also not so good to recommend online resources without following up your recommendations. That would be just like setting homework and never marking it. Who's going to do it if no one's interested in what you've done?

One other exciting development is the planned release of a myCompass app, which is designed as a tool to help manage distress before it reaches the level of needing treatment. The exercises on the app are fun to do and will lead into the myCompass treatment program if that seems necessary. Online treatment programs such as myCompass can identify the user's need for further or more intensive therapy by monitoring progress then making recommendations to that effect. It's a good example of what's known as 'stepped care' in mental health – matching the intensity of the intervention to the severity of symptoms – the aim being to try to catch people before they fall.

On a more serious note, for young people with a history of self-harm or suicide attempts, there is an app recently released by the beyondblue organisation called **BeyondNow**: www.beyondblue.org. au. The app is based on a concept called 'Safety Planning', which is used in clinical practice to provide people at risk with help when self-harming urges arise. It allows practitioners to help people develop a clear plan for staying well by identifying warning signs, avoiding triggering circumstances and managing self-harming impulses. Using this app results in a Safety Plan in your pocket. Best done in collaboration with a health professional, this may be a very useful addition to a young person's survival toolkit.

Online resources are not the whole story in mental health care but are clearly a very useful addition to the tools we have to help people, young and old, manage their psychological wellbeing.

JACK'S STORY

Fifteen-year-old Jack is in Year Nine. He was recently sent to the school counsellor by his English teacher after an angry outburst in which he shouted at one of the other students and left the classroom without permission. His teachers have noticed that he has become withdrawn and scruffy over the preceding few weeks and, on checking his records, the counsellor noted that he has often been late and that there has been a number of unexplained absences in the last term, which were out of character.

The school counsellor found that Jack was pretty uncommunicative. He had difficulty explaining what was going on for him and how he was feeling. He was not keen for the counsellor to speak to his parents but agreed to attend a meeting with them.

At the family meeting, Jack's parents revealed that they were worried about him too. They had taken him to the family doctor, who thought he might be getting depressed and had recommended that he see a psychologist, but Jack had refused to go. They weren't sure what to do next.

After some discussion, Jack agreed to see the counsellor weekly and work through the MoodGYM Training Program with the counsellor's help. This required that the counsellor enrol herself in the program as she had not had any experience using it with a student before and was not completely familiar with its content. She also realised that she needed to talk to Jack about the logistics of looking at the program, e.g. what time he would do it, on what days, and how he would keep a record of what was good about it, what was difficult and any questions he might want to ask her about it.

Jack's counsellor wrote a note to the family GP to let him know what was happening and saw Jack weekly for five weeks while he worked his way through the program, helping him out and keeping an eye on him.

At the end of the MoodGYM program, Jack said he had learned a bit but realised he probably needed to talk to someone about how he was feeling. He agreed to follow up with the GP's referral to a psychologist, as now he knew what was involved in therapy and talking to someone no longer seemed so scary.

In passing, Jack also mentioned that his mother, who had suffered from depression, had done the MoodGYM program too and felt it had been useful for her as well.

TAKE-HOME MESSAGES FOR PARENTS, TEACHERS AND SCHOOL COUNSELLORS/YOUTH WORKERS

A variety of reliable online resources exist that can help young people build their psychological resilience, including educational websites and mental fitness-building programs.

Evidence-based Australian-developed online treatment programs are also available for young people experiencing mild to moderate stress, anxiety and depression.

Mental health education and resilience-building programs are safe for adolescents to use alone or with minimal adult supervision.

If adolescents are already unwell, using online treatment programs should not be seen as a standalone option but used in most cases in conjunction with personal support or face-to-face therapy from a mental health professional.

Parents, teachers and carers can also benefit from the use of online self-management programs and using the programs may put them in a better position to guide and advise the young people in their care.

Few online programs for younger children exist but a number are currently in development and will be available in the near future.

When recommending eMH resources, be sure to be familiar with their content.

Author biography

Dr Jan Orman MBBS MPsychMed is a Sydney GP with a special interest in mental health and a GP educator with Black Dog Institute, a mood disorders research institute in Sydney, Australia. She has an interest in the use of online resources to help people improve their mental health. Most recently she has led the e-Mental Health in Practice (eMHPrac) project team at the institute, designing and delivering education programs for GPs about the use of online mental health resources.

www.blackdoginstitute.org.au/emhprac

See also:

Chapter 3: Understanding the Teenage Brain

Chapter 4: Online Grooming and Cyber Predators

Chapter 5: Healthy Habits for a Digital Life

Chapter 6: Online Time Management

Chapter 19: The Commercialisation of Childhood

Chapter 20: Sexualisation: Why Should we be Concerned?

Recommended websites:

BiteBack: www.biteback.org.au

Chilled Plus Online: www.chilledplus.org.au

Cool Little Kids Online: www.coollittlekids.org.au

e-Headspace: www.eheadspace.org.au

Headspace: www.headspace.org.au

MindSpot Clinic: www.mindspot.org.au

Mindspot Indigenous Wellbeing: www.mindspot.org.au/indigenous-wellbeing-course

Mood Mechanic: www.mindspot.org.au/mood-mechanic

myCompass: www.mycompass.org.au

Reach Out: www.au.reachout.com

The Desk: www.thedesk.org.au

The BRAVE program: www.brave4you.psy.uq.edu.au

ReachOut Apps:

Breathe: www.au.reachout.com/reachout-breathe-app

Worry Time: www.au.reachout.com/reachout-worrytime-app

Music Escape: www.itunes.apple.com/au/app/music-escape/id971949389?mt=8

 We also recommend the very popular companion volume **GROWING HAPPY, HEALTHY YOUNG MINDS** – resilience, bullying, depression, anxiety, body image and many more important issues.

 For more online resources visit: **generationnext.com.au/handbook**

THE MENTAL STILLNESS APP
Kabir Sattarshetty

Every year Mission Australia conducts its large survey of Australia's young people to identify their major concerns. Over the past several years, the issue of stress has featured high on the list of issues that young people feel they need help with. While everyone might experience periods of stress from time to time, prolonged stress and even sometimes extreme stress for short periods are often precursors to more serious mental health problems. So stress is really something that we ought to help young people manage, and it is something that young people want and need help with.

Over the past decade meditation and mindfulness have become increasingly fashionable as ways of reducing stress, improving mood and generally enhancing wellbeing. To better understand meditation, our research has focused on the ancient ideas from which these practices have arisen. We have found that one relatively less known part of the meditation tradition, the experience of mental silence, is in fact particularly important. This is because clinical trials have consistently shown that the mental silence component of meditation yields stress-reducing and mental wellbeing-enhancing benefits that are significantly greater than placebo.

Why is mental silence so important? As we each grow more aware of our inner environment, many of us have come to realise that there is a constant background mental chatter that seems to accompany us virtually wherever we go, whatever we do. While we all seem to accept it as a normal part of our inner life, mental health professionals also recognise that this rumination can often have a major impact on how we think and feel. In fact, the ruminations can themselves both worsen, as well as be the source of, stress. Often, during times of mental illness, these ruminations can become overwhelmingly negative.

Meditation, particularly mental silence, is aimed at specifically addressing this mental noise and its toxic effects on our wellbeing. During the mental silence experience, that inner noise is neutralised and yet the meditator is fully alert, fully aware and in full control of themselves and their faculties, and can think if they want to; however, for the duration of their meditation session they experience no unnecessary mental activity. This is 'mental stillness' or 'mental silence'. It is inherently refreshing, destressing and at the same time energising.

The experience of mental silence, we have found, is specifically associated with beneficial effects on mental and sometimes even physical health. Studies conducted by researchers from Sydney University found that in schools, just five to ten minutes of practice, once or twice a day, was enough to improve mental health and reduce the risk of mental illness. Teachers also reported improved engagement and better mood and associated behaviours in those children who engaged with the techniques.

To make this important method more available, we have developed The Mental Stillness App. This is a free, evidence-based resource that is available to the public, professionals and also to young people. It provides simple guided-meditation sequences on video that can be used on demand. These sequences have been developed over several years of rigorous research and testing. They can be used by anyone from age five to ninety-five.

Find out more about the research and evidence at

www.mentalstillness.org

Kabir Sattarshetty

Kabir is a registered nurse. His research and development of the mental stillness guided meditation sequences was done under the auspices of the Department of Psychiatry, Sydney University, as part of his Masters of Medicine degree.

LEARNING AND DEVELOPMENT

16. COULD IT BE ASPERGER'S?

Professor Tony Attwood

This chapter will explain the defining characteristics of 'Asperger's syndrome', a form of autism. The characteristics can change from early childhood to the adult years and vary according to gender and the person's adaptations to the recognition of being different to peers.

INTRODUCTION

The diagnostic term 'Asperger's syndrome' has been in clinical and common usage since the early 1980s, but the 2013 edition of the *Diagnostic and Statistical Manual of Mental Disorders* (DSM-5) has replaced this eponymous term with the new diagnostic category of Autism Spectrum Disorder (ASD) Level 1. According to DSM-5, the essential features of ASD are persistent deficits in reciprocal social communication and social interaction, and restricted, repetitive patterns of behaviour, interests or activities.

PERSISTENT DEFICITS IN SOCIAL COMMUNICATION AND SOCIAL INTERACTION

Deficits in social-emotional reciprocity

The underlying assumption in the DSM-5 criteria is that someone who has an ASD has difficulty 'reading' social situations. Clinical experience indicates there are three adaptations to this characteristic. The most conspicuous is a tendency to be withdrawn, shy and introspective in social situations, avoiding or minimising participation or conversations; or, conversely, actively motivated for and actually seeking social engagement, but being conspicuously socially clumsy, intrusive and intense, often dominating the interaction and being unaware of social conventions such as acknowledging social hierarchy or personal space. In each example, there is an imbalance in social reciprocity.

There is a third strategy for coping with difficulties with reading social situations, and that is to avidly observe and intellectually analyse social behaviour and to achieve reciprocal social interaction by imitation, and using an observed and practised social script based on intellectual analysis rather than intuition. This is a compensatory mechanism often (but not exclusively) used by girls and women who have ASD. They are able to express superficial social abilities that can be confusing to the conversation partner or diagnostician. In addition, adults who have ASD can gradually learn to read social cues and conventions, such that the signs of deficits in social-emotional reciprocity may not be conspicuous during a short social interaction.

ASD Level 1 (Asperger's syndrome) also has a signature language profile. This can include impaired pragmatic language abilities (i.e. the art of conversation) such as attentive listening, with a tendency to engage in monologues and a failure to follow conversational rules. There may also be literal interpretations, with a tendency for the person to become greatly confused by idioms, figures of speech and sarcasm. There may also be unusual prosody: for example, a child may consistently use an accent based on the voice of a television character, or an adult may speak with an unusual tone, pitch and rhythm. All these characteristics affect the reciprocity and quality of conversation.

A deficit in emotional reciprocity can be explored by examining whether the person shows reciprocal affect in facial expressions, body language and tone of voice. The clinician can tell a story of personal experiences and assess whether the person was in tune and resonated with the clinician's feelings and experiences by the use of nodding, reciprocal smiles and appropriate facial expressions, and complimentary sounds or utterances.

Deficits in nonverbal communicative behaviours used for social interaction

A distinct characteristic of ASD at all three levels is a difficulty with non-verbal communication: that is, reading someone's body language, facial expressions, gestures and voice to indicate specific thoughts and feelings and then incorporating that information in the conversation or interaction. An example might be not reading the nonverbal signals that indicate 'Not now, I am busy', or 'I am starting to feel irritated'. The diagnostician can note whether the person consistently gives eye contact at key points in the interaction and whether he or she is able to accurately read facial expressions and tone of voice that indicate clear as well as subtle emotional states.

Deficits in developing, maintaining and understanding relationships

The diagnostician needs to explore the number, quality and duration of friendships and relationships throughout childhood, adolescence and the adult years. There is often a desire to establish friendships without a complete or realistic idea of what friendship entails.

Children who have ASD Level 1 display a particular developmental sequence in making and keeping friends. In the early school years, the child may not be motivated to socialise with peers, having discovered aspects of life (such as collecting batteries or reading about ancient Rome) that are more enjoyable than socialising. The child may be content with long periods of solitude, preferring to be engaged in a special interest. For those who do actively want to play with their peers, social play in the early school years tends to be more action than conversation. Friendships between typical children tend to be transitory, and social games are relatively simple, with clear observable rules that must be followed. The child who has ASD Level 1 may appear to be able to make and maintain these more superficial friendships of early childhood. However, brave attempts to increase social integration are often ridiculed by peers, and the naive and socially immature child with ASD Level 1 may be deliberately excluded. Children who have ASD Level 1 are extremely vulnerable to being teased, rejected, humiliated and bullied by their peers.

In adolescence, friendships are based on more complex interpersonal rather than practical needs, someone to confide in rather than someone with whom to play ball or make believe games with dolls. It is at this stage of development that the gap in social understanding and integration with peers becomes the most conspicuous. The adolescent who has ASD Level 1 can be overwhelmed by the changing and increasingly complex nature of friendship, leading to feelings of isolation and loneliness. A teenager who has ASD Level 1 explained that 'I would rather be alone, but I can't stand the loneliness'.

There can be a delay of several years in the occurrence of romantic experiences, and a lack of progress in the dating game compared to peers. However, some adults who have ASD Level 1 can succeed in achieving a lifelong relationship. Their partner may have a natural understanding of ASD, which contributes to the success of the relationship.

Restricted, repetitive patterns of behaviour, interests or activities

Stereotyped or repetitive motor movements, use of objects or speech are characteristics usually associated with more severe autism, that is, Levels 2 and 3, and are not usually observed in those who have ASD Level 1.

Insistence on sameness, inflexible adherence to routines or ritualised patterns of behaviour. Routines and rituals are imposed in daily life, with the person showing great agitation if prevented from imposing and completing a particular routine or ritual. Variety is not the spice of life for someone who has ASD Level 1. There is a determination to maintain consistency in daily events, and high levels of anxiety if routines are changed. One of the characteristics of ASD that is not in the diagnostic criteria is high levels of anxiety. This can be Generalised Anxiety Disorder and other expressions of anxiety such as phobias, often for specific sensory experiences such as the sound of a dog barking, social anxiety, fear of making a mistake and selective mutism. Clinical experience indicates the imposition of routines and rituals may actually be a mechanism for coping with high levels of anxiety as they are soothing and relaxing. Specific events may have been associated with, or perhaps have led to, anxiety and are to be actively avoided, hence the tendency to insist on sameness.

Highly restricted, fixated interests that are abnormal in intensity or focus. The diagnostician makes a note of the person's range of interests, collections and hobbies, as well as the acquisition of information on a specific topic, throughout childhood and the adult years. An example of an interest that is unusual in terms of focus is the collecting of photographs of drain covers, and one that is unusual in intensity is an interest in horses that is so intense that the person has a desire to have her mattress in the stable and sleep there.

The special interests all have a use-by date, ranging from hours to decades, and have many functions, such as being a 'thought blocker' for anxiety, an energy restorative after the exhaustion of socialising, or an extremely enjoyable activity that is an antidote to depression. The interest may involve the creation of an intricate alternative world that may be more accommodating of the characteristics of ASD. The special interest can also create a sense of identity and achievement as well as provide an opportunity for making like-minded friends who share the same interests. The sense of wellbeing associated with the interest can become almost addictive, sometimes leading to concern that it is dominating the person's time at home to such an extent that it is preventing engagement in other activities.

Hyper- or hypo-reactivity to sensory input. The new DSM-5 includes reference to sensory sensitivity as one of the hallmark characteristics of ASD. This has been a characteristic of ASD that has been clearly and consistently described by those who have an ASD, and recognised by parents. Sensory sensitivity is also a dimension of autism previously examined in the published diagnostic assessment scales and may play a central role in distinguishing ASD from other clinical conditions.

Sensory sensitivity can be a lifelong problem, with sensitivity to distinct sensory experiences that are not perceived as particularly aversive by others. These can include specific sounds, especially sharp noises such as a dog barking or someone shouting; tactile sensitivity on a specific part of the body; and aversive reactions to specific aromas, light intensity and other sensory experiences. In contrast, there can be a lack of sensitivity to some sensory experiences such as pain and low or high temperatures. The child or adult can feel overwhelmed by the complex sensory experiences in particular places or situations, such as shopping malls, supermarkets, birthday parties or school playgrounds. Sometimes, social withdrawal is not due to social confusion, but to an avoidance of sensory experiences that are perceived as unbearably intense or overwhelming.

Symptoms must be present in the early developmental period (but may not become fully manifest until social demands exceed limited capacities, or may be masked by learned strategies in later life).

Young children, and especially girls with ASD Level 1, may be able to use constructive coping and adjustment strategies to camouflage their deficits in social interaction and communication. They may achieve social success by observing and imitating others, creating an alternative persona, or escaping into the world of imagination in solitary fantasy play, reading fiction or being with animals rather than peers. These mechanisms may mask the characteristics of ASD Level 1 for some time, such that the child tends to slip through the diagnostic net during the primary or elementary school years. However, there is a psychological cost that may become apparent only in adolescence. It is emotionally exhausting to be constantly observing and analysing social behaviour, trying not to make a social error or being perceived as different. Adopting an alternative persona can also lead to confusion with self-identity and low self-esteem. The stress, strain and exhaustion can result in the development of a clinical depression. The clinician diagnosing or treating the mood disorder may subsequently identify the characteristics of ASD Level 1.

COMPENSATORY AND ADJUSTMENT STRATEGIES TO BEING DIFFERENT

Clinical experience has identified four compensatory or adjustment strategies developed by young children with ASD Level 1 as a response to the realisation that they are different from other children. The strategy used will depend on the child's personality, experiences and circumstances. Those children who tend to internalise thoughts and feelings may develop signs of self-blame and depression, or alternatively use imagination and a fantasy life to create another world in which they are more successful. Those children who tend to externalise thoughts and feelings can either become arrogant and blame others for their difficulties, or view others not as the cause but the solution to their problems and develop an ability to imitate other children or characters. Thus, some psychological reactions can be constructive while others can lead to significant psychological problems and a secondary diagnosis of a mood or personality disorder.

A reactive depression

Social ability and friendship skills are highly valued by peers and adults and not being successful in these areas can lead some children with ASD Level 1 to internalise their thoughts and feelings by being overly apologetic, self-critical and increasingly socially withdrawn. The child, sometimes as young as seven years old, may develop a clinical depression as a result of insight into being different and perceiving him- or herself as socially and irreparably defective.

Intellectually, the child has the ability to recognise their social isolation, but lacks social skills in comparison to intellectual and age peers, and does not know intuitively what to do to achieve social success. Brave attempts by the child to improve social integration with other children may be ridiculed and the child deliberately shunned. Teachers and parents may not be providing the necessary level of guidance and especially encouragement. The child desperately wants to be included and to have friends but does not know what to do. The result can be a crisis of confidence.

There can be increased social withdrawal due to a lack of social competence that decreases the opportunities to develop social maturity and ability. The depression can also affect motivation and energy for other previously enjoyable activities in the classroom and at home. There can be changes in sleep patterns and appetite, and a negative attitude that pervades all aspects of life and, in extreme cases, talk of suicide, or impulsive or planned suicide attempts. The signs of depression can continue into the adult years with a third of adults with ASD Level 1 experiencing cyclical or chronic depression.

Escape into imagination

A more constructive internalisation of thoughts and feelings of being socially defective can be to escape into imagination. Children with ASD Level 1 can develop vivid and complex imaginary worlds, sometimes with make-believe friends. In their imaginary worlds with imaginary friends, children with ASD Level 1 are understood, and successful socially and academically. Another advantage is that the responses of the imaginary friends are under the child's control and the friends are instantly available. Imaginary friends can prevent the child from feeling lonely.

Having an imaginary friend is typical of the play of many young children and is not necessarily of clinical significance. However, the child with ASD Level 1 may only have friends who are imaginary, and the intensity and duration of the imaginary interactions can be qualitatively unusual, with this characteristic extending to the adolescent years.

Searching for an alternative world can lead some children to develop an interest in another country, culture, period of history or the world of animals and nature. The interest in other cultures and worlds can explain the development of a special interest in geography, astronomy and science fiction, such that the child discovers a place where their knowledge and abilities are recognised and valued.

Sometimes the degree of imaginative thought can lead to an interest in fiction, both as a reader and author. Some children, especially girls, with ASD Level 1 can develop the ability to use imaginary friends, characters and worlds to write quite remarkable fiction. This could lead to success as an author of fiction for children or adults.

The escape into imagination can be a psychologically constructive adaptation, but there are risks of other people misinterpreting the child's or adolescent's intentions or state of mind. Under conditions of extreme stress or loneliness, the propensity to escape into an imaginary world and imaginary friends can lead to an internal fantasy becoming a reality for the person with ASD Level 1. The person may be considered as developing delusions and being out of touch with reality. This could result in a referral for a diagnostic assessment for schizophrenia.

Denial and arrogance

An alternative to internalising negative thoughts and feelings is to externalise the cause and solution to feeling different. The child can develop a form of overcompensation for feeling defective in social situations by denying that there is any problem, and by developing a sense of arrogance such that the fault or problem is in other people and that the child is above the rules that they find so difficult to understand. The child or adult sees themselves as an omnipotent person who never makes a mistake, cannot be wrong and whose intelligence must be worshipped. Such children can deny that they have any difficulties making friends or reading social situations or someone's thoughts and intentions. They consider they do not need any programmes nor to be treated differently from other children. They vehemently do not want to be referred to a psychologist or psychiatrist, and are convinced that they are not mad or stupid.

Nevertheless, the child does know, but will not publicly acknowledge, that they have limited social competence, and are desperate to conceal any difficulties in order not to appear stupid. A lack of ability in social play with peers and in interactions with adults can result in the development of behaviours to achieve dominance and control in a social context; these include the use of intimidation, and an arrogant and inflexible attitude. Other children and parents are likely to capitulate to avoid yet another confrontation. The child can become intoxicated by such power and dominance, which may lead to conduct problems.

When such children are confused as to the intentions of others or what to do in a social situation, or have made a conspicuous error, the resulting negative emotion can lead to the misperception that the other person's actions were deliberately malicious. The response is to inflict equal discomfort, sometimes by physical retaliation: 'He hurt my feelings so I will hurt him.' Such children and some adults may ruminate for many years over past slights and injustices, and seek resolution and revenge.

The compensatory mechanism of arrogance can also affect other aspects of social interaction. The child may have difficulty admitting being wrong and be notorious for arguing. There can be a remarkably accurate recall of what was said or done to prove a point, and no concession, or acceptance of a compromise or a different perspective. Parents may consider that this characteristic could lead to a successful career as a defence lawyer in an adversarial court. Certainly the child has had a great deal of practice arguing their point.

Unfortunately, the arrogant attitude can further alienate the child from natural friendships, and denial and resistance to accept programmes to improve social understanding can increase the gap between the child's social abilities and that of their peers. We can understand why the child would develop these compensatory and adjustment strategies. Unfortunately, the long-term consequences of these compensatory mechanisms can have a significant effect on friendships and prospects for relationships and employment as an adult.

Imitation

An intelligent and constructive compensatory mechanism used by some children, and especially girls who have ASD Level 1, is to observe and absorb the persona of those who are socially successful. Such children initially remain on the periphery of social play, watching and noting what to do. They may then re-enact the activities that they have observed in their own solitary play, using dolls, figures or imaginary friends at home. They are rehearsing, practising the script and their role, to achieve fluency and confidence before attempting to be included in real social situations. Some children can be remarkably astute in their observation abilities, copying gestures, tone of voice and mannerisms. They are developing the ability to be a natural actor.

Becoming an expert mimic can have other advantages. The child may become popular for imitating the voice and persona of a teacher or character from television. The adolescent with ASD Level 1 may apply knowledge acquired in drama classes to everyday situations, determining who would be successful in this situation and adopting the persona of that person. The child or adult may remember the words and body postures of someone in a similar situation in real life or in a television programme or film. They then re-enact the scene using borrowed dialogue and body language. There is a veneer of social success but, on closer examination, the apparent social competence is not spontaneous or original but artificial and contrived. However, practice and success may improve the person's acting abilities such that acting becomes a possible career option.

There are several possible disadvantages. The first is observing and imitating popular but notorious models, for example, the school bad guys. This group may accept the adolescent with ASD, who wears the group's uniform, speaks their language and knows their gestures and moral code; but this in turn may alienate the adolescent from more appropriate models. The group will probably recognise that the person with ASD is a fake, desperate to be accepted, and is probably not aware that they are being covertly ridiculed and set up. Another disadvantage is that some psychologists and psychiatrists may consider that the person has signs of dissociative identity disorder (often known as multiple personality disorder), and fail to recognise that this is a constructive adaptation to having ASD.

When adults with ASD Level 1 have used imitation and acting to achieve superficial social competence, they can have considerable difficulty convincing people that they have a real problem with social understanding and empathy; they have become too plausible in their role to be believed.

Having worked as a clinician for almost forty years, I have seen some young adults who had the classic, clear and conspicuous signs of ASD Level 1 in early childhood achieve, over decades, a range of social abilities and improvements in behaviour such that the diagnostic characteristics are sub-clinical; that is, the person does not have a clinically significant impairment in social, occupational or other important area of functioning. There may still be very subtle signs of ASD Level 1, but when the diagnostic tests are re-administered, the person achieves a score below the threshold to maintain the diagnosis. There is now longitudinal research that is starting to confirm clinical experience that about 10 per cent of those who originally had an accurate diagnosis of ASD Level 1 in childhood no longer have sufficient impairments to justify the diagnosis.

Author biography

Professor Tony Attwood is a clinical psychologist who has specialised in autism spectrum disorders since he qualified as a clinical psychologist in England in 1975. He works in private practice, and is also adjunct professor at Griffith University, Queensland, and senior consultant at the Minds and Hearts clinic in Brisbane. His book *Asperger's Syndrome: A Guide for Parents and Professionals* has sold over 350 000 copies and has been translated into over twenty-five languages. His subsequent book, *The Complete Guide to Asperger's Syndrome*, is the primary textbook on Asperger's syndrome.

See also:
Chapter 1: Understanding Teen Sleep and Drowsy Kids
Chapter 3: Understanding the Teenage Brain
Chapter 7: Problematic Internet Use and How to Manage It
Chapter 8: Computer Game Addiction and Mental Wellbeing

Recommended websites:
Child Autism UK: www.autism.org.uk
Autism Education Trust: autismeducationtrust.org.uk
Asperger Syndrome.me.uk: www.asperger-syndrome.me.uk
National Autistic Society UK: www.autism.org.uk

Further reading:

Attwood, T, 1998, *Asperger's Syndrome*, Jessica Kingsley Publishers, London.

Attwood, T, 2004, *Exploring Feelings Cognitive Behaviour Therapy to Manage Anger*, Future Horizons, USA.

Attwood, T, 2007, *The Complete Guide to Asperger's Syndrome*, Jessica Kingsley Publishers, London.

Attwood, T, Evans, C & Lesko, A, 2014, *Been There. Done That. Try This!*, Jessica Kingsley Publishers, London.

Attwood, T & Garnett, M, 2013, *CBT to Help Young People with Asperger's Syndrome to Understand and Express Affection*, Jessica Kingsley Publishers, London.

Attwood, T & Garnett, M, 2013, *From Like to Love for Young People with Asperger's Syndrome*, Jessica Kingsley Publishers, London.

Attwood, T & Garnett, M, 2016, *Exploring Depression, and Beating the Blues. A CBT Self-Help Guide to Understanding and Coping with Depression in Asperger's Syndrome*, Jessica Kingsley Publishers, London.

Manocha, R (Ed), 2017, *Growing Happy, Healthy Young Minds: Generation Next*, Hachette Australia, Sydney.

We also recommend the very popular companion volume **GROWING HAPPY, HEALTHY YOUNG MINDS** – resilience, bullying, depression, anxiety, body image and many more important issues.

For more online resources visit:
generationnext.com.au/handbook

17. DYSLEXIA AND LEARNING DIFFICULTIES

Mark Le Messurier

This chapter will help you to understand the needs our dyslexic children face and how they can be met by parents, teachers and GPs.

INTRODUCTION

Dyslexia is a specific learning disability that is neurological in origin. It is characterised by difficulties with accurate and/or fluent word recognition and by poor spelling and decoding abilities. These difficulties typically result from a deficit in the phonological component of language that is often unexpected in relation to other cognitive abilities and the provision of effective classroom instruction. Secondary consequences may include problems in reading comprehension and reduced reading experience that can impede the growth of vocabulary and background knowledge.

AUSPELD (The Australian Federation of SPELD Associations) believes this definition best reflects current research evidence on the defining features of dyslexia. This definition has also been adopted by the International Dyslexia Association, and the National Institute of Child Health and Human Development.

Dyslexia falls under the broad umbrella of Specific Learning Disorders (affecting 15 to 20 per cent of the population). It is referred to as a learning disability because it can impede life socially, emotionally and academically. Dyslexia affects about 10 per cent of the population, although it is being underdiagnosed. That's two or three children in every Australian classroom and its severity is on a sliding scale. It attempts to explain why a person can do relatively well (even really well, because some dyslexics are gifted) in some areas of learning, but encounter unexpected problems in reading, writing and spelling.

The exact causes are not clear, but researchers agree there are structural brain differences in dyslexics that are likely to account for the way the brain develops and functions.[1] Dyslexic genes have been identified and the data suggests that if a dad or a mum is dyslexic, their sons have about a 75 per cent chance of being dyslexic too, while girls will have a 25 per cent chance. However, current information suggests too many girls are slipping under the radar and not being identified.

IN THE BEGINNING

Ask most children as they head off to school what they want and they'll tell you they want to learn to read. Many have watched their mum or dad do it, and most have gained pleasure as they've listened to stories being read to them. Now they want to do it themselves. Soon after starting school they realise their learning is not the same as their classmates'. The others scoot through the glorified levelled reading boxes, while they struggle to recall sounds, letters and word patterns. They burn with frustration because they can't access this highly prized currency. This wasn't their dream.

A dreadful shame slowly replaces the dream to read and write. A few turn their shame inwards. They disengage and stop trying. Some become sad, withdraw from friends and refuse to go to school. For those with a propensity to act out their humiliation, the script plays out with great speed. They perfect eruptive emotion and errant behaviour. Not being able to crack the print/alphabetic code still hurts, but at least they gain recognition for something.

There is now more than enough clinical evidence to show that both male and female dyslexics carry elevated negative perceptions about their capacity to learn, about themselves and their futures.[2]

The result is heightened levels of behavioural turbulence and mental health difficulties.[3] Every dyslexic can tell you about embarrassing or soul-destroying experiences that have occurred at school. There's plenty of sadness, anxiety, anger and despair. And why shouldn't there be? After all, the myths and inaccuracies about dyslexia still thrive in our community:

'Dyslexia does not exist.'

'There is no way to truly diagnose it.'

'It can't be diagnosed until a child is eight years old.'

'If you're doing okay at school, you can't be dyslexic.'

'Can't be – no one else in the family has it.'

'Face up to it, he's a slow learner.'

'Face up to it, she's lazy.'

'Repeating a school year helps.'

'More reading practice helps.'

'There's no cure. So why resource or fund it?'

'He'll outgrow it.'

'They all write backwards or reverse letters.'

'When he tries he can read so it isn't dyslexia.'

This condition is too easily misread and underappreciated. Whether or not a child learns to read should not be a matter of chance. Illiteracy and low literacy must not be tolerated.

CASE STUDY – TIM'S STORY TOLD BY HIS MOTHER, SUZIE

Our Timothy had been very flat for most of the summer holidays, but over the last couple of weeks he cried a lot about having to go back to school. A day did not pass without him questioning why he 'really' had to go. With a few days of the holidays left it seemed he had resigned himself to return to school. His younger brother and sister were asleep, Timmy was watching the television in the lounge and I was in the kitchen. *Thud.* A couple of seconds passed. *Thud.* A few more seconds passed. *Thud* is the only way to explain the sound. It was like nothing I'd heard before. *Thud.* It got the better of me, so I went to investigate. Not often did I need to check on Timmy, as we had been blessed with a calm, thoughtful child. I made my way into the lounge, and there I saw Timmy doing a handstand high on the back of the couch.

'Timothy, how many times have I told you and your brother?'

Thud.

'No. No. No. No. Stop!'

He was lifting himself up as high as he could, and then jerked his hands away so his head crunched into the couch seat below. The 'thud' was his feet hitting against the wall, helping to propel him with all the more force into the seat. I grabbed him and pulled him onto my lap.

'You could break your bloody neck if you keep doing this!' I screamed.

'I know,' he calmly responded.

'If you know why on earth are you doing it?'

'I don't want to be here. I want to die,' he said, staring into my eyes.

He continued, 'I don't want to go to school and if I am dead I won't have to go. You can't help me, Mum. I'm never going to read.'

I hugged him and sobbed. I couldn't let him go.

Timothy had spent eighteen months in preschool, eighteen months in Reception and twelve months in Year One and had stalled on the readers from the orange box. Each of them had just a word or two to a page. His best friends were beginning to read the Harry Potter books. A few months after this incident Timothy was identified with dyslexia. Timothy was seven and a half when he tried to escape the world because he couldn't read.[4]

COULD WHAT HAPPENED TO TIM HAPPEN TO ANY CHILD?

Years ago Rudolf Dreikurs, an Austrian psychiatrist and educator, alerted us to a poignant fact: when children are not able to achieve an anticipated social status, they climb a 'ladder of discouragement' until their faulty logic allows them to believe they've reached a status worthy of them.[5] Each rung on the ladder represents a deeper level of discouragement that drives more complex and worrying behaviours. Tim jumped past the three lower rungs on the ladder: the need to seek attention, the quest for power and control, and the desire to seek revenge. He jumped to the highest rung: hopelessness. Feeling this way, he could only see one solution. Tim's situation highlights our call to duty. Children who are struggling to meet their anticipated social status are reliant on us to show them a way to hop off this 'ladder of discouragement'. The research tells us clearly that literacy underachievement (especially in reading) has high overlap between tricky behaviour, anxiety, disengagement from learning, truancy, reduced physical health, poor self-esteem, depression, suicide and a tendency towards anti-social behaviours and crime in the future.[6] Literacy is fundamental to a child's success, happiness and capacity to participate as a contributing adult member of society.

WHAT ARE THE TELLTALE SIGNS OF DYSLEXIA?

Early on, children likely to have dyslexia show problems pronouncing longer words. At first, they might say hos-tab-ble instead of hos-pi-tal. In the beginning it's cute, but it doesn't go away and soon becomes socially embarrassing. Word-finding difficulties are common too. This is when a child might say, 'Mum, it's outside there, just through the thing.' The thing is, in fact, the door. The number of dyslexics with a history of 'glue ear' and ear infections is significant and the existence of continuing ear infections in early childhood appears to deliver a major impact on the development of language and literacy.

At preschool, or within the first few months of school, good teachers notice the poor association between sounds and letters. The child's phonological skills do not develop as it does for others. Their reading lacks fluency and speed. They trip over small common words like 'was' for 'saw', and 'they' for 'that'. They read words that are not there, keep forgetting simple words and lose their place. They sound out syllables as they read, but forget them before they can blend the word together. It is so frustrating for them. Yet their reading comprehension is often better than their reading.

Some dyslexics can learn for a spelling test and get reasonable results while others struggle to get one or two words correct, especially when they are not grouped in word families. When retested on the same words three weeks later, little has stuck. A common observation is that dyslexics spell words phonetically. In addition, dyslexics have issues with planning, organisation and coordination. Some find it difficult to express themselves clearly, or to completely grasp what others mean when they speak. These ongoing language issues can reach well beyond the classroom, and affect social and emotional connections as well as self-image and confidence.

CAN A PERSON HAVE MORE THAN ONE KIND OF LEARNING DISABILITY?

Yes, dyslexia may be in the company of:

Dysgraphia – A writing impairment. Those with dysgraphia are often slow to learn to write; may experience prolonged letter reversals; produce inappropriately sized letters; mix upper and lower case letters; forget word spaces; and produce untidy, spidery and inaccurate bookwork. They just can't seem to get their ideas on paper and the speed of writing is also reduced. Children with dysgraphia may have only impaired handwriting, only impaired spelling (without reading problems), or both impaired handwriting and impaired spelling.

Dyscalculia – A mathematical impairment may be present as well. Indicators include persistent number reversals (e.g. 37 becoming 73), copying inaccuracies and continual misreading of written information so that mathematical outcomes are ruined. These students often say, 'That's an add sign, isn't it? Or is it a multiply sign?' They have difficulty retaining simple formulas, remembering the sequential steps involved in basic maths operations and recalling number patterns, especially the multiplication tables – many will never be able to learn them all.

Interestingly, studies have shown that as many as 60 per cent of those diagnosed with a learning disability have also been diagnosed with ADHD.[7] We need to be mindful of links between dyslexia and other conditions.

DOES AUSTRALIAN EDUCATION HAVE A UNIVERSAL EARLY READING SCREENING SYSTEM IN PLACE FOR CHILDREN?

No. Yet one of the most compelling findings in the reading research is that the poor reader in the early years is likely to be the poor reader in middle school because appropriate reading instruction/ intervention is unavailable in most schools.[8] This is a big barrier to the success of many students and this wrong could be righted by having quality reading instruction available to all kids in all schools, well beyond the early years.

Early identification to prevent and alleviate reading problems is critical. Back in 2008 in her book, *Proust and the Squid*, Professor Maryanne Wolf, Director of the Center for Reading and Language Research and international authority on reading, emphasised that students at risk of reading difficulties can be detected at four years of age. Given this, the relative ease of testing and the benefits of early literacy screening, the current system in Australia is a disgrace. It is not good enough to allow children to fail the first several years of school and wait until Year Three to assess their literacy and numeracy skills with NAPLAN (National Assessment Programme tests).

WHAT CAN I DO TO SUPPORT A CHILD'S WELLBEING WHEN THEY'RE STRUGGLING WITH DYSLEXIA?

Putting the data together from many studies, we see that males and females tend to cope differently with their dyslexia.[9] Generally speaking, we learn that dyslexic girls are prone to suffer inwardly. Issues such as anxiety, poorer self-esteem, subtle avoidance-based behaviours, self-harm and depression are common. Girls often hit a brick wall later on in secondary school, surprising both teachers and parents, because they've masked the difficulties for a long time. Boys, on the other hand, are more likely to get fed up, give up and disengage from learning/school.[10] So what's to be done?

Start by considering the child's personality and coping capacity. How does this young person feel about having dyslexia? Are they more likely to blame others, let it eat away at them, fall into defeat, or be angry? Are they a positive problem-solver? Do they show good determination? What about their family's ability to cope? A dyslexic child will have a lot to deal with no matter how well things unfold. Are their parents positive problem-solvers? Does depression or anxiety also run in the family? Does the child really understand what dyslexia is? Do their parents really understand it? Does it run in the family? This disability requires big doses of resilience from everyone in the equation.

Linking up with sensible, grounded parents with a dyslexic child may help. Having a sensible parent who has been through this can be sustaining for parents beginning to find their way. Similarly, linking a child with a teen who is positive and practical and has long had a dyslexic diagnosis can be a wonderful support. You could also refer them to a psychologist who can counsel the parents and/or the child – even if only to set them on the right road with the right kinds of resources, understandings and contacts.

Traditionally, counselling in schools has had a low priority for the treatment of dyslexic children and adolescents. Yet many students are very receptive to counselling as it helps them to make sense of the issue, forge practical ways to succeed and reduce despair. We've also learned that a counselling approach in conjunction with quality structured reading instruction is more successful than using a quality structured reading programme in isolation. The research tells us that counsellors do not need to be highly skilled. Any adult who can be warm, practical and hopeful working within the education sector can fulfil a mentoring role.

WHAT DOES A 'DYSLEXIA-SENSITIVE' TEACHER LOOK LIKE?

They're a delightful mix of ordinary, optimistic, practical and compassionate. These are teachers who initiate sensitive conversations with students:

- 'Hey, I know you're dyslexic. Together we'll make it work.'
- 'Just in case you're worrying I won't ever ask you to read in front of the class.'
- 'If you don't get something, just ask me, and if you can't ask me, ask your mum or dad.'

These are teachers who make it clear to students that they want to go on the learning journey with them and are keen to discover how they learn best. Teachers who use the words 'learning preference' rather than 'learning disability'. Teachers who choose to make students and parents feel safe, supported and hopeful. Teachers who are able to reassure their student that many dyslexics do really well with their lives, and have a great selection of YouTube clips and past students to reinforce this. They are empathic adults who help young people to recognise their strengths, and then move from what they can do to the things they find more challenging. Dyslexia-sensitive teachers actively set up special provisions and work with kids so they understand their entitlements, such as:

- Exemption from reading out loud in front of the class.
- Handouts instead of copying notes from the board.
- Extra time in tests and exams.
- Use of a word processor in lessons and tests.
- Use of a calculator in lessons and tests.
- Work to be marked without penalty in relation to spelling and grammar.
- A variety of assessment options – private discussions, PowerPoint, a reader or a scribe in tests and so on.

They also teach students how to break their work down into manageable chunks so they can find a way into it and get to the end of it, because anxiety, procrastination and disorganisation are often a big part of this condition. Dyslexia-sensitive teachers know these kids learn differently, and no matter how well they are taught, many will never cope with rudimentary reading, spelling and writing skills. These students excel when taught how to use some of the brilliant little organising options in smartphones, from taking photos of task sheets, homework, formulas or notes on the white board to recording (video and audio) the teacher giving specific information. Also consider:

- *Free Natural Reader Version 11* – talks text from anywhere out loud to listen to. Simple and free!
- *Free 7 Sticky Notes* – great way to help students plan, stay on task and remember.
- *Speak Selection tool* on smartphones, iPhones, iPads and iPods – it can speak from any text and can gather information from web pages.
- *Dragon Naturally Speaking Premium Edition* – voice recognition software remains tricky to train, but can be brilliant.
- *Audacity* – free recorder to record ideas, teacher instructions or to record homework that's set.
- *Echo Smartpen* – wirelessly transfers written notes and audio to a computer or tablet.

Not only do these options allow young learners to access their higher-level thinking skills more easily, but they help to buoy motivation as well.

WHAT DO 'DYSLEXIA-FRIENDLY SCHOOLS' LOOK LIKE?

A number of dyslexia-friendly schools with dyslexia-sensitive staff do exist. Schools with committed leadership and skilled staff offer a beacon of hope to dyslexics and to those with different learning preferences. But you'll have to do your homework and get out there and hunt them down! A good place to start is to visit the British Dyslexia Association website (www.bdadyslexia. org.uk/parent/bda-services-parents). There you will find a link to their Local Dyslexia Associations (LDAs) that should be able to supply you with some good leads about these kinds of schools in your area.

Keep in mind that dyslexia-friendly schools do not need to be exclusive or showy – they work for students because dyslexia is understood and talked about in positive ways. There's no stigma about having a different learning preference and requiring other ways of expressing and retrieving information. These are educational environments where the hurdles students face are openly acknowledged, and ways are actively found to help them learn, progress and succeed.

What you'll find are teachers who have chosen to participate in specialised training about how to teach reading and spelling, how to compensate for poor memory and organisation, and how to help kids attack text successfully. In dyslexia-friendly schools, quality reading instruction isn't confined to the early learners. It's continuous, with appropriate and targeted reading programmes capturing young teens as well.

Parents in dyslexia-friendly schools are, as a matter of course, provided with mainstream information about dyslexia and how they can work with the school to support their child. The progress of students is continuously tracked and shared with parents to ensure no student slips through the cracks. As well, there's encouragement and training so students feel confident to access text-to-speech and predictive-typing software.

WHAT'S SPECIAL ABOUT TEACHING A DYSLEXIC TO READ?

There is a gold-standard approach to teaching reading. And when we use this many more students, dyslexics and non-dyslexics, will find reading success. Australian teachers, for the most part, are not aware of this. This is not a criticism about the dedication of teachers, but a comment on the deep systemic failure to impart what has long been available in the reading research to teachers.

Dyslexic children require a specific kind of reading instruction. The Orton-Gillingham Multisensory Method was developed in the early 1930s by Samuel Orton and Anna Gillingham, and provides a legacy as an effective dyslexia treatment. It provides a focus on:

- Explicit training in phonological awareness.
- Strong emphasis on decoding, or word work.
- The reading of progressively more difficult texts incorporating the skills taught.
- The practice of reading attack and comprehension strategies while reading texts.

The truth is nothing has changed since an Australian government inquiry into the teaching of reading in 2004. It concluded that all students benefit from methods that explicitly teach reading. Methods that highlight the relationship between phonology and orthography in language that help students to break the code and master text-attack skills to aid in comprehension. This, of course, is the gold standard legacy Orton-Gillingham has left us with.

AS A PARENT, CAN I TEACH MY CHILD TO READ?

Yes, you can. Specialist early intervention, usually with a skilled teacher or speech pathologist, has been a well-trodden path for families in Australia. It's a great way to go, but takes a big commitment and can be expensive. The heartbreak is that quality reading remediation has had to be sourced outside of school systems simply because it has not been available in most schools. This is a big barrier against reading success, and it's morally unforgiveable.

These days, an increasing number of parents are researching how to teach their dyslexic child to read, and it doesn't take them long to discover the evidenced-based programmes mentioned above. Some parents embark on teaching their children independently. Others decide to work with a skilled teacher or speech pathologist and use them as a coach, while using a recognised reading programme to reinforce and stimulate their child's learning.

A WORD OF WARNING

Not everything that glitters is gold! There is a group of aggressively marketed programmes (often computer-based) claiming to 'rewire the neural language circuits' and alleviate dyslexia, autism, ADHD and more. Sadly, a few have ended up in schools and by doing so they have morphed into looking as though they have some legitimacy. They continue to con teachers, parents, allied professionals and children despite independent studies showing they have very poor or no transfer effects. If in doubt about the effectiveness of any programme or intervention, visit the Macquarie University website – MUSEC Briefings – for the fact sheets.

A FINAL WORD

It is easier to build strong children than to repair broken men.

Frederick Douglass, 1817–1895

Perhaps this sounds whimsical, but it is wise to coach children to accept their learning preference or difference. After all, it will always exist. This is a much better option than a child wishing they were dead because the emotional burden of dyslexia feels too heavy to carry. Help them to see their strengths, find interests and satisfaction and feel hopefulness.

We need to see the success of our dyslexic students as a litmus test about the quality of reading instruction within schools. Sadly, international assessment programmes, such as PIRLS, provide evidence of declining literacy and numeracy standards in Australia.[11] The number of students achieving at the lowest proficiency levels is unacceptably large and compares unfavourably with many other countries participating in these assessments. Clearly, Australian children are being short-changed. It remains unacceptable that such a significant number of Australian children can barely read and write. It is a national disgrace. When we truly get our reading practice right for dyslexic students, we'll get it right for all students.

Author biography

Mark Le Messurier is a teacher, counsellor, author and presenter. He works in schools and in private practice in Adelaide as a coach to young people, parents and teachers. Mark is the co-author of the What's the Buzz? social skills/friendship programme now assisting children with diverse abilities around the globe. Already in sixty countries, it is currently being rolled out in Chinese schools. He is the author of: *Archie's Big Book of Friendship Adventures, Raising Beaut Kids, Parenting Tough Kids, Teaching Tough Kids* and *CBT: A how-to guide for successful behaviours.*

www.marklemessurier.com.au

See also:
Chapter 2: Emotions and Relationships Shape the Brains of Children
Chapter 3: Understanding the Teenage Brain

Recommended websites:
British Dyslexia Association: www.bdadyslexia.org.uk
BTN Dyslexia 2014: www.youtube.com/watch?v=_aZo2B28N3o
Channel 7 ADA Interview about dyslexia (Australian):
    www.youtube.com/watch?v=DYhUcZKqerg
Dyslexia: A Hidden Disability: www.youtube.com/watch?v=8m1fCz3ohMw
Sir Richard Branson on dyslexia: www.youtube.com/watch?v=_CehY6TsoLc
Steven Spielberg discusses his dyslexia for the first time ever:
    https://www.youtube.com/watch?v=4N6RKHOHMJQ
What is dyslexia? – Kelli Sandman-Hurley: www.youtube.com/watch?v=zafiGBrFkRM

Further resources:

Wordshark 5 and Numbershark 5 (software) – www.wordshark.co.uk

Further reading:

Manocha, R (Ed), 2017, *Growing Happy, Healthy Young Minds: Generation Next*, Hachette Australia, Sydney.

 We also recommend the very popular companion volume **GROWING HAPPY, HEALTHY YOUNG MINDS** – resilience, bullying, depression, anxiety, body image and many more important issues.

 For more online resources visit:
generationnext.com.au/handbook

18. FRIENDSHIP AND SOCIAL SKILLS

Madhavi Nawana Parker

Getting along with others and knowing how to handle difficult feelings leads to healthier friendships, contributing to stronger mental health and wellbeing. Social and emotional literacy skills include empathy, self-awareness, reciprocity and coping with emotions constructively.

INTRODUCTION

While siblings and parents are a strong source of love and connection, providing wonderful opportunities to develop social and emotional skills, friends outside of the family are an important part of growing up and becoming your own person. For children who struggle with making and keeping friends, developing skills in social and emotional literacy gives them a better chance at friendship, resilience and wellbeing.

WHY ARE FRIENDSHIP AND SOCIAL AND EMOTIONAL LITERACY IMPORTANT?

Academic achievement has commonly been seen as a sign of success. A vital underpinning of academic achievement and self-confidence is a person with solid friendships and good social skills. People who belong to a social group tend to be much better at handling their feelings and behaving in ways that other people feel comfortable with. Friendships enable self-exploration, trust and empathy. Socially isolated young people miss out on building these skills and are more likely to experience anxiety and loneliness.

Teaching social and emotional skills from an early age helps children fit in with their family, school and community. For anyone struggling socially and emotionally, focused social and emotional skills training is vital. In Professor John Hattie's groundbreaking book, *Visible Learning*, he emphasised that social skills programmes offering explicit skill building, direct modelling and emotional coaching not only improve the social and emotional climate but strengthen the quality of learning that takes place in classrooms.[1]

WHAT HELPS THE DEVELOPMENT OF HEALTHY FRIENDSHIPS AND SOCIAL AND EMOTIONAL LITERACY?

One important influence in becoming a good friend and having good social and emotional literacy is the quality of caring relationships early in life. Children who enjoy warm, affectionate parenting with firm but fair boundaries have a better chance of forming strong, reciprocal relationships with others.

Children with emotionally connected families tend to have higher self-esteem, increased confidence and deeper empathy. As a result they enjoy healthier friendships and have stronger social skills. Warm, reciprocal relationships are valuable throughout all stages of development and encourage ongoing emotional development, greater self-worth and a stronger motivation to learn.

Connecting children to groups outside of the family through sports, hobbies and other community activities builds their social network and their sense of belonging. Spending time with people outside of the family is important for a young person's mental health and wellbeing. Through these connections, children can experience the benefits of a broader community who can help them out when immediate family is not available. Across a broad range of reciprocal relationships, children learn to cope with their emotions, build resilience and problem-solve the everyday ups and downs of friendship. Caring adults such as teachers and parents as well as siblings and friends provide the guidance and practice necessary to continue to improve on social and emotional literacy.

WHAT CAN CAUSE PROBLEMS IN DEVELOPING HEALTHY FRIENDSHIPS AND SOCIAL AND EMOTIONAL LITERACY?

During childhood, social and emotional resilience can vary, affecting a child's ability to be a good friend. Illness, change, conflict or stress can make it harder to get along well with others. Usually these phases do not last long and, over time, these experiences can serve well as an opportunity to build flexibility, develop problem-solving skills and become more resilient.

When a child does not seem to have the skills to keep up with other children their age during play, specific social-skills training may be needed. For some children, these skills do not come easily and may be delayed or impaired due to neurological or developmental obstacles such as autism spectrum disorders, anxiety disorders and developmental delay. Social-skills coaching from parents, educators and health professionals can help children gain the necessary skills to belong to a friendship group.

WHAT TO DO IF SOMEONE IS STRUGGLING TO MAKE FRIENDS

Social skills can be taught. Social and emotional literacy programmes, like What's the Buzz? by Mark Le Messurier and Madhavi Nawana Parker, offer families and schools an opportunity to focus directly on values, getting along with others, problem-solving, conflict resolution and handling difficult emotions.[2] There are many more programmes that teach these skills to young people and one programme alone is rarely enough. Resources to direct professionals to a broad range of helpful programmes can be found at PSHE Association (www.pshe-association.org.uk).

Social and emotional literacy programs built around the SAFE criteria below have a better chance at improving social skills and academic performance.[3]

SAFE:

Sequenced: follow a logical breakdown of skills.

Active: allow students an opportunity to practise the skill
through role play and practice.

Focused: time is dedicated to teaching specific skills.

Explicit: specific skills are taught in each session.

Focusing on strengths is especially important when a young person
is struggling to get along with others. Giving too much feedback to a
child about what needs improving without balancing it by celebrating
existing and developing strengths will weaken the impact of any
intervention.

SOCIAL LITERACY SKILLS TO TEACH YOUNG PEOPLE TO MAKE AND KEEP FRIENDS

While there are many skills at play in strong and balanced friendships;
empathy, keeping calm, friendly facial expressions, good listening and
social problem-solving are among the most valuable skills that can be
taught. They can all improve over time with practice and maturity.

Showing relaxed and welcoming facial expressions builds trust
and helps other people feel comfortable and interested. A child with
confident facial expressions and a happy demeanour easily places other
people at ease. A child with a blank, agitated or intense expression
on the other hand can make others feel uncomfortable, which may
interrupt forming a new bond. Children can learn to show a friendlier
face through role plays and by practising these expressions in front of
a mirror.

Good listeners tend to be better companions and often give as
much as they take in a friendship. Listening skills take time, practice
and maturity to develop. Most children need reminders to listen –
particularly when they are experiencing feelings such as anxiety,
frustration and excitement. Listening skills can be developed by
playing games that focus on tuning into what is going on around
you. Consciously noticing sounds in nature together, meditation

and mindfulness are all great ways to build attention span and listening ability. Games that require listening and memory are also helpful. Drama games and plays where children have to focus on others and what they are saying and doing in a script are enjoyable and helpful ways to develop confidence and listening ability.

Children who problem-solve through friendship ups and downs tend to have the confidence of their peers. They look for solutions instead of focusing on the problem and, over time, can become more light-hearted with their approach to getting along with others. Problem-solving is another way to develop empathy – another essential skill for making and keeping friends. Part of the friendship process is being able to endure and solve different opinions and needs. These differences allow for the development of greater empathy for others and deeper self-awareness. Conflict also provides an opportunity to build skills in repairing hurt, accepting differences and learning how to compromise. Children who are able to engage in social problem-solving often thrive as they learn to prevent and resolve disagreements in a way that satisfies both parties. Children without these skills tend to see things from their own perspective, misinterpreting behaviour and sometimes damaging relationships. Teaching young children as early as possible to understand other people's feelings and perspectives is an important foundation in the formation of friendships. When conflicts occur, being solution focused is more helpful than repeating complaints, disengaging from the friendship, punishing the other person or arguing. Provide problem-solving frameworks like the one at the end of this chapter (BOSS from The Resilience and Wellbeing Toolbox), so they can use this to guide them to find a solution.

EMOTIONAL LITERACY – TEACHING YOUNG PEOPLE ABOUT FEELINGS

Another important skill in friendships is being able to regulate emotions – in other words, know how to handle difficult feelings well. This is not always easy, even for adults. Young people who are emotionally balanced most of the time tend to be more likeable.

Children who struggle to manage feelings such as anger, frustration, impulsivity or excessive excitement can make other children feel uncomfortable and anxious, lowering their chances of building new friendships. Emotions are contagious and may be quickly absorbed by others. A child who struggles to keep calm often puts their playmates into a state of discomfort without even knowing it.

Teaching children from an early age about feelings and how to handle them helps young people get along well with others, especially when conflict arises between friends. This ability is rarely automatic, although some personalities may develop the skill easier than others. These social-emotional responses take time to practise and brain development has a role to play too. The prefrontal cortex that governs these abilities continues to develop well into early adulthood.

HOW TO TEACH EMOTIONAL LITERACY

Reading and reflecting upon books about social situations together is a useful way to build emotional literacy and empathy.[4] Some great books for supporting emotional learning include:

Enemy Pie by Derek Munson
Should I Share My Ice Cream?, *Can I Play Too?* and *My Friend is Sad* by Mo Williams
Those Shoes by Maribeth Boelts and Noah Z Jones
The Name Jar by Yangsook Choi
Feelings by Aliki
Each Kindness by Jacqueline Woodson and EB Lewis

Preparing children for situations that make them anxious by teaching coping strategies can help them feel more confident. If a child is known to struggle with a particular skill, prepare them ahead of time in an encouraging way about what to expect and how they might handle it. For example, a child who becomes anxious about losing can be reminded before playing that while winning feels good, the most important thing is to play in a way that makes people want to play with you again. A reminder of what to say and do when losing as well as winning helps children feel prepared. Simple comments like, 'Good game!' or gestures like friendly eye contact, a handshake or a high-five can help distract from the disappointment of losing, while keeping children connected in a positive way.

Role-plays allow children to objectively practise social-emotional skills without being present in play or conflict where the stakes are high. Coming up with situations that are relevant to the child and role-playing them helps the child practise skills in a relaxed and enjoyable way. Problem-solving is an important part of learning in role-plays that focus on handling conflict and difficult feelings. Most social-skills programmes offer plenty of role-plays to teach a range of social-emotional skills. Young children may also enjoy puppet shows that explore the ups and downs of friendships. Productions like these can provide a great opportunity to learn through observation and reflection. This can be especially helpful for children who struggle with finding the confidence to role-play.

Labelling feelings is important when teaching children how to cope with difficult feelings. Emotions can quickly overwhelm even the most courageous of children. Labelling feelings, whether it's anger, worry, excitement or joy, provides children with a sense of emotional security. When a child has become very angry, for example, naming the feeling and pointing out the incident it is related to helps build social-emotional literacy. It can be useful to say something like, 'You feel angry. You didn't win the game.' By practising this, children can become more comfortable talking about their own feelings and recognising feelings in others. This often means they are liked and accepted more by peers.[5] Another way to label feelings is to cut out pictures from magazines of different people experiencing different emotions. Encourage the child to label the feelings and, together, try to come up with different reasons and perspectives that might be behind the emotions.

Distraction and diversion can boost a child's ability to calm down when they are emotionally overwhelmed. Keeping a 'calm/happy box', which is filled with interesting and calming activities, photographs and books can be a great distraction for a child when they are too stressed to calm down with another person. Encourage the child to help put the box together with objects that interest them. Ensure these cannot be used at other times so they maintain their effectiveness. Other distractions include introducing a different person to the situation, pointing out something of interest to the child, asking them to help with something they are skilled at, turning on some upbeat music or even pretending to struggle and need help with something unrelated.

Laughter can help circumnavigate difficult emotions into something more constructive. Many young people with social-emotional challenges are under constant stress from conflict and the exhaustion of trying to keep up with their more socially savvy peers. Being prepared to play the clown and lighten up when a child is emotionally drained can energise them and help them feel connected to you. Laughter lowers blood pressure and reduces stress hormones, making difficult situations easier to handle. Making sure that young people have plenty to laugh about each day and that they aren't taking life too seriously can contribute to a healthier and more positive outlook.

Stress management techniques such as diaphragmatic breathing can be taught ahead of emotional flare-ups, providing a vital skill for maintaining calm. The '6 tricks for keeping calm' guide sheet from The Resilience and Wellbeing Toolbox provides a simple snapshot for young people to keep calm.[6]

HOW TO TEACH SOCIAL LITERACY SKILLS

Empathy is another essential part of getting along with others. The process of induction can increase perspective and prosocial behaviour when there has been a conflict between young children. When a child hurts someone's feelings, the adult calmly explains the impact their behaviour has upon the other person while showing empathy. The caregiver might say, 'You kicked Jack's bag angrily when you passed him. Jack is confused and feels bullied.' Through induction, children can take responsibility for their actions and the impact their actions have on others. When a child blames others for their actions or is not encouraged to see things from another person's perspective, it will become harder for them to maintain positive relationships. Children with limited empathy and social perspective can be challenging playmates. They tend to interact in ways that are focused on asserting their own importance and meeting their own needs rather than the needs of the friendship pair or group.

These days, children are conversing more than ever through email, text messages and social media. This reduces opportunities to practise listening, eye contact and reciprocity face to face, which are vital aspects of healthy relationships. Skills strengthen through repetition. Too much time on technology means less time building social skills through daily interactions. The prefrontal cortex (which is involved in planning complex cognitive behaviour, personality expression, decision-making and moderating social behaviour) appears to be profoundly influenced by interpersonal relationships.[7] Making relationships between others a priority and reducing the amount of time friendships develop through technological means can make a long-term difference to the development of a healthy brain and, ultimately, healthier relation-ships with others.

Compromise and accepting different perspectives are other important foundations for getting along with others. Through compromise, children can learn to work out what is most important to them and what they are willing to give up to reach a reasonable solution with a friend. Teaching young people that problems can be solved and relationships repaired through compromise is one way to help them secure and sustain long-term friendships with others. It also builds empathy, as the child explores the other person's needs. This is much more fruitful than staying focused on their own needs and placing all their energy into getting what they want rather than meeting their friend halfway.

Learning to cooperate together in play increases empathy and social skills, deepening the bond between friends. Teaching young people simple statements and questions like, 'I've got an idea – do you want to hear it?' 'Have you got some ideas?' 'How would you like to do/play this?' 'We can use your idea first' and 'Let's work this out so we all get some of what we want' help develop good cooperation and play skills and ensure that young people feel included and cared for.

HOW TO TELL IF A YOUNG PERSON MAY NEED HELP WITH THEIR SOCIAL AND EMOTIONAL LITERACY

- Frequent, ongoing conflict with other children that does not occur in phases but dominates most of their friendships.
- Difficulty seeing other people's perspectives, often feeling they are hard done by and misunderstood by their peers.
- Excessive moodiness that cannot be explained by what is going on in their environment.
- Difficulty handling feelings – often overreacting or having meltdowns when things do not go their way. While this can be developmentally appropriate for toddlers and preschoolers, by school age most young children can cope with difficult feelings with their peers most of the time.
- Expressions of loneliness or feeling disconnected from others.
- Social anxiety – spending too much time warming up to interactions so that they miss the chance to play and interact.
- Poor empathy – unable to notice, understand and accept other people's differing emotions and perspectives.
- Frequently avoiding parties and play dates.
- Struggling to use friendly ways to get another person's attention.
- Choosing to spend more time alone during breaktimes than with peers.
- Getting along better with adults than with children their own age.
- Ongoing difficulty with winning and losing well into the primary years.

WHERE TO FIND HELP

Seeing a GP can be a great start to discussing where a child's development might be at.

Paediatricians can help put a child's developmental milestones in perspective to assess whether they are reaching necessary milestones.

School counsellors often have training in social and emotional literacy programmes and can help build these skills in small groups at school.

Psychologists and health professionals often offer social and emotional literacy programmes for young people to participate in.

Organisations such as ELSA Support have useful links to social and emotional literacy information and resources.

'Solutions for kids' on Facebook offers free weekly tips to build social and emotional literacy, resilience and wellbeing.

HOW FRIENDSHIP CAN MAKE A DIFFERENCE TO A PERSON'S WELLBEING AS WELL AS OVERALL ACHIEVEMENT

When students are offered social and emotional literacy alongside the academic and sporting curriculum throughout their education, friendship, caring, empathising and handling difficult emotions will become part of who they are. Academic or sporting achievements alone cannot provide the richness and strength of a solid and healthy friendship. They certainly cannot provide children with an antidote for loneliness.

When people feel connected and enjoy a sense of belonging, they have the platform to contribute to themselves, their peers, their families and communities in ways that impact positively throughout their lifetime. They also behave and perform better. Positive relationships with others are at the core of our happiness. Happiness offers limitless potential in those who experience its true joy.

TAKE-HOME MESSAGES FOR TEACHERS AND SCHOOL COUNSELLORS/YOUTH WORKERS

Having clear and prosocial policies in schools as well as providing a selection of social and emotional literacy programmes provides an important foundation for promoting students' abilities to get along well with others. Cooperative classrooms support social and academic growth. Encouraging students to work together and take on roles that benefit each other's learning enables students to contribute to their school community, even when they struggle socially. When bullying occurs, it is important schools respond promptly to support both the victim (to cope and recover) and the bully (to improve their behaviour and repair the damage). This way schools maintain high expectations around how all students should treat each other, further embedding values essential for making and keeping friends. A socially and emotionally skilled, connected, friendship-oriented school provides a strong foundation for overall achievement.

TAKE-HOME MESSAGES FOR PARENTS

Learning social and emotional literacy skills is a process that takes time and practice. A child will not be able to use those skills immediately or all the time without plenty of encouragement and gentle reminders. Nor will they suddenly become social when this doesn't fit in with their true nature. Some children not only like to be in places such as the library instead of the playground, but need that time away from the hustle and bustle of school life to recharge their batteries. Others simply enjoy time alone or time away to observe and consider.

Siblings can provide a helpful backdrop for developing and practising these important skills. Allow plenty of time for them to play together and enjoy shared interests like beach-combing, time with pets and playing sports. Through fun as well as conflict, they can problem-solve together towards a shared goal. Children without siblings can develop these skills when school friends join family outings from time to time, through extended family and by being part of social clubs and other friendship groups. In time, most children will find their way and develop friendships that can last a lifetime.

Author biography

Madhavi Nawana Parker is a published author of social and emotional literacy programmes. She has co-authored three books with Mark Le Messurier. Madhavi and Mark's social skills programme is used across the globe to teach social-emotional literacy to young people. Madhavi's latest book, *The Resilience and Wellbeing Toolbox: A guide for educators and health professionals*, was published in 2017. Madhavi's weekly tips and framework for encouraging relationships based on social-emotional literacy and resilience in young people can be found on Facebook and Twitter at 'Solutions for kids'. Madhavi speaks regularly to parents, teachers and health professionals on the topics of resilience, anxiety, positive discipline and social-emotional wellbeing.

www.madhavinawana.com.au

www.theresilienceandwellbeingtoolbox.com.au

www.whatsthebuzz.net.au

See also:
Chapter 2: Emotions and Relationships Shape the Brains of Children
Chapter 3: Understanding the Teenage Brain

Recommended websites:
Collaborative for Academic, Social and Emotional Learning: www.casel.org
Mark Le Messurier: marklemessurier.com.au
ELSA Support: www.elsa-support.co.uk
Seasons for Growth: www.seasonsforgrowth.co.uk
The Resilience and Wellbeing Toolbox: www.madhavinawana.com.au
What's the Buzz? A social skills enrichment program: www.whatsthebuzz.net.au

Further reading:
Baumeister, R & Tierney, J, 2012, Willpower: *Rediscovering the greatest human strength*, Penguin Books, USA.
Hattie, J, 2013, *Visible Learning for Teachers : Maximizing Impact on Learning*, Routledge, London.

Le Messurier, M & Nawana Parker, M, 2014, *Archie's Big Book of friendship adventures: A guide to solving social hitches and friendship glitches*, available: www.whatsthebuzz.net.au

Manocha, R (Ed), 2017, *Growing Happy, Healthy Young Minds: Generation Next*, Hachette Australia, Sydney.

Moore, GA, Cohn, JF & Campbell, SB, 2001, 'Infant affective responses to mother's still face at 6 months differentially predict externalising behaviours at 18 months', *Developmental Psychology* 37, pp 706–714.

Siegel, DJ & Bryson, TP, 2012, *The Whole-Brain Child: 12 Revolutionary Strategies to Nurture Your Child's Developing Mind, Survive Everyday Parenting Struggles, and Help Your Family Thrive*, Bantam, USA.

Werner, EE & Smith, RS, 2001, *Journeys from childhood to midlife. Risk, resilience, and recovery*, Cornell University Press, Ithaca, New York.

MEDIA, CULTURE AND YOUNG MINDS

19. THE COMMERCIALISATION OF CHILDHOOD

Christopher Zinn

Our children are conditioned, and often delighted, to be among the most materialistic and consumer-focused in history. While research underlines the cost of such consumerism to young people's wellbeing, growing awareness of the issues and family and societal interventions can help.

HIDING IN PLAIN SIGHT

Parents and teachers face many headline issues including drugs, mental health and obesity but they may overlook related and relevant questions around consumption. What if the demands and desires fostered in the young, through our increasingly commercialised world, actually contribute to these and other problems?

Apart from the obvious annual excesses at Christmas, the commercial forces encroaching on the young are often taken for granted or even normalised.

Advertising and marketing are accepted as an inevitable part of the prosperous modern world where children are lavished with material goods unimaginable a generation earlier. The impact of the online outreach of brands through techniques such as sales images implanted in games and other digital persuasions to buy are only getting stronger. There are legitimate concerns about issues such as the sheer amount and placement of junk food advertising and the use of overt sexuality to sell to children. But the broader fallout on children and adolescents of our acquisitive culture – measured in an excess of burgers, digital devices or branded clothing – is often overlooked.

While there are many tangible benefits to the consumer-led economy such as choice, competition and quality of life, it would be naive not to consider the downside. For the bounty of the consumer world, which gives us such plenty and pleasure, can also be detrimental to our tech-savvy kids' wellbeing. Over time, clerics such as the current pope, philosophers and environmentalists have railed against the waste, inequity and challenges of rampant materialism. But using evidence, child psychologists, paediatricians and researchers have unearthed other uncomfortable effects on our children of this fast-changing world.

From their general wellbeing and sense of self to more specific symptoms such as depression, anxiety and loneliness, the findings are in. Children are targeted online and via social media to buy more stuff, and encourage their families to do likewise, in ways more powerful, inventive and intrusive than ever. Governments have tried but many would argue their efforts have been largely impotent in controlling the spread of entreaties to kids to eat, buy, spend and own via traditional media such as TV.

Concerns once raised about youngsters' exposure to television commercials now seem quaint compared to the almost unquantifiable intrusion of digital channels into their lives. So, what hope do we have around recognising, regulating and counterbalancing the omnipotent commercial push of the internet and its compelling screen culture?

I'll argue we can no longer rely solely on government interventions and need to use some of the learnings outlined below to assist young people in vulnerable and formative stages. Families and society need to call out self-serving commercialism where it doesn't help our children and encourage them to see there is more to life.

But, of course, we have to start by being prepared to practise at least a little of what we preach.

PROBLEM – WHAT PROBLEM?

For some years I have worked with consumer groups on campaigns including those focused on securing clearer food labelling and improved toy and product safety. It's valuable to encourage healthier diets and reduce the toll of avoidable injury, and even death, but the forces bringing many of these products to market were rarely mentioned.

Consumerism, the excessive, endless and dissatisfying acquisition of more and more stuff, and its unforeseen consequences, especially for the young, were just not talked about. The question of why consumer groups don't seem to want to explore this area led me to enquire further afield and find evidence of often surprising and negative effects on youth. As the father of two teenage boys with rooms cluttered with toys, video games and clothes, and exposed to relentless yet subtle marketing messages, I had a vested interest.

I have no agenda against the consumer world, which has given us so much, but merely seek to ask and share some questions about its excesses. In a similar vein, some have focused on consumerism's effect on the environment or on the spirit and even the waistline. My focus is consumerism's effect on the young. My intention is not to unduly disturb the reader but alert them to what is confronting our children, and help empower both parties with facts as to what can be done about it.

In my research one image stuck in my mind: a photo of a little boy called Xavier and his first birthday party. It was complete with a petting zoo, cowboy and Indian photo booth, and doubtless many presents. It was a small sign of how quickly the staging of a simple but significant event had become so lavish as adults spent big on their kids.

Consumerism – and we are talking about the excesses – is not to blame for all our children's woes but it could be contributing to many of them. Adults face their own challenges around what's been called 'affluenza' but surely we owe our children more support to navigate the marketing and materialistic maelstrom.

For starters, our acquisitiveness for new cars, bigger homes and the latest devices is not lost on our offspring and their own appetites to possess more and more. In a wicked equation, parents generally have more stuff but less time and are prone to guiltily giving their kids presents to compensate for their lack of presence.

Australian data shows that the key explanation for seeking longer working hours is heightened levels of consumerism and the need to service household debt.[1] It's a paradox identified, especially in the compulsive consumption of the English-speaking parts of Europe, by marketing expert Dr Agnes Nairn in a report for the United Nations' children's agency UNICEF. 'While children would prefer time with their parents to heaps of consumer goods, [their] parents seem under tremendous pressure to purchase a surfeit of material goods for their children.'[2]

It was a preference borne out in a second-grade ethics class I attended at Bondi Public School. A class of fourteen was asked to choose between being given the latest iPad or spending a weekend with their dads, camping. In a finding that might surprise some parents, and might not apply to teenagers, all but three (all boys) opted for the camping weekend. And, on reflection, even one of the three relented, opting for the experience instead.

Over recent years the cost of toys, electronics and other childhood distractions has come down while their availability has shot up. The same UNICEF research says even comparatively poor families and their children can suffer from an overabundance of cheap, often unopened and broken stuff. The influence of peers and parents is, of course, crucial and may counterbalance media messages' and research can indicate the relative impacts.[3]

So let's look more closely at the cause and effect of consumerism on kids. It's been described as akin to a chronic disease that has crept up so stealthily and is such a part of the wallpaper we hardly know it is there.

CAUSE – THE MEDIA HAS THE MESSAGE AND IT CAN BE SPEND, SPEND, SPEND

Poor little Barbie. The doll remains a lightning rod for issues around gender but in the mid-1950s her manufacturer, Mattel, used her to pioneer advertising direct to children through their favourite TV shows. They sold the toy and the brand name direct to the fledgling consumer, in this case the child, with access to requisite funds, and effectively bypassed the parent. Even by 1960 Dr T Berry Brazelton, one of the USA's leading paediatricians, was quoted as saying acquisitiveness and consumerism were root causes of parents and children not knowing each other.

During the next half-century in both the US and Australia the marketing techniques aimed at children grew more and more sophisticated, as did the explosive growth of a consumer culture. Much of the evidence and analysis of this phenomenon comes from the US, UK and Europe, but there's much common ground in many countries around the world.

In her groundbreaking 2004 book, *Born to Buy*, Juliet Schor found that children recognised logos at eighteen months old, could ask for products by name at two years old and by three and a half, believed certain brands made them cool, strong and smart. By first grade they could name 200 brands. She defined US teens and 'tweens' then as the most brand-orientated, consumer-involved and materialistic generation in history.[4] At the same time the American Academy of Pediatrics found the average young person was exposed to 3000 ads on TV, the internet, magazines and billboard every day.[5]

Digital devices and the music, games and videos held on them might have reduced the physical clutter of CDs, DVDs, etc., but the desire for ownership remains just as strong. And despite the presumed sophistication of even young children, they are still vulnerable to the sales pitch.

The American Psychological Association has found that children under eight can't critically comprehend TV ads and are prone to accept the commercial messages as truthful, accurate and unbiased. It recommended such advertising aimed at these age groups be restricted but, as has been the case with many such reform proposals, after consultations nothing happened.[6]

In Australia, Sharon Beder from the University of Wollongong blew the whistle with her 2009 book, *This Little Kiddy Went to Market*. She claimed the decline in young people's wellbeing was aligned with corporate interference in their lives, with marketing designed to foster discontent and turn them into consumers defined by what they had and not who they were.[7] Since then, of course, there's been an exponential growth in the internet, social media channels, apps, screen-time and digital devices.

Compared to their European counterparts, Australian children aged nine to sixteen are among the youngest and most prolific users of the internet in the world. Figures just out from the UK, which mirror changes here, show that on average schoolkids aged between five and fifteen are online fifteen hours a week, up 78 minutes in just a year, with declining viewing of TV.[8]

Three- and four-year-olds are online for an average 71 minutes a day and this figure rises to four hours if you include watching TV and playing video games. University of Sydney business school marketing researcher Teresa Davis found 561 full, associated and implied brand images in one minute embedded in one game app aimed at five-year-olds.[9]

Whatever you may think of such changes – and there are proponents who believe iPads and tablets might actually be good for kids' minds – they offer multiple and powerful channels for marketing direct to kids. Online sites now contain 'native ads', which feature stories and pictures that, even for an adult, can be hard to distinguish from editorial.

There's a code of conduct in Australia for advertisers, which says that if such ads are targeted at children it should be made clear they are advertising. Innovative marketing, especially social media, uses behavioural techniques to target young consumers with data derived from their profiles and web-browsing history.

There's also much interest around online 'influencers' such as bloggers, who are paid in cash or goods to provide what's called 'promoted content' in ways that aren't always transparent. Needless to say, regulation around the marketing of many products, such as junk food, is limited at best and ineffective or almost nonexistent online. It's a loophole that is frequently exploited.

The conundrum is highlighted by Flinders University law professor Elizabeth Handsley. She contributed a report to the World Health Organization calling for intervention to redress such targeted marketing of high-fat, -salt and -sugar foods to children. 'Parents hand over these digital devices to their children but are not having the capacity to track what is happening to their children online and what their children are exposed to . . . yet these [marketing] companies are tracking very closely what their children are up to,' she said.[10] Apart from their own spending power, children aged six to thirteen have about 650 million dollars in personal savings, and are targeted for the influences they bring to bear on adults.[11]

Roy Morgan Research is particularly interested in those aged six to thirteen because they are the primary decision makers or key influencers on their parents for buying decisions around cars, holidays, technology and food.

The data and insights around this market segment are valuable. It costs $14,950 to buy the full report called 'Understanding Young Australians'. One 'interesting fact' they give you for free is that children aged between six and nine are 27 per cent more likely than the average young Australian to agree with the statement, 'I would rather be rich than happy when I grow up'.[12]

EFFECT – THE EVIDENCE ON HOW EXCESSIVE COMMERCIALISATION CAN AFFECT CHILDHOOD

What is called the internalisation of consumer culture ideals – that's to say, a focus on getting stuff – has been linked by research with lower wellbeing in children. The theory is that by focusing on external or extrinsic values, such as materialism and how you look, less attention is paid to internal or intrinsic values. They include more positive ideas about relationships and who you are, and so the focus on the opposite extrinsic values can lead to lower satisfaction with life.

Consumerism tends to focus far more on extrinsic values. While there have been studies on adults and adolescents, until now there's been little work into the formative years of childhood. Evidence suggests children with higher self-esteem are less likely to be materialistic and vice versa – those with lower self-esteem are more likely to be materialistic.

And the good news is that interventions involving priming other, more positive feelings can bring about real change. Researchers from the United States have found even simple actions to raise the self-esteem of younger consumers can dramatically impact on their expressions of materialism.[13]

In other experiments, children given signals that primed them for higher self-esteem, for example, by showing them videos that made them feel better about themselves, tended to score lower on measures of materialism than their peers who were not primed this way.[14]

At the University of Sussex in southern England they've been running The Children's Consumer Culture Project. It's said to be the first systemic examination of the impact of this environment on kids aged eight to fourteen and their personal and social wellbeing. They found children who immerse themselves in consumer culture, despite the promise of advertising, feel worse about themselves and not better. And there was clear evidence of a negative downward spiral where those with lower wellbeing adopted more consumer values, which then lowered their wellbeing further.

The Sussex research looked at 'ideals' of money, costly possessions and looking good to see how much children are driven by external motives, such as peer pressure and social recognition, which are more likely to result in lower wellbeing. A longitudinal survey of 1000 children over almost three years found the adoption of consumer culture values and wellbeing are closely linked. Lower wellbeing leads to greater consumer value adoption, which in turn lowers wellbeing even further.

It also showed that those who felt rejected by their peers are more likely to adopt consumer values to compensate. But this 'win friends' strategy was ultimately counterproductive as it predicted for more rather than less peer rejection.[15]

Priming techniques, which were used with full ethical clearance, debriefing and support, evaluated various influences on children's feelings. Those who were primed around their appearance and materialistic ideals scored lower on body esteem and higher on materialistic motives. In short, the outcomes were more negative. Children who were primed for intrinsic values, which focused on the activities in life they really enjoyed, scored more highly in wellbeing measures.

The academics pondered the following key finding of their pioneering work. If the one-off and brief priming or manipulation of extrinsic consumer culture values can so affect a child's feelings and thoughts, what is the impact of a 'daily bombardment of advertisements and associated peer pressure'?

And it's not just the advertisers who are to blame; we parents are well in the frame too. The US Journal of Consumer Research carried a study that showed adults whose parents rewarded their good behaviour or grades with gifts were more likely to base their self-worth on material goods. They were also more likely to be judgemental about other people based on what possessions they had. The researchers identified what they called 'material parenting' to express love and shape behaviour.[16]

If you have been raised with such strategies, which are hardly rare in the home or school, you are more likely to grow up with materialistic values, and if your possessions are taken away, you are going to be more insecure.

WHAT'S BEING DONE TO MINIMISE THE EFFECT ON CHILDREN?

Australia has hardly been a pioneer in interventions to protect children from marketing but comparable nations have sought to, if not always succeeded, in taking action.

In the late 1970s in the US the Federal Trade Commission, after holding hearings and reviewing research, concluded it was unfair and deceptive to advertise to those under six years old.[17] No ban eventuated but at different times various European and Scandinavian nations have regulated this area. In 1991 Sweden and Norway banned all advertising for those aged under twelve and Denmark and Belgium severely restricted it. In Greece no toys could be advertised on TV before 10 p.m.

In 2011 an ambitious UK government proposal called for a total ban on all TV, radio, billboard and online advertising aimed at children under sixteen despite the market being worth A\$200 million a year.[18] But Reg Bailey, the chief executive of The Mothers' Union, who published an independent review of the commercialisation and sexualisation of childhood, said insidious online marketing simply made any such ban ineffective. His report found no need to cut children off from the commercial world completely but let them manage it themselves while supported by proportionate regulation and responsible business practice. He called for comprehensive and effective regulation across all media to protect children from excessive commercial pressures.[19]

The review also asked that marketers not exploit any gaps in advertising regulation to unduly influence the choices young consumers may make. It wanted to see parents and children given access to a sound knowledge of both marketing techniques and the applicable regulation.

A slightly earlier report called 'The Impact of the Commercial World on Children's Wellbeing', commissioned by the UK government, took a different tack, arguing the young are neither helpless victims nor savvy consumers. It saw the evidence for much of the detriment felt by kids as very limited. 'We need to look at children's consumption in the round, in relation to broader changes in the economy and family life, without succumbing to nostalgia for a mythical golden age,' it said.

It claimed it was difficult to separate commercial factors from other influences such as parents and peers, and as consumer culture was not going to disappear, families needed to better understand how it worked and how to deal with it.[20]

More recently a worldwide survey into the subjective wellbeing of 53000 children aged eight, ten and twelve across fifteen varied countries including Ethiopia and England found no correlation between their life satisfaction and the lack or otherwise of material possessions.[21]

Children tend to be happy no matter what, but when the relative rankings of their reported happiness were compared with their grown-up counterparts, the impact of materialism on wellbeing is more apparent. The effects of commercialisation do not just reside in the individual but can also affect the whole of society.

The UNICEF report previously mentioned said a key cause of the London riots in 2011 was obsessive consumerism as seen in the looting of shops with designer goods.[22] The UN agency's sad conclusion about British households it studied was: 'Most children agreed that family time was more important to them than consumer goods, yet we observed within UK homes a compulsion on the part of some parents to continually buy new things for their children and for themselves. Boxes of toys, broken presents and unused electronics in the home were witness to this drive to acquire new possessions. Most parents realised that what they were doing was often "pointless", but seemed somehow pressured and compelled to continue.'[23]

WHAT CAN WE DO?

Before being too disappointed in the role of government to address many of these issues, remember that in 1874 the British Parliament legislated to protect children from the efforts of merchants to induce them to buy.

But as the UK Mothers' Union report found, even with heavy regulation, the 'insidious' advertising online makes bans and controls largely redundant.[24] So while lobbying efforts for better codes of conduct from business and government oversight must continue, what can we do as parents, teachers and citizens?

Firstly, we might recognise that there are some signs the tide is turning, with more people questioning and turning their backs on 'all-you-can-eat' consumerism. In terms of excessive birthday parties for the young, there's also a trend for do-good parties where guests give to charity instead of handing over gifts to expectant and unappreciative kids.

Trends forecaster and author of *Stuffocation*, James Wallman, says buy-nothing and buy-less campaigns and anti-consumer movements are growing. He suggests 'peak-stuff' might have been reached as experiences are being valued more highly than materials, but it might take fifty years to get back to any kind of normality.[25]

In the meantime, there are some tips as to how we can help our children navigate the world of plenty we have helped deliver and on their own terms, help themselves too.

TAKE-HOME MESSAGES

- The first clear bit of advice is that children clearly prefer being given adults' quality time and attention instead of goods. Being given these gifts is more likely to help them grow up to be less materialistic and judgemental of others and their possessions. In turn kids, at least of a certain age, really value experiences, such as that camping trip with Dad, over and above even the latest technology. Take them at their word.

- Value giving and gratitude – Apart from their intrinsic worth, actions like this are only good for children's wellbeing at levels that reduce the adoption of consumer values. Try to flip the negative spiral – more consumer values leading to lower wellbeing – into a positive one of enhancing wellbeing to reduce consumer values. They are never too young to start. Xavier of the lavish birthday party will only have photos to remind him of what happened. Try not to engrain 'material parenting' too early by rewarding good behaviour with gifts. Use praise instead.

- Practise what you preach – Many of the models of excessive materialism have come from parents as kids either soak up our own acquisitiveness or are showered with gifts to compensate for time lost while working away from them. Beware what adult behaviours, such as envy for another's house or car, they may subconsciously internalise.

- Try to limit screen-time and exposure to advertising. The very hardest comes last. You may have your strategies but check out other ones too. Anything you can do to reduce the sheer mass of messages that suggest that buying stuff leads to happiness will help, especially since the opposite is true. Do not let advertisers dictate to you or your children or students what might be considered normal.

- Finally, we must realise that the evidence shows well-tailored and targeted interventions at the individual or group level can make a difference. To quote two leading experts in the field, Chaplin and John from the Journal of Consumer Research in 2007: 'Our results indicate that simple actions to raise self-esteem among young consumers can have a dramatic impact on expressions of materialism.'

CONCLUSION

The issues raised by the commercialisation of childhood pose real questions for society, only some of which have been raised here. It may be necessary to protect younger children from the worst excesses with more vigour than we've seen to date. But, ironically, older kids, through their grasp of new technologies and social media, can be empowered to make better choices and see through the hollow claims of consumerism. The University of Sussex study put it thus: 'Children can be helped, both at home and school, and may even be able to help themselves and their peers to put consumer culture into perspective.'[26]

Author biography

Christopher Zinn is a consumer advocate, campaigner and media commentator who works in the marketplace of consumer empowerment. A father of teenagers, he is concerned about the invisible toll consumerism takes on society. He developed these themes in a series of talks to Generation Next audiences around Australia in 2015.

www.determinedconsumer.com.au

See also:

Chapter 7: Problematic Internet Use and How to Manage It
Chapter 20: Sexualisation: Why Should we be Concerned?
Chapter 21: Porn as a Public Health Crisis

Further reading:

Manocha, R (Ed), 2017, *Growing Happy, Healthy Young Minds: Generation Next*, Hachette Australia, Sydney.

We also recommend the very popular companion volume **GROWING HAPPY, HEALTHY YOUNG MINDS** – resilience, bullying, depression, anxiety, body image and many more important issues.

For more online resources visit:
generationnext.com.au/handbook

20. SEXUALISATION: WHY SHOULD WE BE CONCERNED?

Maggie Hamilton

This chapter explores the impact of the sexualised world teens and tweens inhabit, how to protect them and positively respond to the dangers they face.

INTRODUCTION

Everywhere kids look there are sexy images in ads, on billboards and in magazine editorials. They observe sexy conversations and scenarios in sitcoms and music videos, DVDs and films, and in porn. With this level of exposure to sexualised content come observable pressures. These pressures are changing the way tweens and teens interact. How they see themselves. How they behave. As Dr Joe Tucci, CEO of the Australian Childhood Foundation, puts it, 'When we expel kids from childhood, we push them into adulthood.'[1]

There has always been pressure on teens. Is the current environment really that different, and if so, in what ways? According to Dr Joe Tucci, a decade ago few children were reported for problematic sexual behaviour. Generally these were ten- to twelve-year-old boys exposing themselves or masturbating in public. In a few short years this landscape has changed rapidly. In one region alone, Dr Tucci tells of how in 2010 there were 220 referrals of children aged seven to fifteen exhibiting problematic sexual behaviour, ranging from low-level incidents to increasing numbers involved in coercive sexual behaviour, including penetration incidents. Some with multiple targets.[2]

Two decades ago problematic sexual behaviour could be traced back to a teen or tween experiencing sexual abuse, then acting out these same incidents on peers. In 2010, 30 per cent of reported cases of problematic sexual behaviour in teens and tweens involved kids who hadn't experienced sexual abuse, or family violence and trauma. A third of these kids were girls. What caused this shift? Where are we at now, and what can we do about it?

SEXUALISATION AFFECTS YOUNG CHILDREN TOO

In 2006, a seven-year-old girl was sexually assaulted over two months by a boy her age at a Queensland primary school. Hitting her and threatening to kill her if she spoke out, the boy repeatedly forced this young girl to perform oral sex. A few weeks later in a New South Wales primary school, teachers struggled to deal with a rash of ten-year-old girls photographing themselves topless, then sending these photos to peers.[3] While shocking, these incidents were soon forgotten, but the problem remained.

Fast forward a decade to police discovery of a website with over 2000 photos of high school students from seventy Australian schools. Most images were selfies. Some were of young girls engaged in sex. One young girl in a low-cut top had her photo copied from her Facebook page, and hailed as a 'win' when reposted on this disturbing site. Successful young 'hunters' – contributors of graphic material to this site – were eligible for 'bounty': access to a cache of pornographic photos. On this same site a 'wanted list' contained the names and images of young desirable teens who this forum would like to see nude. Encouraged to 'Go get her boys', members were doing just that.[4]

Today, sexual incidents are prevalent in schools, including primary schools. Sexting, for example, is something children as young as eight now participate in, once they get their first (camera-enabled) phone. At age eight inappropriate photos centre around bare bottoms and breasts. By high school the images would make any X-rated movie proud.

THE CURRENT GENERATION GAP
MAKES OUR KIDS VULNERABLE

Life has changed radically in a few short years, and our young people are at the cutting edge of these changes. This is happening at a time when many parents lack confidence, while others simply want to be cool. The current generation gap has possibly never been greater, which makes our kids even more vulnerable to the sexualised material they are subjected to. Teens and tweens are also acutely aware of how ill informed adults are about their world, their challenges, and find this endlessly frustrating. That's why they turn to their peers, the media or the net for answers. While the information they get may be misleading or inaccurate, it's accessible and immediate, something we as adults generally are not.

How parents can help

- Don't assume life's pretty much the same as it's always been.
- Make regular time to chill out with your children, and allow issues to arise.
- Keep up to date with what's happening – subscribing to online blog Collective Shout (www.collectiveshout.org/blog) is a good start.

THIS IS NOT A TIME TO BE COMPLACENT

Early childhood professionals and parents are now reporting unacceptable sexual behaviour and language at preschool. They speak of tongue-kissing, and children's inappropriate and determined exploration of each other's bodies, of the use of such words as 'sexing' when talking about love and affection. One mother of a five-year-old told of her daughter's distress at constantly being pressed by a little friend to play 'vagina to vagina'. A day later the mother of another small girl in a different city confided how her daughter was battling the same harassment. The Australian Bureau of Statistics point to a 20 per cent rise in young people under twenty sexually assaulting others from 2008/09 to 2013/14. In 2014, a quarter of these under-twenty offenders were ten to fourteen years old.

THE NEW TECHNOLOGIES HAVE CREATED RADICALLY DIFFERENT CHILDHOOD EXPERIENCES

When we assume the lives of our children are much the same as they've always been, we leave them vulnerable. Our children and young people inhabit a highly complex landscape with ready internet access and mobile phones, webcams and camera-enabled phones, and phones able to download direct from the net. With these and other devices, they can access a world of information and experiences in seconds. Most of this material is beyond parental supervision. Some is harmless, much is not.

SEXY IMAGES ARE GOOD FOR BUSINESS, NOT SO GOOD FOR OUR KIDS

With these technological developments, manufacturers can now access kids direct. The highly competitive tween and teen market is literally worth billions, and sex is an important part of the selling formula as kids view it as forbidden, enticing and grown up. There's a proliferation of sexy images and content on billboards, clothing, product wrappers, on screen and in newspapers and magazines, promising young people they can be everything they long to be: attractive, popular, sophisticated. For many kids, the combination of sex and shopping is irresistible. The seductive images and language targeted at young people are all the more potent because major companies employ cultural anthropologists and child psychologists. They know our children's lives intimately and which buttons to press. How then, if at all, does this hypersexualised environment affect our tweens?

How parents can help

- Explain clearly why certain content is harmful – discuss, don't lecture.
- Create open discussions at home around the pressures of this sexualised environment.
- Use situations in the media, films and sitcoms to help frame the way your child might view tricky situations, using such openings as: 'I wonder why X did that?' 'How would they feel?' 'What should they have done?'

PUBERTY ISSUES ARE HAPPENING YOUNGER

'Some girls are now fashion conscious as young as three or four,' reflects Debra, a community liaison officer and mother of two girls. With this focus on fashion comes a desire to act in a more adult way. Sexy behaviour is sold as desirable, and necessary if kids want to be cool. The fallout is less glamorous. 'We're now seeing six-, seven- and eight-year-olds involved in coercive, manipulative sexual behaviours, because there's a confusion around what sexuality means,' says Dr Joe Tucci of the Australian Childhood Foundation. 'This can be very traumatic to the child they're doing this to.' Victims often have to undergo intensive counselling to deal with their trauma, he explains.[5]

How teachers can help

- Media education is essential from early primary school onwards.
- Visit the website of the National Society for the Prevention of Cruelty to Children (www.nspcc.org.uk) for information to support in-class personal safety curriculum.
- The UK Safer Internet Centre (www.safeinternet.org.uk) helps with online safety.

THIS GENERATION'S IMMATURITY LEAVES THEM VULNERABLE AROUND HIGHLY SEXUALISED CONTENT

British neuroscientist Susan Greenfield warns that contemporary lifestyles and computers keep boys and girls childlike – in need of constant reassurance, instant gratification and assuming the world revolves around them. This growing immaturity among our young comes at a time when they have ready access to a world of information, including porn. Without the maturity to deal with disturbing sexual material, they become ever more vulnerable.

How parents can help

- Work on your child's resilience.
- Create a rich culture in the home of friends and family of different generations, of interesting and unusual pastimes.
- Encourage an interest in nature, different culture, sports and/ or the arts.

WHEN GIRLS SEE THEMSELVES AS OBJECTS THEY BECOME VULNERABLE

A growing number of professionals who work with girls are concerned about the objective way in which many girls now view themselves. 'What troubles me is that it's like girls don't feel they have any rights,' one high school teacher tells. 'It's like they want to be objects to be desired.'[6]

Professionals are also concerned that there is little dialogue around a girl's right to say no. Increasingly, girls simply accept that they will have to perform sexual acts that may be embarrassing, painful and humiliating, because that's what they're meant to do. 'You just do all this sex stuff with boys,' explains Poppy, aged twelve, 'you don't have to love them or anything.'

Other professionals report a deteriorating sexual climate around teen girls. 'When I first started teaching in 2000, there was a sense of wanting to be sexy, but it wasn't common for girls to be having sex at twelve – it was more likely at fourteen,' one young teacher explains. 'Now it's [having sex] more common at twelve. It's like girls want to be wanted and loved in that moment, and that's enough.'[7]

With the shrinking of childhood and the collapsing of valuable life experiences, girls are even more willing to do whatever it takes to fit in. This same teacher spoke of one student, aged fourteen, who took off with a friend in a car full of boys. During the ride, the girl was pressured into taking her top off. She complied because she didn't want to look 'silly'. The boys then took a photo with their mobiles and sent it to other kids. When the girl told her teacher, she had no sense of being violated. 'Girls are terrified of being isolated and not being seen as cool,' this teacher explained. 'It was like the girl could only see herself as how boys were seeing her.'[8]

Another teacher told how one girl she was counselling admitted to having sex with several boys and her stepfather. The way the girl related her experiences, she had no sense of being violated by her stepfather. Agreeing to sex, she believed, was what you were meant to do.

How parents can help

- Teach your kids that their body is theirs and not to be messed with.
- Help them by giving them examples of where they might be vulnerable.
- Assist them to recognise toxic situations, and how to extract themselves.
- Work out with your kids scripts to say no in language they would use.

WORRYING TRENDS IN ATTITUDES TOWARDS SEX

A recent UK study of anal sex among youths aged sixteen to eighteen from diverse backgrounds sheds further light on the concerning dynamics surrounding sex. Sometimes inspired by pornography, sometimes not, the male teens in this survey mainly initiated anal sex, sometimes pushing girls to participate. They expected to enjoy the experience, and to sometimes have to take a coercive role to get what they wanted, while most girls expected to endure pain and/or damaged reputation, as that was what they thought they were meant to do.[9]

How parents can help

- Teach your kids that coercion is never okay.
- Help them understand the difference between love and exploitation.
- Assist them to fully understand what makes a good relationship.

SEXY IMAGES ARE HAVING A SERIOUS IMPACT

Some professionals see clear links between the hypersexualised imagery girls are constantly exposed to and their sexual behaviour. 'There is a huge desensitisation around sexualised images,' says one clinical psychologist, who heads up a sexual assault team at a major New South Wales hospital. 'The boundaries have become blurred not just for girls, but their parents, and the whole of society. You can't drive down the street without seeing this material. If these images were put up at work, they'd be seen as sexual harassment, but we constantly see women in pornographic poses on buses and billboards. So, why are we surprised that young girls are participating in rainbow parties and having anal sex? It's been sold to them as empowerment, it's a great con job.'

How teachers can help

- Create a multimedia competition, supported by local business, for kids to explore the pressures.
- When kids research their own landscape, the results can be powerful, as kids like to learn themselves.

'We're seeing a collapsing of childhood,' warns another psychologist who supports victims of sexual assault. 'Younger and younger children becoming victims of sexual assault. In our performance culture, "performance" is part and parcel of what's going on with girls.' In their desire to perform for peers, girls are putting themselves in increasingly risky situations. 'Oral and anal sex are now just like kissing. To girls it's not really sex. When their relationship with a boy begins at this level, then the expectations are that they'll be up for a whole lot more.'

ADULTS CAN UNWITTINGLY END UP CONTRIBUTING TO THE PRESSURES

'Young girls grow up with their lives captured on camera and video by friends and family,' one psychologist pointed out. 'It's only a relatively small step for them or their peers to capture more intimate details of themselves and their life.' She goes on to explain, 'We're seeing a growth in girls being encouraged to take photos of themselves, which can then be used for bribery. With threats to tell their parents or new boyfriends what they've been up to, these girls can then be groomed to take more and more explicit photos of themselves. The trauma from these situations can be as bad as physical assault for girls, causing sleeplessness, flashbacks, not wanting to go out – the symptoms of post-traumatic stress.'

How parents can help

- Think about how, where and why cameras are used in the home.
- Are there better, more enriching ways to celebrate/capture the moment?

TEEN CULTURE SUGGESTS GIRLS NEED TO BE PRIMED FOR SEX AT ALL TIMES

Competition in this new performance culture is fierce, so sexual boundaries continue to be pushed, helped along by girls keen to extend their repertoire by access to porn. Along with faux lesbianism, teachers talk of a growing interest in threesomes. 'From what the girls say, the boys will think nothing of asking, "Can I have sex with your friend at the same time as well?",' one teacher says. 'The way things are, it's like it's prudish to say no.'[10]

How parents can help

- Help kids recognise when situations are harmful.
- Teach them about body boundaries and what behaviour isn't acceptable.

While sexual abuse of girls has always existed, according to experts, this too is taking new forms. 'We're now seeing girls vulnerable to the same range of risks adult women face – being harmed on their way home, by taxi drivers, by boyfriends,' one professional says. The objectification of girls doesn't help. 'Sexual offenders have less empathy,' one psychologist explains. 'They see their victims as objects. So the more we encourage girls to view themselves as objects without depth or difference, the more we place them at risk.'

Certainly the language used by many teen girls suggests they're inhabiting a war zone. Teen girls speak of a night out of sticking together and watching out for each other, making sure their drinks are never left unattended and that they're never alone. They tell of pretending to drink to look part of the scene so they won't be made fun of, and of making sure they all leave together.

Those at the cutting edge of teen issues are in no doubt as to the vulnerability of this generation of girls. 'Personally, I have huge concerns. Young girls are now being targeted by older boys,' says one senior clinical psychologist, who heads a sexual assault support team at a major hospital. 'We see a lot of twelve- to fourteen-year-olds, targeted by boys seventeen to eighteen years. These are young girls wanting to be grown-up, who're still very young and trusting, who fall prey to pre-planned situations. They're plied with alcohol, and possibly drugs, and often raped anally. In the past it was rape by one boy, but now it's two or three boys, and often filmed. The severity of assaults is also growing.'

OLDER TEENAGERS SEE THE RAMPING UP OF SEXUALISED BEHAVIOUR IN YOUNGER TEENS

'You're now seeing guys and girls together at twelve and thirteen with serious commitments and doing crazy [sex] stuff,' Daryl, aged seventeen, says. 'They're just kids, but it doesn't surprise me, because we're made to grow up faster.' Some see these changes as inevitable, others are concerned by them. 'I see younger kids doing stuff at thirteen and fourteen, like sex, alcohol and drugs, and I am appalled,' says Gary, aged seventeen. 'Young teens have sex, because that's what you do. You've got young girls reading things like how to give the perfect blow job at thirteen,' Dylan, aged eighteen, says. 'That stuff's everywhere. You can't escape it.'

What teachers can do

- Create a culture in older students at school that looks out for younger school kids.

The way girls are talked about does have an impact, as Sara, a high school teacher, points out. 'It all starts with the language – how sex is referred to. Young boys talking about "f**king a girl", "having a **ck". They wander around the school grounds saying, "I'd tap that", or "I wouldn't tap that". Or they talk openly about "fingering her". It's this grotesque, yet casually demeaning way they talk about girls as sex objects.'

WHAT'S THE POINT OF VIRGINITY?

When the lines are blurred and few boundaries exist, our children end up making their own rules, or imitating what's seen in pop culture. As it's not cool for a teen, even a young teen, to be a virgin, what are teens meant to do about this pressure to 'come across'? In one coastal town, professionals were dealing with the fallout of girls as young as thirteen who were going out and getting drunk, then finding someone to have sex with, so they could say they were no longer a virgin. The boys they had sex with were picked at random. Others find f**k buddies.

So where is all this pressure leading girls? In a major study into the impacts of sexualisation on girls, the American Psychological Association Task Force found that when girls engage in objectified behaviour and are anxious about their appearance, their ability to focus is diminished, making it harder to think logically and to compute. This in turn impacts their decision-making and their ability to do well in such subjects as mathematics, which requires focused reasoning.

The APA Task Force found clear links between sexualisation and the three leading causes of mental health issues in girls, namely depression, low self-esteem and eating disorders. It concluded that a sexualised environment encourages sexism towards girls; that fewer girls are likely to take up careers in engineering, science, technology and mathematics; and that there are likely to be higher rates of sexual harassment and sexual violence.[11]

IT'S HARD FOR TODAY'S BOYS AND GIRLS TO HAVE RELATIONSHIPS WITHOUT SEX

When you're living in a sex-saturated environment, there's a lot of pressure. Increasingly, sex is seen as part of the deal. A number of teens I interviewed admit to liking someone, but not even considering going out with them, because of the expectation they would have to have sex. Interestingly, it's not just girls who are under this pressure. 'Yeah, sex is now expected as part of relationships,' Dylan, aged eighteen, says. 'Young males are starting to expect it, because that's what's shown on films and stuff.' These expectations can leave girls vulnerable to assault, and boys to assault charges.

BOYS ARE VULNERABLE TOO IN THIS CLIMATE

With this level of full-on attention to sex, it's hard for boys to resist temptation, despite their better judgement, and as a result they may well wear the consequences for years. 'It's a concerning scenario,' explains Sam, a youth worker. 'Boy meets girl. Girl likes him, so takes explicit photos and sends them to the boy. They get together. The relationship splits up. The boy is hurt and angry, so he circulates the photos. Then he's in trouble. If she is under sixteen and, depending on where he lives, he can be up for a whole range of charges from indecent treatment of a child under sixteen, to circulation of child exploitation material. Just to hang on to the explicit photos means he can be charged with child exploitation.'

What parents can do

- It's essential boys learn clear boundaries.
- Boys need to have the pressures they are under recognised, then see why porn is a bad idea.
- Strong, clear, good role-modelling by dads and other men in boys' lives is essential.

BOYS AND PORN

These days a boy's access to porn is a given. For some it starts as young as six and seven, for others porn comes later. 'There's the porno aspect of the internet now,' explains Harrison, aged fifteen. 'Kids don't have to buy it off older boys like they used to do. It's readily accessible. Some boys use it quite regularly. There's quite a culture of it. Inside jokes and words. A lot of boys talk about it in an open and relaxed manner. Most of my peer group admit to doing it. What they know about sex becomes quite sensationalised. They realise sex isn't exactly like that, but it's quite pleasurable. It can change the way boys talk in groups.'

Boys just being boys?

Remarkably, some parents still regard boys accessing porn purely as a sign their boys are growing up. There's also the view that if porn is accessed in the privacy of the home, it doesn't affect anyone else, but this clearly is not the case. 'When we go into a boy's background after a sexual offence it's clear the majority have been accessing porn,' explains Sam, who works with troubled youth. 'You can see this also from the kinds of acts they have performed – it's an obvious imitation of something they've seen.'

What parents can do

- Give boys a clear sense of what makes a great guy and what makes a creep.
- Encourage open discussion about difficult subjects.
- Help him to see a situation where he might be vulnerable and how to react.
- Ensure your son knows he need never battle along on his own.

ONCE BOYS GET INTO PORNOGRAPHY, THEIR WHOLE WAY OF RELATING TO GIRLS CHANGES

Boys themselves are aware if this. 'Some boys will definitely see girls differently after looking at pornography. It doesn't have a good impact at all,' admits Lucas, aged fifteen. In one local incident, a thirteen-year-old girl went off to meet a schoolboy she'd met a few days before in a park. To her surprise they were joined by several of his friends. Over a number of hours she was sexually assaulted and repeatedly raped. Forced to perform oral sex on a number of the boys, she was repeatedly told to 'just smile like you're enjoying it'. The incident was filmed and circulated. Those reporting the court case remarked on the complete lack of remorse shown by the boys, who were said to come from good homes. In a paper on adolescent sex offenders in Australia, Dr Ian Nesbit points out that teens are responsible for 'approximately 20 per cent of adult rapes and 40 per cent of child sexual assaults'.[12]

THE BRAIN SCIENCE

We now know porn rewires the brain, leading to addiction, obsessively seeking out certain sexual experiences, needing increasingly heightened levels of stimulation, and experiencing withdrawal symptoms when porn isn't available. In *The Brain That Changes Itself*, psychiatrist Norman Doidge tells how he noticed, in his male patients, interest in making love was replaced by simply 'needing a f**k', that their 'sexual creativity' was dying, as increasingly they needed to experience the scenarios they'd downloaded to become aroused. The end result was a decrease in interest in their regular partners, potency issues and handling their ever-increasing hardcore tastes.[13] Norman Doidge sees teen access to porn as particularly problematic. Young people's minds are especially plastic, and still in the process of forming sexual tastes and desires. Because softcore pornography is no longer hidden, it can have an enormous influence on these young people who also have limited sexual experience.[14]

PORN IS ABUSIVE TO BOYS

It is easy to blame boys for accessing porn. Yet increasingly experts are realising just how abusive early access to porn can be, as porn shuts down a boy's emotions and distorts his views on sex. 'Pornography has given boys a shared language, a sense of entitlement around sex, and a belief that the sexually explicit material seen in pornographic material is what girls want to do,' explains one psychologist who works with sexual assault victims. 'Seeing it in their living room normalises pornography. It gives young guys a way of relating to each other, which in turn reinforces abuse.'

In one Canadian study of boys aged thirteen to fourteen in urban and rural areas, more than a third of the boys said they had viewed pornographic movies and DVDs 'too many times to count'. Just over seven out of ten of these boys accessed pornography on the net. More than half saw it on a speciality TV channel.[15] In this same study, two out of ten boys aged thirteen to fourteen viewed porn at the home of a friend. Dr Joe Tucci, who heads up the Australian Childhood Foundation, points out that while only a small proportion of child sexual assault offenders had accessed porn in the past, now every case they deal with has experienced exposure to porn. An important point to note is that with the right assistance, perpetrators can move on from this unhelpful behaviour.

What teachers can do

- Develop a school code that keeps boundaries clear.
- Visit The Mix website (www.themix.org.uk/sex-and-relationship/porn) for information to support in-class discussion.

The measure of a healthy society is one that nurtures and protects its young. Our current sexualised climate is abusive to boys and girls. What will this new generation be like as adults, when increasingly sexual acts centre around performance? How will their relationships fare, when boys and girls witness the torture of women and girls for pleasure? Already we are seeing increasing numbers of victims of domestic violence. There is growing evidence that porn does change the brain's pathways, and behaviour. We also know those addicted to porn are unable to connect meaningfully with those they care about, to sustain healthy relationships, and even when successful in other aspects of their lives, they end up living on the fringes.

The current generation is struggling in this hypersexualised environment. Struggling for intimacy, for meaningful connections, with what it means to be a boy or girl right now. The wider questions are: What kinds of men and women will this generation become? How will our young people experience the nuances of relating? What hope have they at true intimacy? What will the sexualised landscape look like for their children, and their children's children? How can we turn the tide?

WIDER CONSIDERATIONS

- An urgent review of advertising in public spaces, and in the products and games marketed to our young.
- Ongoing education of parents about this new climate, including parents of preschool and primary school children.
- The social impact of goods and services need to be added to the bottom line, so companies with products that negatively affect our children and teens are made accountable.

Author biography

Writer, publisher and social researcher Maggie Hamilton gives regular talks, lectures and workshops, is a regular media commentator and a keen observer of social trends, and presents at parents' evenings, professional development forums and at conferences. Her books have been published in Australia, New Zealand, Holland, Italy, Korea, China, the Arab States, Lithuania and Brazil, and include *What Men Don't Talk About*, which examines the lives of boys and men behind the stereotypes; *What's Happening to Our Girls?*, and *What's Happening to Our Boys?* which look at the twenty-first century challenges of our girls and boys respectively; and *Secret Girls' Business*, a fun, funky, empowering gift book for girls. She has addressed over 50 000 Australian parents, and countless professional forums, adding additional dimensions to her work.

www.maggiehamilton.org

See also:
Chapter 3: Understanding the Teenage Brain
Chapter 13: Talking to Young People about Online Porn and Sexual Images
Chapter 19: The Commercialisation of Childhood
Chapter 21: Porn as a Public Health Crisis

Further reading:
Manocha, R (Ed), 2017, *Growing Happy, Healthy Young Minds: Generation Next*, Hachette Australia, Sydney.

We also recommend the very popular companion volume **GROWING HAPPY, HEALTHY YOUNG MINDS** – resilience, bullying, depression, anxiety, body image and many more important issues.

For more online resources visit:
generationnext.com.au/handbook

21. PORN AS A PUBLIC HEALTH CRISIS

Liz Walker

This chapter examines how the pornography industry is shaping culture and why we need to respond. It considers the impact on the adolescent brain; how it places young people at risk for addiction; conditions users towards sexual acts and templates that mirror porn images; contributes to sexual problems; and links to other mental health concerns. Suggestions are provided as to how to frame a response and engage community for change.

INTRODUCTION – THE NEW FRONTIER

Over the past few decades, ease of access to the internet has changed almost every aspect of our lives. This includes access to pornography. Pre-internet, pornography was the brown-paper-bag variety. Users typically read a magazine or watched a video and when finished, tucked it away for next time. Pin-up-style images have given way to endless genres and availability. Now, it's a click away – any amount, any time, any variety.

The internet has completely overpowered previous legal limitations to protect children and young people from sexualised content. The most concerning aspect from a child and teen developmental perspective is that mainstream free online pornography is hardcore. While not all porn falls within the hardcore genre, what is most commonly available online is broadly defined by researcher Linette Etheredge as demanding 'violence and inequity as its core script line'.

This definition came from analysing material found on free websites such as Pornhub, RedTube, YouPorn and the most extreme teen porn. Etheredge found that 'degradation, humiliation, punishment and extreme submission appear to be the general objective of the power dynamics or behaviour depicted'.[1]

Professional practice and research shows that free and easy access to sexually violent online pornography is contributing to myriad challenges for users, more so for children and young people. Not only has consumption become normalised, the toll on relational, emotional, mental, sexual and social development for young people demands a proactive response. However, first we must understand how an abyss of exploitation, abuse and misogyny became normalised online.

INDUSTRIALISED PORNIFICATION

A well-oiled machine, the porn industry and associated lobby arms such as The Free Speech Coalition, work diligently at convincing the public that their product – commodified sex – will provide a manual for a cutting edge, fun and creative sexuality. The profits of the porn industry would suggest that they have been successful in their PR. It is estimated the industry is worth $US97 billion – a staggering growth rate in view of the approximate yearly gross of $7 billion in the late 1990s.[2]

The industry churns out every imaginable scene and genre, overtaking fantasies of countless users. Survey rates vary as to how many people watch pornography regularly. One estimate is that 9 to 16 per cent of women and 27 to 40 per cent of men aged eighteen to thirty-nine use pornography in an average week; while another report found that 16 per cent of women and 46 per cent of men in the same age range do so.

These figures tell us that pornography viewing is common and frequent for a significant number of the population. Accordingly, this translates to high levels of web traffic. Traffic statistics by Similar Web in January 2017, rank Pornhub as the twenty-second most popular website globally.[3] Pornhub's 2016 year-in-review revealed an astonishing 23 billion visits – up from 21.2 billion in 2015. That's 64 million visits per day, 2.6 million per hour, and 44 thousand per minute. 4 559 000 000 hours of porn were watched on Pornhub alone in 2016 – this equates to 5 246 centuries. Globally, Australia ranks eighth in the top 20 web traffic countries.

Pornhub has an estimated worth of $2.5 billion, yet is topped by Xvideos, at approximately $3 billion. Pornhub keeps its edge by combining with another seven free porn sites to lead the industry under the ownership of MindGeek. Dr Gail Dines, internationally acclaimed expert on how pornography shapes our identities, culture and sexuality, has shown in her research how MindGeek dominates the market and monopolises the marketplace. A revolving door exists between MindGeek's paid and free sites. Free sites expand the consumer base and generate enormous ad revenue. A percentage of users are then diverted to pay for premium porn.

Dines notes a rise of lobbying groups and industry associations. These groups, funded by the industry, have the capacity to engage in public relations campaigns, legal battles and research and, in turn, influence political activity.

The accessible, affordable, anonymous and addictive characteristics of pornography combine with a relentless marketing machine intent on normalising violent, abusive and exploitative sexual interests. Industrialised pornification is a global phenomenon that leaves no part of culture unscathed.

THE ROLE OF TECHNOLOGY

Normalisation of the porn industry owes much to Hugh Hefner; however, *Playboy* magazine has now become commercially unviable in the sexual revolution it promoted. Playboy's influence pre-internet peaked in popularity with a 5.6 million readership, eventually dropping to 800 000. With the rise of technology, Playboy CEO Scott Flanders announced in October 2015 that the magazine would no longer publish nude photos. He is quoted as saying, 'That battle has been fought and won . . . You're just one click away from every sex act imaginable for free. And it's just passé at this juncture.'[4]

Ease of access jumped with porn 'tube' sites that launched in 2006, the year after YouTube commenced. Smartphone ownership led to another jump in the ease of access to pornography. Given that 91 per cent of teens go online multiple times per day from their smartphones, it is essential for parents to be aware of how to put measures in place to reduce access to porn on mobile devices. Regular, honest and open conversations should complement device monitoring, as young people also have access to sexualised and pornographic content through apps, dating sites and social media.

All technology has a range of benefits and pitfalls, with the latest being virtual reality. The American Organisation Protect Young Minds explains that virtual reality (VR) is the creation of a completely synthetic, digital environment, accessed via a headset or goggles. VR porn is already here, compatible with the PlayStation VR, and is being aggressively marketed by Pornhub. Without a shred of evidence, it is already being touted that VR porn is '20 percent sex, 80 percent therapy'.[5] Technology combines with porn to trick the brain and body into thinking it is having a real sexual experience. Concerns have already risen as to what impact this will have long term on the brain and sexual function. What is certain, however, is that a VR porn experience is totally disconnected from actual reality and meaningful intimacy.

> No matter which technology is delivering porn, kids need an internal filter in order to reject it.
>
> Protect Young Minds

THE ADOLESCENT BRAIN

Pornographers rely on biological responses of arousal, desire and orgasm, commercialising what can potentially be the most intimate of human experiences. The porn industry, like all predatory industries, knows that if they hook young people to become regular users, the stronger their consumer base will be and the greater their profits.

One of the reasons why it's so important to speak with children and young people early is that pornography holds greater implications for the developing brain than it does for the adult brain. Each of the following areas make the adolescent brain more vulnerable to brain changes, including altered sexual tastes and addiction.

Stronger desire for pleasure

During adolescence, the reward-seeking (limbic) region of the brain tends to be more emotionally reactive and develop at a faster rate than the area responsible for decision-making. Young people are drawn to activities that have high rewards of fun, novelty and pleasure, and will preference those feelings over boring or less enjoyable activities.

Decreased sensitivity to aversion

Research suggests that even when a substance, behaviour or situation produces a negative effect, if there are other positive factors in play – such as peer approval or the pleasure reaction to pornography – aversion to the stimuli may be ignored in preference for the pleasure reward. This helps explain why some teens can have an increased capacity to sit through a film that totally grosses them out, yet at the same time, they rave about how much they enjoyed it.

This person's recollection of the compulsive escalation to content they found 'sick' illustrates this point.

> I started looking at internet porn when I was 11. I immediately became hooked, and spent hours daily viewing porn. Simply seeing a pair of exposed breasts was enough to get me off. But desensitization soon kicked in, and I began developing fetishes to get the same hit from porn. It started out with different ethnicities, then lesbians, then watersports, then scat/bestiality/BDSM/tranny, and then any combination of the above to create the sickest porn imaginable. I can remember sitting in school fantasizing about sick porn that I could search for that night.[6]

Weaker 'brakes'

The development of the prefrontal cortex (PFC) influences decision-making, and is the brain region involved with forward-thinking, planning, attention span, judgement, organisation, risk assessment and impulse control. The PFC also houses the conscience and helps people stay on track with goals. The PFC often takes a back seat to emotional and reward-seeking motivators. During the developmental phase, young people are less equipped to apply regulatory brakes and temper heightened emotions. Young people benefit from exercising rational decision-making, self-control and learning to manage emotions while the prefrontal cortex is in the development phase, much like muscles strengthen with regular use.

Neural growth and pruning

Adolescence is a critical period of neural development. Neural pathways can be understood as the groove the brain becomes accustomed to functioning within. For instance, if a person consistently has coffee first thing in the morning, neural pathways are accustomed to this groove. Throughout adolescence, young people have experiences that drive the formation of neural pathways. Regularly used pathways that are strengthened. Pathways not used are pruned while grooves become deeper. Throughout adolescence, the brain is highly impressionable and more vulnerable to forming addictions.

The influence of hormones

Along with brain changes, hormonal changes are heightened throughout adolescence and may interact with other areas of the brain and the surrounding environment to influence emotional and risk-taking responses.

With malleable brains, teens are less able to foresee outcomes beyond the immediate rewards of arousal, desire and orgasm to pornography. Given the brakes required to regulate behaviour and critical thinking skills are still under construction, the appeal of porn overrides rational decision-making for a significant cohort of young people.

Changing tastes

Sexual tastes are socially conditioned and somewhat fluid. That is, intense stimulation can shape and alter sexual tastes. As illustrated by the young person sharing their story of compulsive escalation earlier, tastes mould over time.

Author of *The Brain That Changes Itself*, Norman Doidge MD, writes that internet pornography 'satisfies every one of the prerequisites for neuroplastic change . . .' He says that the porn epidemic demonstrates that sexual tastes can be acquired, and that while pornographers may say that they are 'pushing the envelope' with new, more hardcore themes, this is because their viewers have built up a tolerance to the existing content – so new material is a necessity.[7]

For at least half of today's users, research published in 2016 confirms that porn is altering users' sexual tastes. One study found:

Forty-nine per cent mentioned at least sometimes searching for sexual content or being involved in online sexual activities (OSAs) that were not previously interesting to them or that they considered disgusting, and 61.7% reported that at least sometimes OSAs were associated with shame or guilty feelings.[8]

Pornographers and supporters of porn often try to suggest that porn helps users to 'find their true sexual tastes'. They argue that any guilt associated with porn use is due to sexual hang-ups and unnecessary shame. Yet this argument fails to account for the increasing number of users seeking support via online forums for unwanted changes to sexual tastes. Their concerns often relate to extreme content that was not part of their desires prior to porn use.

Forums are filled with people sharing stories about porn-induced fetishes and the development of sexual obsessive compulsive disorders. It's little wonder that these conditions surface, given adolescence is a time when brain connectivity is very sensitive to both the environment and experiences that streamline future behaviour. Research in the neuroscience arena has found that experiences seemingly quite harmless can have a profound effect by altering the organisational structure of the brain, both during development and in adulthood. Given the brain's neural plastic capability, it is also reported that these porn-induced fetishes are often reversible with the removal of pornography and/or professional treatment.

To respond to this, it has been suggested that instead of asking the question, 'Should I feel bad about my fetish (or compulsion)?' the better question is 'What is my true sexual nature?' From a neurological perspective, if desires are not authentic and are triggered and fuelled by pornography, continuing to watch porn trains personal sexual responses to that stimulus, driving and reinforcing previously unwanted desires. From a sociological perspective, porn culture sets the norms for what is true and, therefore, everything it produces requires critical analysis.

CHANGING BEHAVIOURS

Toxic decisions seem rational in toxic environments.

Dr John Briere

Research demonstrates that pornography influences sexual scripts. Rather than sexuality being purely a construction of biology, it is strongly influenced by social norms, attitudes, values and personal experiences. In demonstrating this theory, research finds that higher frequency porn viewing correlates with an increased number of sexual partners and a higher incidence of hooking up. It also shows it is more common for men to watch porn during sex to maintain arousal, and for increased requests to perform particular pornographic acts during sex.

In the absence of alternative reliable information, young people are more likely to develop sexual scripts influenced by pornography. For example, accepting a sexual script that 'sex is purely casual/ recreational' can lead to changed behaviours. Queensland practitioner Dr Wendell Rosevear, indicates that he 'quite frequently' treats patients who have between four and ten sexual partners per day;

they face significant risks if they're having unsafe sex.[9] This trend is attributed to hook-up culture and is resulting in a significant rise in sexually transmitted infections.

Writing in a comment on a 2015 blog post the director of a sexual violence counselling service has this to say about the sexual scripting of intimate partner violence:

> In the past few years we have had a huge increase in intimate partner rape of women from 14 to 80+. The biggest common denominator is consumption of porn by the offender. With offenders not able to differentiate between fantasy and reality, believing women are 'up for it' 24/7, ascribing to the myth that 'no means yes and yes means anal', oblivious to injuries caused and never ever considering consent. We have seen a huge increase in deprivation of liberty, physical injuries, torture, drugging, filming and sharing footage without consent.[10]

Hook-up behaviour and a rise in aggressive behaviours among children and adolescents are tangible examples of how pornography is influencing young people's sexual scripts.

SEX AND PORN ADDICTION

The term 'porn addiction' is hotly contested, yet excessive porn use is problematic, foremost for the person involved and, secondly, for their loved ones. This condition is also known as internet pornography disorder or compulsive sexual behaviour.

In a recent cross-sectional (males and females) representative sample study of 6000 (average age: 45), participants were asked if they self-identified with addictions to alcohol, drugs, gambling, eating, gaming and sex. Just over 50 per cent identified one or more of these substances or behaviours as problematic. Nine and a half per cent reported excessive sexual behaviour – having sex in a way that creates problems in life, and/or inappropriate use of pornography, whether online or offline.[11] While this cohort is not separated into differing categories of sex and porn addiction, it's clear there is a remarkably high number of people who struggle in this area.

There is overwhelming evidence to support framing pornography as an addiction. The Your Brain on Porn site says that currently '29 neurological studies on pornographies effects are consistent with 180+ internet addiction "brain studies", many of which also include internet porn use. All support the premise that internet porn use can cause addiction-related brain changes, as do 10 recent neuroscience-based reviews of the literature.'[12]

While it's certainly not the case that all people who watch porn will become addicted, the addiction process progresses through stages: Binge/intoxication – withdrawal/negative affect – preoccupation/anticipation.[13]

A simplified explanation of what is happening in the brain is that pornography triggers a rush of neurochemicals, starting with dopamine to activate the reward centre of the brain. People love the feeling that dopamine induces – a fast car, more chocolate, a bigger rush and, of course, more porn. Nonstop stimulation from pornography is not a natural state of the brain – online porn is a supranormal stimulus. Continued overconsumption triggers dopamine to release DeltaFosB – a protein that activates certain genes, which in turn initiates brain changes. With DeltaFosB strengthening connections between the nerve cells, neuroplastic changes take place. Connections become stronger with each intense experience and the groove formed in the brain leads to automatic behaviour.

The typical process of an addict is that sensitised pathways trigger high-reward circuit activity – cravings that happen before the addict uses (sensitisation). This is followed by desensitisation that has the opposite effect and leads to tolerance – while using, the same initial rush doesn't occur due to low dopamine receptors. Novelty increases dopamine.

To illustrate, the alcohol addict experiences sensitisation with the smell of alcohol. Walking past a pub leads to cravings, before using. However, when the alcoholic drinks he needs more than before because his reward system has down-regulated dopamine, opioids and their receptors. This is the 'consuming' or 'tolerance' phase.

With a porn addict, turning on the computer (or even thinking about a past porn scene or something sexual) causes cravings – sensitisation. But when they use they need something shocking or novel to get the same effect – that's desensitisation leading to tolerance.

As already outlined, the adolescent brain is particularly sensitive to new experiences. Neuroplastic changes inspired by porn use reinforce pathways and can become problematic. For some, this occurs over time and for others, it can happen quite quickly. Often people don't realise they are addicted until they experience the withdrawal symptoms that can accompany stopping use.

> Detailed explanations of the concepts and science related to porn addiction can be found at Your Brain on Porn: www.yourbrainonporn. com and The Reward Foundation: www.rewardfoundation.org

Ben explains:

> I had no idea I was addicted, which is funny considering I would spend hours a day in front of the computer watching increasingly novel video after video. If my internet was running slowly and I couldn't watch, I would go into rages and fits. I could do nothing else but wait until the video started again.[14]

Symptoms of withdrawal reported by users include:

- Anxiety, chest tightness, panic attacks, high heart rate and blood pressure.
- Feelings of impending doom. Depression to the point of suicidal thoughts.
- Chronic fatigue symptoms.
- Inability to take pleasure in anything whatsoever: eating, reading, watching a film, playing music or creating artwork.

- Severe insomnia.
- Increased urge to masturbate – up to ten times in a day.
- Sexual fatigue, loss of libido, loss of interest in life, testicular and groin pain, but still a strong urge to masturbate.
- Incoherent speech.
- Digestive problems.
- Headaches and brain fog.

For anyone stuck in an addictive cycle, free online forums, information sites and apps can be a huge source of encouragement and support (see resource list at the end of this chapter).

REDUCED DESIRES

Increased availability of streaming porn has coincided with a tremendous increase in youthful sexual dysfunction. With regular and consistent porn use, sexual tastes alter and profound brain changes can occur, resulting in reduced desire for the real thing.

Young people are reporting that pornography reduces sexual interest towards potential real-life partners, and that they are experiencing problematic sexual responses. These include porn-induced erectile dysfunction (PIED), difficulty climaxing with a partner, low desire and arousal disorders. Historically, risk factors for these conditions include smoking, alcoholism, obesity, diabetes, cardiovascular disease and similar, with 2 per cent prevalence rates in men under forty.

However, a 2014 study of sexually experienced adolescents aged sixteen to twenty-one reports that 51.1 per cent experience a sexual problem (similar proportions of male and females). Rates of erectile dysfunction were at 26.3 per cent – a massive increase from the 2 to 3 per cent reported in 2002. Half of those experiencing abnormal sexual responses indicate significant levels of distress associated with it. It is reported that when porn is taken away, these conditions reverse.

Young people are typically wired to be sexually curious; however, porn hijacks the neural connections and places the focus on the screen, not the person. People who have stopped using porn report huge benefits, including increased energy, mental clarity and the ability to express empathy, be present and authentically connect. Quitting porn restores human dignity on so many levels.

OTHER IMPACTS ON MENTAL HEALTH

I've had youth and social workers contact me, asking me to make sense of how porn is affecting the young people they work with. One such instance was a query from a worker suspecting that porn was contributing to a fifteen-year-old's mental health issues. He was watching porn three times a day and had other mental health problems – he was diagnosed with acute stress disorder and his father had died a couple of years prior. With consent, the worker contacted the young client's mental health team to let them know, yet the team completely dismissed any suggestion that watching porn was a contributor to ongoing issues.

Given the influence of pornography as a supranormal stimulus on the brain, mental health professionals would be well advised not to dismiss porn as a factor influencing mental health.

This is an excerpt from Reddit user David's personal experience:

I started watching porn when I was about 14 . . . All of my friends were doing the same so I didn't think I was doing anything harmful . . . I am now 28 and I still find myself in the same situation more or less that I was in when I first started out watching porn. I always felt like it was a dirty habit but I guess knowing that the majority of men in our society were also watching porn enabled me to ignore my fears and continue.

I found that if I watched porn more than usual, for example, if I had a day off, I would notice that the type of porn would change, I would find myself watching more extreme porn. This is the part of my story that I think has affected me the most. I was brought up in a loving family, I was taught how to treat women with respect, so what I found so hard to deal with [was] why I was able to watch porn where a woman would be mistreated. I would never treat a woman like that in 'real life', so why did I allow myself to watch these videos? I would get bored of normal porn I guess because I had watched so much of it but even though this is a logical reason why I would end up watching extreme porn, it didn't make me feel any better about doing it and after watching an extreme porno I would feel sick and really disgusted with myself. I would also find that if I didn't watch porn for a couple of days then my taste would go back to 'normal' porn but the effects of watching the extreme porn would still be there in my real life.

Since I was about 18 I have found it difficult to make eye contact with people, I have suffered from low self-esteem and in turn an inability to connect with people. Stupidly I didn't really connect the dots between porn and my sociability till recently and one of my main drives to quit porn is to reconnect with society.

About 1 year ago I tried to take my own life, I had watched some stuff that I couldn't erase from my mind and the guilt was eating me alive. Thankfully I was unsuccessful . . .[15]

The graphic nature of pornography in and of itself can be distressing, yet the associated arousal, orgasm and addictiveness can be a significant drive in continued use, despite negative consequences. David's use drove him to attempt suicide. Astute professionals will benefit from including problematic porn use as a trigger for suicidal ideation, as well as being aware of links to other mental health issues.

Research indicates that low self-esteem and depressive traits are linked to compulsive use of mainstream pornography. Users report greater depressive symptoms, poorer quality of life, more mental- and physical-health diminished days, and lower health status than compared to non-users. Associations have also been found between internet porn use and loneliness.

It should be of concern to parents and professionals that pornography use interferes with decision-making; decreases a person's ability to delay gratification; diminishes working-memory; and, with increased use over time, impacts academic performance.

It appears that any addiction-related behaviour can impact on the brain's ability to focus on important life-skills tasks, more so with respect to sexual arousal and adolescent development.

Much of the research mentioned has been in relation to the impact of pornography on boys however the literature indicates that problematic or addictive porn use has similar impacts on girls' brain development and mental health. In addition, a meta-analysis found that evidence consistently indicates that 'everyday exposure to [sexualised] content is directly associated with a range of consequences, including higher levels of body dissatisfaction, greater self-objectification, greater support of sexist beliefs and of adversarial sexual beliefs, and greater tolerance of sexual violence toward women'.[16] Other impacts of young people using pornography include decreased self-confidence; higher rates of conduct problems and delinquent behaviours; difficulties with social integration and bonding with caregivers; higher rates of anxiety; earlier onset of sexual experimentation; and sexual preoccupation.

Each of these points is worthy of further focus, with significant evidence indicating that pornography negatively impacts young people's mental health.

Framing a response

Between stimulus and response there is a space.
In that space is our power to choose our response.
In our response lies our growth and our freedom.

Viktor E. Frankl

The challenge when speaking with teens (or anyone) about porn, is to not project shame (external projection of 'there is something wrong with you'). Instead, we need to be clear about how the porn industry has targeted users, and be empathetic about the hook that pornography has become for a significant population group.

At the same time, it's important to create a new framework of understanding from as many angles as possible. This includes teaching about the impact of porn on mental health, how it becomes an obstacle for intimacy for many users, and the cost of porn on society.

One response to pornography has been to push for porn literacy. At worst, this approach argues for showing power-balanced (feminist-friendly) porn in the classroom; and at best, it advises increased access to sexual information, promoting sexual pleasure, productive solutions to sexual harm, and greater conversation about gender, race, consent, and power.

However, if we as a society have any hope of raising kids to stand against the onslaught of porn culture framed by a multi-billion-dollar industry and the tsunami of misogynistic messages it ushers with it, we need something stronger than porn literacy. Instead, we need critical porn analysis, which is a much tougher conversation. This approach asks how porn is affecting individuals, relationships, families, communities and nations. And it asks kids and teens to play a conscientious role in healing the harms done thus far. Critical porn analysis also deconstructs the prevailing norms around porn so kids can develop an analysis that is counter to the hegemonic discourse.

Critical porn analysis teaches kids online protective behaviours; the impact of pornography on the brain that triggers arousal and orgasm to scenes that are not a part of most adult relationships; the addictive nature of pornography; high rates of erectile dysfunction and arousal disorders experienced by long-term users; body-image issues and performance anxieties; and pornography's contribution to relationship breakdowns and divorce.

Critical porn analysis contextualises porn within an industrial setting to reveal how these images are not simply images of sex, but carefully choreographed scenes that deliver to the consumer images of degradation, brutality and abuse against women as a way to keep an increasingly desensitised user population interested. Critical porn analysis exposes the multi-billion-dollar industry that shapes sexuality and hijacks preferences in the direction of previously unwanted desires. It stresses how porn promotes acceptance of attitudes that endorse inequality, racism and sexual degradation – and refuses to call this 'entertainment' or 'sex'. Critical porn analysis provides an in-depth, reflective conversation about increasing sexual violence towards partners, triggered by porn users who insist they need to get off by replicating what they repeatedly watch online. Critical porn analysis is honest about how porn manipulates a significant minority of young people into self-exploitation and behaving in harmful ways towards themselves and others.

Challenging the dominant discourse is no easy feat. For many, speaking about pornography invokes personal discomfort. Some still imagine porn from yesteryear as the naughty magazine stashed under the bed. Some are offended by the 'P' word, uncomfortable at its mention. Some have loved and lost a partner to its grips. Some are oblivious to signs of addiction or ensuing brain changes. Some claim empowerment and liberation with its use. Some are vocal on the issue of violence against women, yet fail to recognise porn as a vehicle of delivery. And some actively use with no conscious awareness of its contribution to a toxic culture where people are stripped of their humanity in exchange for debasement.

As the research mounts and the harms become too obvious to ignore, a cultural revolution emerges from the voices of young people themselves. The first generation raised on high-speed internet porn inspires an unlikely new breed of hero, including people such as Gabe Deem from Reboot Nation, Alexander Rhodes from NoFap, Jessica Harris from Beggar's Daughter, and Noah Church, author of *WACK: Addicted to Internet Porn*. These young people have stepped through recovery from addiction and porn-induced sexual issues. They emerge from the fog having counted the cost, with an acute awareness of the level of violence in porn they once freely participated in. They now choose to lead the way for others to turn their back on porn.

Others leading the charge are brave young voices. Through open conversation and critical analysis, pockets of young activists are intent on proclaiming that 'people deserve to be valued as people' rather than commodified sex objects. With the tide against them, the exchange is authentic connection – intimacy – and a personal version of sexuality rather than one constructed by the porn industry.

Engaging the government, schools and community on this insidious epidemic is as difficult as it is necessary. For a growing number of people, self-awareness of what porn viewing contributes to, in turn, motivates behavioural change. It is hoped that with increased conversation and education (and perhaps collective awakening), more people will be empowered to be a voice for change.

Author biography

Liz Walker is an accredited sexuality educator, speaker, author, and Director of Health Education at Culture Reframed: the global lead in solving the public health crisis of the digital age. Liz is an exceptional communicator and passionate advocate for children and young people, and chairs the Australian organisation Porn Harms Kids: addressing the harms of children and young people accessing online pornography. Well-connected internationally, Liz regularly provides consultancy to government, non-profit and professional organisations.

www.lizwalkerpresents.com
contact@lizwalkerpresents.com

See also:
Chapter 7: Problematic Internet Use and How to Manage It
Chapter 13: Talking to Young People about Online Porn and Sexual Images

Recommended resources:
Culture Reframed – Solving the Public Health Crisis of the Digital Age. Research-driven education to prevent, resist and heal the harms of violent mainstream pornography and hypersexualized pop culture. www.culturereframed.org
Youth Wellbeing Project – holistic relationships and sexuality education with a focus on providing skills for Critical Porn Analysis. IQ4porn equips Primary & Secondary Schools to implement policies and learning materials for students, and directs staff and parents to further support. www.youthwellbeingproject.com.au
Liz Walker Presents – Find support specific to porn addiction through apps, forums, websites and books. www.lizwalkerpresents.com/support-for-porn
Childline has information suitable for children over the age of twelve concerning online porn. See the link www.childline.org.uk/info-advice/bullying-abuse-safety/online-mobile-safety/online-porn

Recommended websites and apps:
Sex & Porn Addiction Help: www.sexaddictionhelp.co.uk
Parents Protect!: www.parentsprotect.co.uk

Brook: www.brook.org.uk (provides wellbeing and sexual health support for young
  people)
Your Brain on Porn: www.yourbrainonporn.com
The Reward Foundation: www.rewardfoundation.org
Alexander Rhodes – NoFap: www.nofap.com
Fortify Program: www.fortifyprogram.org
Quit Pornography Addiction: www.bit.ly/quitpornographyaddiction
Brainbuddy App: www.brainbuddyapp.com
Recovery Tribe App: www.rtribe.org

Further reading:

Amen, DG, 2005, *Making a Good Brain Great,* Three Rivers Press, Random House, USA,
  pp 16, 37.
Beyens, I, Vandenbosch, L & Eggermont, S, 2014, 'Early Adolescent Boys' exposure
  to Internet pornography: Relationships to pubertal timing, sensation seeking,
  and academic performance', *The Journal of Early Adolescence* 35(8), pp 1045–1068.
  DOI: 10.1177/0272431614548069
Braithwaite, SR, Coulson, G, Keddington, K & Fincham, FD, 2015, 'Sexual Scripts –
  The Influence of Pornography on Sexual Scripts and Hooking Up Among Emerging
  Adults in College', *Archive of Sexual Behavior* 44, pp 111–123. DOI: 10.1007/s10508-
  014-0351-x
Casey, BJ, Jones, RM & Somerville, LH, 2011, 'Braking and Accelerating of
  the Adolescent Brain', *Journal of Research on Adolescence* 21(1), pp 21–33. DOI:
  10.1111/j.1532-7795.2010.00712.x
Cooper, A, 1998, 'Sexuality and the Internet: Surfing into the new millennium',
  CyberPsychology & Behavior, Mary Ann Liebert, Inc. 1(2), pp 187–193. DOI:10.1089/
  cpb.1998.1.187
Jenson, K, 'Virtual Reality: What No One is Telling Parents', Protect Young Minds,
  17 November 2016. www.protectyoungminds.org/2016/11/17/virtual-reality-parent-
  guide
Kolb, B & Gibb, R, 2011, 'Brain Plasticity and Behaviour in the Developing Brain',
  Journal of Canadian Academy Child Adolescent Psychiatry 20(4), pp 265–276. PMCID:
  PMC3222570
Manocha, R (Ed), 2017, *Growing Happy, Healthy Young Minds: Generation Next,* Hachette
  Australia, Sydney.
Park, BY, Wilson, G, Berger, J, Christman, M, Reina, B, Bishop, F, Klam, WP & Doan,
  AP, 2016, 'Is Internet Pornography Causing Sexual Dysfunctions? A Review with
  Clinical Reports', *The Journal of Behavioral Sciences* 6(3), p 17. DOI:10.3390/bs6030017
Pizzol, D, Bertoldo, A & Foresta, C, 2016, 'Adolescents and web porn: A new era of
  sexuality', *International Journal of Adolescent Medicine and Health,* 28(2), pp 169–173.
  DOI: 10.1515/ijamh-2015-0003
Regnerus, M, Gordon, D & Price, J, 2016, 'Documenting Pornography Use in America: A
  Comparative Analysis of Methodological Approaches', *The Journal of Sex Research* 53(7),
  pp 873–881. DOI: 10.1080/00224499.2015.1096886
Sun, C, Bridges, A, Johnson, JA & Ezzell, MB, 2016, 'Pornography and the Male Sexual
  Script: An Analysis of Consumption and Sexual Relations', *Archives of Sexual Behavior*
  45, pp 983–994. DOI: 10.1007/s10508-014-0391-2

Walker, L, 'Young People Need Critical Porn Analysis; "Porn Literacy" Is Not Enough',
    Generation Next, 9 December 2016, www.generationnext.com.au/2016/12/young-
    people-need-critical-porn-analysis-porn-literacy-not-enough
Yoder, VC, Virden III, TB & Amin, K, 2005, 'Internet Pornography and
    Loneliness: An Association?', *Sexual Addiction & Compulsivity*, 12(1), pp 19–44
    DOI: 10.1080/10720160590933653

BOYS BECOMING MEN

22. HOW BOYS ARE TRAVELLING AND WHAT THEY MOST NEED

Maggie Hamilton

This chapter will encourage parents, teachers and counsellors to help bring out the best in boys by helping them develop a strong sense of belonging, a powerful nuanced vision for themselves and what they can offer others.

INTRODUCTION

We all want this new generation of boys to have a strong sense of self and what they uniquely have to offer; to become well-rounded adults; and to be confident about taking their place in the world. We also want boys to fully engage with those around them – with employers and potential partners, and others.

To achieve this, boys need to know themselves, their strengths and their weaknesses, to know how best to work with what they've got, to understand and respect others, to deal effectively with complex people and situations, and to look beyond themselves and their current need for entitlement and contemplate what they can offer their community, their nation, their world.

If boys are to achieve this, they need strong narratives that support this vision. Currently most of the stories we hear are about boys who are a danger to themselves and others; about boys who have come adrift from the social fabric; boys who are vulnerable, angry, isolated, depressed, out of control. At worst these narratives suggest that boys and men are in crisis, at best they indicate there's room for improving their lives. Is it any surprise that parents, teachers and other professionals working with boys talk of the growing challenge of communicating and engaging with boys, of boys understanding their true worth?

So how are boys travelling? How do they feel about where they are at? About the future? Why the extreme behaviour? What does this tell us? What can we do about it? What most boys ache for is to experience a real sense of belonging, to be part of their tribe. And why not? Who among us wants to live on the fringes?

What, then, do we offer today's boys in terms of belonging? Almost from birth advertisers encourage boys (and/or their parents) to spend up big, to purchase the right gear, to have the right look so boys can 'belong'.[1] 'Lucky' boys grow up in rooms full of the branded toys and gear while the rest ache for these possessions because they want to belong, because belonging's an essential part of being human.

Only a few decades back, belonging was about being useful to family and community; a boy's greatest achievement was to be able to take care of himself and others; giving was more important than getting; the lives of others were of equal concern to his own. Now a boy's belonging is tied to looks and possessions, to how he packages himself. Yet there's nothing in these shallow attributes to help boys with the business of living, no developmental benefits, no opportunity to explore and expand their knowledge of themselves and their world.

It doesn't help that as a society we increasingly regard boys as flawed, as problems needing to be solved, without taking any responsibility for the ways in which we constantly disenfranchise them. Most boys ache to be heroic, to do something significant and to be acknowledged for this; possibly boys always have. In the past, boys learned how to help protect the town or village, to hunt and help grow food. Today, aside from sport, there are few opportunities for boys to be heroes, except online. With numerous video games to choose from, boys need hardly ever leave cyberspace. It is sobering to discover how many hours boys spend in such pursuits and in the toxic content they so readily immerse themselves in.[2,3] How is it we allow boys almost unlimited access to cyberspace, where they can bully, gamble, take on other identities, view live sex acts, and the worst kinds of violence, knowing there are few pointers here on how to be a real man in the real world?

Video games offer boys a degraded form of heroism. They encourage boys to hunt down and kill those who are different; to avail themselves of sexual opportunities, however casual, brief or violent; to partake in torture; to inhabit a landscape where mercy has no place. One reviewer described the Red Steel Hands-On game as offering 'plenty of chances to practice the noble art of beating the living crap out of a guy, then letting him live so you can earn Respect points and become a kinder, gentler yakuza murderer'.[4] When they're playing video games, boys get the chance to be everything they're not in real life – powerful and in charge. It's just a pity there are so few positive life skills to be gained here.

Growing up in a world awash with highly sexualised messages, visuals and narratives, and the increasing use of porn, it's hard for boys to understand what's appropriate and what's not. How do you gain a positive and life-affirming sense of your sexual self when sexting begins for some at age eight; when boys are now watching porn in groups the way they would football; when increasingly torture is an integral part of porn?[5] Our pornified culture offers boys none of the nuances needed for sustained satisfying relationships, presenting instead a world that is violent, predatory and impersonal.

What is clear is that the masculine ideal of the strong silent type, which we continue to perpetuate, is an outmoded and harmful ideal that in no way aligns with the twenty-first-century lives our boys will lead. It doesn't serve boys or men well to be silent when they need to speak up, to be strong at a time when they need to admit to being vulnerable. But still we continue to socialise our boys to keep their feelings to themselves, to be a man when they're not even sure what this means.

Noted American psychologist Dan Kindlon, who works with disenfranchised boys in the judicial system, describes this process as the 'emotional mis-education' of boys. In his compelling book *Raising*

Cain he states that the more out-of-control a boy is, the less able he is to deal with emotions and by extension, situations that challenge.[6] Child and family psychologist Michael Thompson observes that while boys are born with the same emotional potential as girls, by preschool a girl is six times more likely to use the word 'love' than a boy. And by age eight or nine, boys are already viewing life one-dimensionally, evaluating everything and everyone around them in terms of strength and weakness.[7]

The pressure on boys not to feel is huge. We do this by shaming boys from early on for daring to express their emotions. Once shamed, a boy will do everything possible not to have this happen again. When we ask boys to be silent, basically we're asking them not to express their humanity, not to feel. Whether or not boys express their feelings doesn't make their feelings go away. These feelings remain buried, creating huge frustration and anger. Years of suppressing their emotions can make it hard for boys to empathise with others, to read what's happening around them. When we deprive boys of the opportunity to develop their emotional intelligence, we diminish their capacity to engage in the world.

Boys don't know what to do with their vulnerability. Who does when they're young, when they're wrestling with a whole range of issues from peer pressure to puberty? Why is it we aren't more effective at helping them join the dots? Parents get upset at teen anger. Yet often a boy's anger isn't personal. It may not even be anger that is causing him to explode, but with limited ways in which to express himself, it may be the only way he can let you know what he desperately wants to say. Tony, twenty-six, summed it up perfectly: 'Anger is the first emotion that comes up [as a boy]. If you feel sad, the first emotion is anger. It's very rarely pure anger for young men. If you're feeling guilt or hurt or weak, then you express it with anger, because if you're angry, you're a man. It has to be aggressive anger, not latent anger, otherwise that's seen as girly.'

Boys need to learn to be comfortable with emotions, their emotions and those of others. We would do well to pay attention to Professor Janet Hyde's landmark study, which found that gender differences in the cognitive abilities and communication styles between men and women were relatively small.[8] Put simply, boys and girls share the same abilities to feel, to compute. Yet still we socialise our boys to be strong and independent, before they have had a chance to get a sense of themselves and their world, then wonder why so many suffer a profound sense of isolation.

To reimagine the role of boys, we need to look to the future, to get an understanding of what is needed in the decades ahead. Already we know the world will be more global in focus, that many boys will have a number of jobs, possibly three or four careers. They will mix with people from across the planet, and experience a level of change we can barely imagine. A future such as this needs good communicators. It needs boys who are engaged, empathetic, self-aware, who are highly adaptable, and not fazed by the challenges constant change brings.

If boys are to be equal to this new world, they will need excellent language and literacy skills. They will also need a new narrative about boys and men. A narrative that empowers, that gives boys a nuanced, detailed vision of what they can become. There's a great role for men to play in this process, by relaying to boys powerfully authentic life stories, which include admissions to moments of vulnerability, doubt and despair, and how these very real human experiences were overcome. Boys need to spend more time with men, real men, good men, for this to happen. They need a powerful sense of belonging, of honouring and being honoured, of being exposed to uplifting ideas and situations designed to bring out their greatness.

A lot has been demanded of men and boys in recent decades in terms of understanding and respecting women and girls, and boys are now growing up with a heightened sense of what is needed here. What we must guard against is neglecting to teach boys how to be aware of their own needs, and how to positively fulfil them. We also need women and girls to fully understand and respect the nuances of what it means to be a boy, a man.

A boy's vulnerabilities manifest in all kinds of ways. They too have become sensitive to messages around presentation. 'Grooming and hair styling is very important,' Angus, seventeen, says. 'It's more accepted now among guys using foundation and stuff, sometimes a bit of eyeliner and natural-coloured lipstick. A lot of guys are very vain.' While keeping up with the latest trends can be fun, it can also be stressful.

'Grooming is important for sure,' admits Toby, sixteen. 'I'm very self-conscious about my body, and the clothes I wear. I try to look the part for the occasion. Most kids do. It's mostly about looking good.' This was Rick's experience also. 'There's pressure from the media, male superstars, teen celebrities, to wear certain clothes. That's what girls are looking for, so guys dress to fit the part,' he explains.

Today boys are much more self-conscious about their bodies, now they too are exposed to endless images of the ideal male bodies in ads and on billboards, in films and magazines. For many boys it's about muscles, trim waists and fabulous abs. They want to be able to take their shirts off. 'There is a worry about body image,' said Lucas, fifteen. 'I see it around a bit, like boys getting worried about the way they look. I see them going to the gym regularly, trying to get big.'

It's only recently we have begun to focus on boys' body issues. 'For a long time we thought boys didn't have problems with body image, because we were using the wrong measures,' explains Naomi Crafti of Eating Disorders Victoria. Traditionally, research on body issues centred around weight loss. The numbers of boys wanting to bulk up tended to cancel out those focused on weight loss, so it was thought boys didn't have significant body issues.

This takes us back to how boys feel about themselves, and about a tangible sense of belonging. It's time we saw feelings as an essential part of being human, not just a female preserve. In the two major pieces of research I undertook on boys, culminating in my books *What Men Don't Talk About?* and *What's Happening To Our Boys?*, I was taken aback at the depth of a boy's feeling. If we want to understand this then we need to learn how boys communicate, how often they will reveal as much about what they don't talk about as what they do, and how their discomfort emerges around certain issues in inappropriate comments and jokes. Understanding these cues are essential to getting where boys are at.

What a difference this level of understanding would make to our boys were we able to get them to open right up. A recent study into men who had experienced non-fatal suicides revealed the extent of pain these men felt at never being able to express their emotions.[9] The men talked of the immense pressure, the fear, the ambivalence around what they were feeling, of the isolation they'd felt as teenagers, and the importance of always keeping their fears bottled up. When this pressure became too great, they chose death over disclosure.[10] Not all boys and men feel this level of despair, but too many are angry, something the teenage boys I interviewed talked of over and over. Many boys simply struggle on, but in more extreme cases they end up harming themselves or others.

There's a real argument for actively nurturing the emotional intelligence of our boys so they can recognise and manage the intensity and differing types of emotions. With the advent of the hot intelligences, boys are now able to learn to be more adept in their interactions with others.[11] Once comfortable with their own emotions then their interpersonal skills, they can begin to work on group dynamics and on what it means to be a leader, at home and at school, in their community and beyond.

For boys to be successful in this new world, we need to teach them about self-management – how to navigate this increasingly complex world with ease, by helping them differentiate between their child and emerging adult selves, by understanding how the child in them tends to react in key situations, and how their adult self might react.

Too often our boys are at sea when dealing with the nuances of everyday life. Pastoral care and other self-development programmes have a vital role to play in exploring these nuances. So boys learn, for example, that saying sorry isn't just about expressing remorse but demonstrating that their response is genuine.

Programmes that allow boys to explore the full complexity of friendship, fear and failure in detail serve them well, as do those that tackle racism, homophobia and misogyny. Given the lack of engagement we see among boys, we have to work harder at pushing through the crust of boredom that has settled over this generation, to achieve a more positive re-engagement in life. This is the perfect place to then begin to explore the countless ways to be a man in today's world.

If we're to turn this generation of boys around, we need to expose them to situations that give them a bigger vision of themselves and their world, by instituting more robust helping cultures at home and school. To achieve this we need to assist boys to let go of any sense of entitlement, this constant emphasis on 'me', because greatness is never just about 'me'. Helping must be seen as a privilege, not a chore. This means exposing boys to a wide range of experiences, from volunteering to learning about how to deal with difficult people and tricky situations, with disappointment, fear and failure, with death and other key life experiences, so that they learn how to connect powerfully with others, to make a difference in other people's lives. There is a great role for Men's Sheds here.

Vulnerability, isolation and loneliness are part of the human experience. Boys need to know it's okay to feel these emotions. What's not okay is for them to bury and deny these feelings, to be encouraged by society to ignore them. True strength is built on self-knowledge, on learning to recognise our vulnerabilities, and getting help to heal those parts of us that need bolstering in some way.

It's vitally important we raise boys whose qualities align with future needs. We need boys who know themselves; who, in understanding and respecting their own needs, are better equipped to relate to others; who are able to deal with life's challenging situations; who have solid emotional intelligence, are good communicators, and are fully and positively engaged with those around them. Put simply, it's time to push beyond the negative narratives around men and boys, this current destructive culture of entitlement, and groom our boys for greatness, for lives that will benefit themselves, their families, their communities.

The stronger a boy's foundation, the better equipped he is to participate in life's moments, both big and small. The media coverage of male violence in its many forms is a call to action, a call to embrace a bigger vision for our boys, to help birth a happier, more empowered generation of tomorrow's men.

Author biography

Writer, publisher and social researcher Maggie Hamilton gives regular talks, lectures and workshops, is a regular media commentator and a keen observer of social trends, and presents at parents' evenings, professional development forums and at conferences. Her books have been published in Australia, New Zealand, Holland, Italy, Korea, China, the Arab States, Lithuania and Brazil, and include *What Men Don't Talk About*, which examines the lives of boys and men behind the stereotypes; *What's Happening to Our Girls?*, and *What's Happening to Our Boys?* which look at the twenty-first century challenges of our girls and boys respectively; and *Secret Girls' Business*, a fun, funky, empowering gift book for girls. She has addressed over 50 000 Australian parents, and countless professional forums, adding additional dimensions to her work.

www.maggiehamilton.org

See also:

Chapter 1: Understanding Teen Sleep and Drowsy Kids
Chapter 2: Emotions and Relationships Shape the Brains of Children
Chapter 3: Understanding the Teenage Brain
Chapter 7: Problematic Internet Use and How to Manage It
Chapter 21: Porn as a Public Health Crisis
Chapter 23: Understanding and Managing Anger and Aggression

Recommended websites:

The Princes Trust: www.princes-trust.org.uk
Reach Out: www.reachoutuk.org
UK Mens Sheds Association: menssheds.org.uk

Further reading:

Biddulph, S, 2013, *Raising Boys: Why Boys Are Different, and How to Help Them Become Happy Well-Balanced Men*, Finch Books, Sydney.
Kindlon, D & Thompson M with Barker, T, 1999, *Raising Cain: Protecting the Emotional Life of Boys*, Ballantine Books, New York.
Lamb, ME (Ed), 1997, *The Role of Fathers In Child Development* (3rd ed), John Wiley and Sons, New York.
Lashlie, C, 2002, *The Journey to Prison: Who Goes and Why*, HarperCollins, Auckland.

Manocha, R (Ed), 2017, *Growing Happy, Healthy Young Minds: Generation Next*, Hachette Australia, Sydney.

Miedzian, M, 1991, *Boys Will Be Boys: Breaking the Link Between Masculinity and Violence*, Anchor, Bantam, Doubleday, New York.

Palmer, S, 2009, *21st Century Boys: How Modern Life is Driving Them Off the Rails and How We Can Get Them Back on Track*, Orion, London.

Rubenstein, A, 2013, *The Making of Men: Raising Boys to Be Happy, Healthy and Successful*, New South Books, Sydney.

Sax, L, 2007, *Boys Adrift: The Five Factors Driving the Growing Epidemic of Unmotivated Boys and Underachieving Young Men*, Basic Books, Philadelphia.

Ungar, M, 2009, *Turning the Me Generation Into the We Generation: Raising Kids That Care*, Allen & Unwin, Sydney.

23. UNDERSTANDING AND MANAGING ANGER AND AGGRESSION

Melissa Abu-Gazaleh

This chapter will highlight what parents and educators can do to support young people to understand and cope with their own feelings of anger and reduce the display of aggression.

INTRODUCTION

Anger and aggression-related problems are prevalent among young people in Australia, with one in five having trouble controlling their anger.[1] These problems can often be symptomatic of underlying mental health issues including depression and anxiety. Our role as parents, educators and mentors is to provide the guidance to enable young people to gain access and support to better manage their mental health, feelings of anger and subsequent aggressive behaviours. All young people face the risk of mishandling angry emotions and behaviours. Aggression, in its simplest form, refers to feelings of anger or antipathy resulting in hostile or violent behaviour. This behaviour can result in physical as well as emotional harm to oneself or others (this includes objects) in the environment. It can take on many different forms – physical, verbal and emotional – and has ramifications for the person involved and those close to them. It is important to note that aggression is often linked to frustration as well as anger. The type of aggression experienced by most people is 'impulsive aggression'. It is fuelled mostly by anger or frustration and is unplanned, often taking place in the heat of the moment.

According to Headspace, Australia's leading mental health service for young people, we need to debunk the myth that anger and aggression are the same thing: 'Anger is a normal feeling that we all experience, while aggression is a behavioural response that can stem from anger, or other emotions such as anxiety. Additionally, aggressive behaviour is not always a sign that someone is angry – it can stem from other strong emotions.'[2]

An important point to make is that anger, in and of itself, is a natural emotion to experience and express. It is a part of our normal mental functioning. However, when anger is experienced frequently or in an intense way that is uncontrollable, this can be problematic. This expression of frequent and intense anger often acts as a sign or symptom of deeper mental health issues, masking feelings of anxiety and depression, among others.[3]

Having worked with thousands of young people and, in particular, boys, we find that the most common emotions that boys feel uncomfortable discussing are sadness and vulnerability. This is because of the stigma around discussing any form of self-care and also how this stigma intensifies when approaching feelings of sadness, anxiety and vulnerability.

We can help young people improve their ability to cope and manage their anger in a healthy way by introducing them to practical strategies to do so. By doing this, we can help guide them to becoming healthier, more independent and happier teens and young adults.

UNDERSTANDING UNHEALTHY RELEASES OF ANGER

Young people can release anger externally by harming others, either physically or verbally, or by damaging and vandalising objects; by impatience, restlessness or difficulty taking responsibility for their angry behaviours, including blaming others for their actions.

Likewise, young people can also express anger inwardly, such as participating in self-harming activities or engaging in negative self-talk, leading them to feel powerless and in constant self-doubt, feeling anxiety and stress and, in some cases, depressive thoughts.

There are a number of warning signs that we may notice if a young person is struggling to deal with their feelings of anger. Some of these include:

- Clenching their jaws or fists.
- Pacing, sweating or physically shaking.
- Making impulsive decisions or behaviours, e.g. swearing, accusing, threats, lashing out.
- Feeling guilt or shame after an angry outburst (because they know that their response was irrational and they recognise this after the fact).

If you want to support a young person to gain a better handle on their own anger, there are a number of steps you can take to support them.

NORMALISE ANGER AS AN EMOTION

When addressing the issue of mental health with young people, the very first barrier we have as parents and educators is to help young people overcome the stigma around expressing emotions. In order to effectively address any anger and potential underlying mental health concerns, parents and educators need to be comfortable discussing emotions. By doing this we can help normalise anger as a valid emotion. Failing to do this means discussions linking our feelings to our behaviour become very difficult. In raising discussions around anger, we must also make the distinction between feeling angry (which is normal) and acting on that anger in various forms of aggression.

To begin the discussion around emotions, we need to help young people expand their understanding of what emotions are. Here are some examples of questions you can ask boys to help them tap into their emotions:

- 'When you're watching your favourite sporting team win a goal or try, how do you feel?' They'll likely say 'incredible, great, pumped up'.
- 'When you're running late for the bus and you're rushing to get there, how do you feel?' The response? Possibly 'stressed then relieved when I get to the bus on time'.
- 'How do you feel when you're having fun with your mates?' 'Awesome.'
- 'How do you feel when someone does the wrong thing by you, like they did something behind your back or they put you down?' 'I feel pissed off.'

To initiate an open and non-judgmental conversation with young people, it's important to go through this process in order for young people to identify and expand their definitions of emotions. We can help show young people how their feelings of anger, if not dealt with at the time, can progress into aggressive behaviours towards others. We often find that young people can easily self-identify issues with managing their feelings of anger or losing control of their behaviour. Often, they tell us that they feel frustrated that in the moment they don't know how to find the language or skills to deal with anger appropriately or know how to identify the triggers to avoid situations where they will feel angry.

HELP YOUNG PEOPLE UNDERSTAND THEIR TRIGGERS

The next step to helping young people change their aggressive behaviour is to deconstruct the process in which they feel and act on anger. We have found that an easy illustration is the anger cycle, a flow chart that demonstrates the typical steps of how one experiences anger. When a young person can understand how anger occurs for them, they can then begin to identify the different stages, giving them an opportunity to understand their own behaviour better and change their course of action.

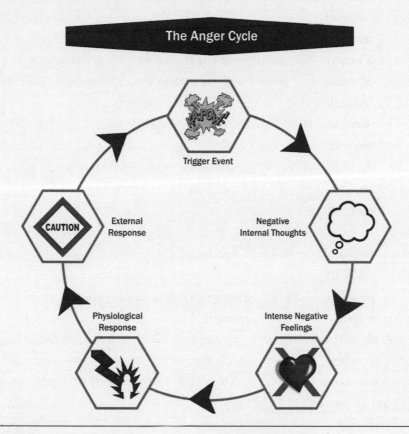

The Anger Cycle

Trigger Event

Negative Internal Thoughts

Intense Negative Feelings

Physiological Response

External Response

Trigger Event

This can be defined as an incident that 'triggers' or initiates an individual's feelings of anger.

Examples:

- Feeling rejected
- Having a bad time at school or work
- Lack of understanding or empathy from friends or family

Negative Internal Thoughts

Following a trigger event that elicits a response of anger, a person may experience negative thoughts about themselves or others.

Examples:

- 'I am a bad friend.'
- 'My parents are really mean.'
- 'The teacher is being unfair.'

Intense Negative Feelings

Negative thoughts can lead to negative emotions. These thoughts can be irrational and the individual may fixate on the trigger event.

Examples:

- Resentment towards friends and others
- Irritation towards a teacher or boss
- Feeling guilty about being a bad friend

Physiological Response

When experiencing feelings of anger there is a physiological response in which the body reacts physically to the trigger event.

- Accelerated heartbeat
- Tensing of muscles
- Perspiration
- Agitation/Trembling

External Response

The external response culminates in a form of behaviour, influenced by the individual's thoughts, feelings and physiological response.

- Raised voice
- Confrontation and Arguing
- Physical Contact or Fighting
- Passive Aggression

The chart on the previous page illustrates the way in which anger not only escalates, but can form a cycle when these feelings of anger remain unaddressed. Feelings of anger can have a build-up effect, meaning that bottling things up can end with getting angry at something small or a person for no reason at all. However, it doesn't need to be this way.

The most effective way to have a young person give this anger cycle some consideration is to try to explain the concept to them, but if they're not showing interest, simply print it off and leave it lying around the house or, if you're a teacher, print and stick it up on the wall in your classroom. Sometimes, the most effective way to deliver a message isn't by explaining it, it's letting the young person discover the information for themselves.

ROLE MODEL POSITIVE ANGER MANAGEMENT

Parents and teachers play a pivotal role in not only showing young people positive ways of managing anger by implementing these strategies themselves, but also showing them that they are open to talking to them about issues troubling them.

Research has shown that how parents manage their own conflict can have a powerful impact on a child. If parents are having a disagreement and they yell, make threats, call each other names or are otherwise aggressive or even violent, they are sending a message to their children that this is how disagreements are managed. If parents instead use good communication skills, if they can demonstrate that they are in control of their emotions and can work towards solving problems and resolving conflict, they are giving their children a much better example to follow.[4]

It is important for parents to think about the type of message they are sending their children. Think about the way you choose to de-stress after a hard day at work. Do you exercise, talk about your day with your partner or listen to music? Or do you use unhealthy means like alcohol to deal with your own anger and stress? Self-reflection is important, as children adopt your behaviour. Children can also learn aggression through the examples of others. When the adults responsible for children's care get angry quickly and often, or when they use reactive, harsh and inconsistent discipline, children are more likely to behave aggressively themselves.[5]

> When we work with boys, you can't go at them with this real kindness, humane stuff. If you try to tell them: 'Well actually, boys, we should all be sensitive image guys and hug each other when we feel sad and talk about our feelings', they'll basically walk outside the room. You can't shift it that much in a short period of time, but what you need to be able to say is that, isn't it bullshit that girls can talk about their feelings and we can't?
>
> Top Blokes Foundation Youth Worker

For parents in particular, help children understand how mismanaged feelings can turn into unhealthy behaviours. Demonstrating this requires modelling consistent behavioural responses. For example, these can include counting to ten before responding if you are angry or upset, using positive expressions in a constructive way and, most importantly, provide positive outlets for emotional release by showing your child that it's okay to admit when we feel lousy and that there are positive ways to deal with these emotions. However, it is not always possible for parents to be the one to whom a child turns to discuss issues of mental health. If you find yourself in this situation, encourage your child to talk to a person they feel comfortable talking to.

Something to try: share a time when you felt angry, or even depressed. What did you do to make yourself feel better? Or, if in hindsight you didn't handle it well, what lessons did you learn that you can communicate with your young person?

WHEN YOU CHOOSE THE BEHAVIOUR, YOU CHOOSE THE CONSEQUENCE

When conducting social education for boys that talks about emotions, the first step we take is normalising all emotions, from sadness to depression to anger and happiness. But there needs to be an important distinction that while it's normal to feel angry, we choose if we want to act on the anger. These are two very different processes. Recently, while working with a group of fifteen-year-old boys at a school, we asked them why street violence and one-punch attacks were so prevalent. One boy asked, 'But what if he didn't mean to kill the person, it just happens sometimes?' We thanked him for his comment and then told the group that while the consequences of actions as a result of feeling angry might be accidental, the person did in fact make a choice to act on his anger, and with that choice comes the responsibility of potential outcomes. It's important to help young people understand that while they may not choose to feel angry, they do choose what they do with that anger.

INTRODUCE THE EIGHT-SECOND RULE

Feelings of anger can lead to impulsive and irrational behaviours, which in a moment of anger can fatally hurt someone. At the Top Blokes Foundation, we encourage young men to enact the eight-second rule – to give themselves eight seconds of breathing time before acting on any behaviours. This serves two important roles: it will provide time needed to delay and distract from the anger-arousing event and, combined with deep breathing, counteracts the fight-or-flight reaction that sometimes underlies anger.

CLARIFY THE DIFFERENCE BETWEEN AGGRESSIVE, PASSIVE AND ASSERTIVE COMMUNICATION

As adults, we often can find ourselves struggling to show assertive communication when in high-conflict situations. If we naturally revert to passive behaviours when dealing with conflict, why do we expect young people to know how to use assertive communication?

Here's a simple way to explain the difference to a young person:

Aggressive – Harsh in words and tone, intimidating, interrupts, patronising, sarcastic, critical, disrespectful, talks over others, doesn't listen to others.

Passive – Talks very little, always agrees with someone even if inside they disagree, avoids telling others how they really feel, puts self down, submissive, always compliant.

Assertive – Will voice opinion in a respectful and mature manner, will tell others how they feel, be firm but polite, respectful towards others, accepts that others will have their own opinions, will stand up for themselves or views without hurting others, will communicate if they are feeling used or taken advantage of.

Help improve their assertive communication when in high-fuelled angry situations. For example, we often role-play a scenario with young men in our Junior Top Blokes Mentoring Programme. We ask boys: 'You're in class and you say "duck" to your friend, but your teacher turns around and accuses you of saying the F word. How do you react?' Most participants will say that they will argue with the teacher, which can land them in additional trouble. So how do we help students to use assertive language when they can traditionally use aggressive language? We help them devise responses that will be effective, e.g., 'Sir, do you mind if we talk about this after class or at break? I would like to explain my side of the story and not take up class time.' Instantly, we see boys' eyes light up, because they've realised that using this form of assertive communication will give them a new sense of respect and self-control, and ultimately a better outcome with the teacher. To reinforce how much more effective this is instead of their usual communication style, we also invite teachers into the workshop and ask how they would react if a boy used assertive communication in a classroom environment. Teachers always respond positively, with one commenting, 'I would really respect and admire their maturity and would be more than happy to address this with them.' We have heard that boys who have a reputation for being angry use this line of language in similar situations with better outcomes.

Useful apps and online resources

At the Top Blokes Foundation, our team of youth workers has tested the following apps and websites and recommend them to young people. If you are wanting to suggest a certain app, download and try them before suggesting to a young person.

Anger Management Techniques and Tips App: This app provides different training and learning styles to suit the user. It includes the top 21 anger management tips, a full version of the Anger Management Wiki, including anger management test guide, quotes about anger, suggested music to assist in relaxation and stress management.

Anger Management: Designed to help the user identify what anger is, why they are experiencing the emotion in the first place and what can be done to control it. Also discusses how substance abuse can affect anger problems.

Breathe2Relax: A portable stress management tool designed to teach diaphragmatic breathing, sometimes called 'belly breathing'. This technique is used as a way of turning on the body's relaxation response.

The Mental Stillness App: A free app that has a variety of meditation programs for all ages. Benefits include reducing distress, anxiety and worries. Helps regulate emotions, develop a sense of empathy and connectedness.

Headspace: A UK-based app that is used by young people and adults internationally. It encourages users to meditate for ten minutes a day and can assist with anger, stress and improving relationships.

MoodGym: A free interactive self-help program that provides cognitive behaviour therapy (CBT) training to help users prevent and cope with depression and anxiety.

PRACTICAL TIPS FOR TEACHERS – A GUIDE

- Ask your student what their triggers are. For example, bullying by certain peers, difficulty with certain teachers, or their academic performance. Knowing this can help identify the problem and create a solution.

- Have an agreed time-out strategy or safe zones to calm down. We find a popular one for boys is to sit outside the classroom for ten minutes. Let the young person create the strategy with your support and take control of their own emotional management.
- Jointly, develop an anger management plan. Look at varying strategies to help your student cope and ensure that all relevant teachers are aware and agree to follow the plan.
- Ask the student to nominate a safe and trusted teacher for them to talk to (don't always assume it's the school counsellor). If the teacher is agreeable, ensure the teacher can set boundaries on the relationship so that they do not feel burdened.
- Encourage them to develop a music playlist to listen to when trying to calm themselves. Encourage them to listen to the music during their time-out, jog around the playground or, in the worst cases, at the back of the classroom during class time.

PRACTICAL TIPS FOR PARENTS – A GUIDE

- Agree on approved ways to express angry feelings. For example, to go for a walk or run around the block, listen to music or remove themselves from the situation.
- Support them to achieve a routine sleeping pattern. Provide incentives for reducing their screen-time before they go to bed.
- Encourage physical activity by increasing the amount of sport or outdoor activities that they do. This will not only improve their mood, but a new social setting can increase their chance of building positive peer networks.
- Agree on a trusted relative or family friend that your child can call when feeling angry or upset. If this is a useful strategy, be mindful to not intrude on their conversation (particularly if your child is a teenager, they will want independence from you). Trust that your relative or family friend will inform you if there is something serious to be aware of.

- Reflect on how you display anger. Role model positive ways to display anger. If you find yourself in screaming matches with your child or that you cope with your own angry feelings with alcohol or other unhealthy outlets, consider that this isn't demonstrating positive behaviours for your child.

WHAT CAN YOU, AS A TEACHER OR PARENT, DO WHEN A YOUNG PERSON IS EXHIBITING ANGRY OR AGGRESSIVE BEHAVIOURS?

- **Stay calm. Be conscious of your tone.** Are you using assertive communication to communicate that their behaviour is inappropriate?
- **State and reinforce the boundaries.** Each parent and teacher will have their own boundaries – set yours and stick to them. For some people, they might say that the police will be called in any circumstance when a young person threatens to hurt themselves or somebody else. For others, this may seem too extreme, but think what you are willing to accept and not accept, and the consequences for each. Communicate this in an assertive and clear manner.
- **Look past the angry behaviour and try to get to the root cause of the problem.** Instead of responding to their angry outburst (which can be hard in the moment), try to understand what they are really hurt about and name it. Helping them to understand the true triggers can help both of you to have an honest and authentic conversation.
- **De-escalate the situation.** If talking with them directly isn't helping, remove yourself from the situation – walk away or ask them to walk away. Giving them space can reduce the immediate angry feelings and help them move to a mood where their anger is under control.
- **Look after your own wellbeing.** If your young person's anger is an ongoing issue, it could have a toll on your family or classroom. While this isn't something that can be

solved overnight, it's important to not let the issue wear you down.

- **Safety plan.** Have a formal plan for what steps to take to keep yourself and others safe. This may be physically leaving the situation, having the young person displaying violent behaviours be removed from the situation or seeking professional intervention (e.g. calling police). Deciding on a safety plan when in a state of calm is more effective as you can think clearer.

- **Help them set goals on managing their anger.** It may be introducing different coping techniques, for example, trying mindfulness techniques for five minutes a day for a week.

ENGAGING PROFESSIONAL SERVICES

If you find that after a considerable amount of time the techniques suggested above are ineffective, and your young person is still displaying severe anger or aggressive behaviours, it may be time to seek external support. The following are starting points. Make an enquiry yourself, and if they're in a position to do so, encourage the young person to seek assistance themselves (if they are at an appropriate age).

We recommend the following:

- **Local GP:** Seeing a GP builds a young person's independence and ability to be proactive about their health. A GP can help a young person build a mental health care plan.

- **Mind** (www.mind.org.uk) is a mental health charity that provides advice and support on a wide range of mental health problems. To learn how to deal with anger in a constructive and healthy way, see www.mind.org.uk/information-sunport/types-of-mental-health-problems/anger. This is also useful for anyone with a friend or family member who has problems with anger.

- **Family Lives** (www.familylives.org.UK) is a charity that supports parents and carers in achieving the best possible relationship with the children they care for. They deal with a range of problems, including teenage aggression at home. (www.familylives.org.uk/advice/teenagers/behaviour/teen-violence-at-home).
- **Childline** (www.childline.org.uk) operates a twenty-four-hour confidential telephone and online counselling service for anyone under the age of nineteen in the UK. Helpline: 0800 1111.**School counsellor:** Young people are usually aware their school has a counsellor. Encourage them to book an appointment (or ask a trusted friend to). Remind the young person that school counsellors are bound by privacy and confidentiality laws.
- **Local youth centres:** Most regions will have a local youth centre that might have specific programmes that deal with young people's anger issues, mental health issues or improve overall wellbeing. These may be mentoring programmes, sports programmes or counselling programmes. Utilising these services can support your young person in conjunction with any other services that they are using.

While it may seem difficult to support a person with anger issues, there are a number of services and online support well regarded by young people. As their role model and guide, you are in a prime position to assist a young person to understand and improve their relationship with their own emotions and subsequent actions. Be persistent and in time they will come to realise that your support was important.

Author biography

Melissa Abu-Gazaleh is the 2016 New South Wales Young Australian of the Year and CEO of the Top Blokes Foundation, a boys' mental health and wellbeing organisation that has delivered social education programmes to over 10000 young men across Australia.

www.topblokes.org.au

www.melissaabugazaleh.com

See also:

Chapter 1: Understanding Teen Sleep and Drowsy Kids

Chapter 2: Emotions and Relationships Shape the Brains of Children

Chapter 3: Understanding the Teenage Brain

Chapter 7: Problematic Internet Use and How to Manage It

Chapter 21: Porn as a Public Health Crisis

Chapter 22: How Boys are Travelling and What They Most Need

Chapter 24: Understanding Boys' Health Needs

Further reading:

Abblett, M & Willard, C, 2017, *Helping Your Angry Teen*, New Harbinger Publications, Oakland.

Bowden, T & Bowden, S, 2013, *I Just Get So...Angry! Dealing with Anger and Other Strong Emotions for Teenagers*, Exisle Publishing, Wollombi.

Gilgun, J, 'Lemons or Lemonade? An Anger Workbook for Teens', www.cehd.umn.edu/ssw/Documents/GilgunPDFs/Lemons-Lemonade-Teens.pdf

Golden, B, 2006, *Healthy Anger: How to Help Children and Teens Manage Their Anger*, Oxford University Press.

Hariton, J, 'What's Normal and What's Not? Adolescents and Anger', www.human.cornell.edu/pam/outreach/parenting/upload/Adolescents-and-Anger-Jo-Hariton.pdf

Kaufman, M, 'The Seven P's of Men's Violence', ecbiz194.inmotionhosting.com/~micha383/wp-content/uploads/2013/03/Kaufman-7-Ps-of-Mens-Violence.pdf

Manocha, R (Ed), 2017, *Growing Happy, Healthy Young Minds: Generation Next*, Hachette Australia, Sydney.

Purcell, M & Murphy, J, 2014, *Mindfulness for Teen Anger: A Workbook to Overcome Anger and Aggression*, New Harbinger Publications, Oakland.

Sells, S, 2002, *Parenting Your Out-of-Control Teenager: 7 Steps to Reestablish Authority and Reclaim Love*, St Martin's Griffin, New York.

Shriver, M, 'Life Ed: Helping Teen Sons Deal with Anger', www.nbcnews.com/feature/maria-shriver/life-ed-helping-teen-sons-deal-anger-n166596

Van Dijk, S, 2011, *Don't Let Your Emotions Run Your Life for Teens*, New Harbinger Publications, Oakland.

For more online resources visit:
generationnext.com.au/handbook

24. UNDERSTANDING BOYS' HEALTH NEEDS

Melissa Abu-Gazaleh

This chapter will examine how social and cultural circumstances impact young men's mental health and wellbeing.

INTRODUCTION

You cannot be blamed if you have tried but faced difficulty in helping boys grow into good men. Our fast-changing youth culture, propelled by evolving technology, presents a number of new challenges when helping boys develop strong values and positive attitudes on issues that will affect them. Factors relating to peer pressure, risk-taking, violence, alcohol and understanding mental health have changed over generations; however, as educators, parents and concerned community members, we are well placed to help boys question and think critically about the social issues and temptations around them. To understand the complexity of young men's health in Australia today, we need to apply macro and micro lenses to the specific issues that affect their sense of identity and worth, and how these are shaped by external influences. Now, more than ever, there is an increased focus on young men's health by researchers and practitioners. This is a positive trend and while physical components of health are equally important to understand, here we will focus on mental, social and emotional aspects of young men's health.

Young men's mental health is perhaps one of the most critical issues that our communities face. On a broader level, 75 per cent of mental health problems emerge before the age of twenty-five[1] and untreated mental illness in young men costs the Australian economy $387 000 per hour in lost productivity (totalling three billion dollars annually).[2] Suicide accounts for 24 per cent of deaths of Australian young men, making it the number one cause of premature death among this group, and when compared to women, men are also three times more likely to die by suicide. In 2014, 2160 men took their own lives, or approximately six per day.[3] There are a number of sub-groups of young males who face additional challenges; for young men from a culturally diverse background, mental health issues are compounded by experiences of racism and other forms of discrimination. In one report, 80 per cent of young people from a CALD (Culturally and Linguistically Diverse) background report experiencing racial discrimination and 20 per cent have been on the receiving end of racist hate speech.[4] For young people who identify as part of the LGBTIQ (Lesbian, Gay, Bisexual, Transgender, Intersex and Questioning) community, up to 80 per cent experience public insult, with 80 per cent of this abuse occurring at school; 50 per cent of young people who identify as trans report considering suicide, and up to 24 per cent of transgendered young people experience major depressive episodes, compared to 6.8 per cent of the general population.[5]

It's not hard for us to picture at least one young man we know who has at some point struggled with their own mental health. These statistics highlight that addressing young men's mental health isn't simple or quick, particularly as they are less likely to access support services than their female peers. Despite a growing number of purposefully designed programmes and services to support the mental health of young people, underrepresentation of young males perhaps stems from wider social and cultural drivers, including how young men perceive their own sense of masculinity.

ROLE OF MASCULINITY IN UNDERSTANDING YOUNG MEN'S MENTAL HEALTH

This ideal of the Australian male begins very early in childhood. Typically, both boys and girls are exposed to messages that often feminise emotions and masculinise violent acts. In boys, this can stunt their empathy and emotional expression, enhance dominance and reinforce links between respect and fear.[6] For example, boys are encouraged not to cry, taught to mask their emotions (as emotions are traditionally seen as a weakness) and are therefore socialised not to ask for help (as this is also perceived as a sign of weakness and vulnerability). These ideals translate later in life to stereotypes like the 'Indestructible Aussie Male' or 'Aussie Battler' – men who are encouraged to conceal their true emotions and deal with problems on their own. This idea of men as 'invulnerable' or 'indestructible' perpetuates the unhealthy relationship between young men and their mental health and emotional self-care. These traditional notions of masculinity – a term referring to the behaviours, qualities and characteristics that are traditionally associated with men – feed into societal issues, as well as impacting the way men and boys understand the importance of mental health. In particular, this stereotype is harmful to male mental health, making it 'difficult for males to make healthy choices and to access the health care and information necessary to achieve optimal health'.[7]

HOW THE FAMILY HOUSEHOLD AFFECTS A BOY'S VIEW OF HIMSELF

If we think about the social and cultural drivers, masculine behaviours are shaped by a number of external influencers including the entertainment industry, media, corporate institutions and the traditionally held beliefs by parents and those directly involved in raising boys into young men. Masculinity, just like femininity, is taught at a young age and boys are socialised to act in a certain (socially constructed) way, which shapes their attitudes and behaviours towards themselves and others. For example, boys are encouraged to wear blue, to engage in rough-and-tumble play and are often given toys considered more masculine (trucks and train sets). The role of socialising boys into traditional ideas of masculinity is often perpetuated within Australian homes. Comments including 'pink is a girl's colour', 'be a big boy and don't cry', 'you throw like a girl' and 'you're such a mummy's boy' are often throwaway comments that people make, which over the years shape how a male adapts his behaviour and emotions to fit within a certain mould. The above comments paint a picture of a type of masculinity that does not leave room for boys to become their authentic self. These comments, however seemingly harmless, do make a difference in how boys and young men come to understand their own masculinity and identity.

THE INDESTRUCTIBLE MALE STEREOTYPE

Over time, a number of unhealthy representations of masculinity have emerged. For example, the 'indestructible male' – that is, the belief that males are immune to illness or defeat – can promote unhealthy risk-taking and reduce levels of self-care, making it difficult for young men to engage with taking care of their mental health or make sensible decisions to improve their general wellbeing. You may have seen similar stereotypes to the indestructible male perpetuated in our culture. Some sociologists refer to this as toxic masculinity. These terms relate to how boys and men are portrayed, perceived and socialised in ways that are unhealthy or harmful to either themselves or others, for example, encouraged to be violent, emotionless or even sexually aggressive.[8] One aspect of toxic masculinity is a belief that dominance is achieved through use of violence. For Australia, youth crime rates show that four out of five young people in the juvenile justice system are male and 80 per cent of youth justice supervision is of fourteen- to seventeen-year-olds.[9] Along with this, 46 per cent of young men take part in physical fights[10] and physical assaults cost the Australian community $1.4 billion a year.[11] Street violence has seen 99 per cent of one-punch attacks committed by men with 96 per cent of victims being male. Out of these, 49 per cent of those attacked were aged between eighteen and twenty-three years old.[12] These figures prompted some Australian states to enforce measures to curb street and alcohol-fuelled violence, including changes to drinks and nightlife entertainment licences.[13] Looking at the role that alcohol plays in this, research highlights that in New South Wales, the rate of hospitalisations from injury due to alcohol-related violence in fifteen- to twenty-four-year-old males was around four times that of females in the same age group.[14] Despite Australia having strong violence prevention and alcohol and drug education both in schools and community settings, we all have a role in helping young men understand how to replace unhealthy ideas of what it means to be masculine with positive behaviours.

RESHAPING THE 'INDESTRUCTIBLE MALE' STEREOTYPE

To be able to shift the perception of men being indestructible, we must look to and understand how key influencers within a young man's life can help reshape what healthy masculinity is. From role models within their peer groups, in the family and community, each has a place in helping young men understand acceptable and unacceptable behaviours.

This forms part of the larger belief in the standards that men are held to. However, if a young man moves away from these behaviours – that is, displays alternative behaviours that don't align with how men are 'supposed' to behave – it heightens the risk of him being criticised and ostracised by their peers. Do you recall instances where boys were called names (for example, 'sissy') or put down by their peers or adults if they didn't appear masculine? This form of social policing is used by both young people and adults in an attempt to regulate a boy's behaviour towards the more masculine. For some boys and young men, this can impact their sense of identity and self-worth and, therefore, their mental health and wellbeing. With alarming statistics around mental health and high suicide rates, it is vital that this perception of Australian masculinity shifts to be more inclusive and accepting of all types of males.

IMPACT OF THE INTERNET: SOCIAL MEDIA AND ONLINE RISKS

The job of raising young men has changed post-internet. Today, boys and young men are a part of the post-PC generation, that is, they are no longer confined to accessing the internet on the one household desktop computer that is fitted with safety features. Nowadays Australian teens own, on average, not one but two portable devices with internet access. This has opened the way for a number of new risks to emerge, including a rise in social anxiety, cyberbullying, inappropriate sexting and accessing online pornography. Similar to conversations you may have with boys and young men about bullying in general, it is also important for them to know about cyberbullying and that they can come to you about these concerns.

Cyberbullying, similar to physical bullying, has negative physical, psychological and social effects, including feelings of fear, loneliness, anxiety, insecurity, depression and academic lethargy.[15] As adults, we all try to keep up with the latest social media platforms, but bullying can occur across any of them, from mobile phone messaging to Facebook, Snapchat, Instagram, Twitter and even through multiplayer video games. While it is becoming increasingly difficult to police young men's devices, a more effective approach is to communicate the risks of online behaviours (such as sexting) and help young men develop strategies to identify and handle these online incidences.

INFLUENCE OF ONLINE PORNOGRAPHY

Pornography use by young males must form part of any conversation about young men's mental health. Today, an Australian boy's first time of viewing porn is at eleven years old. Young males aged twelve to seventeen years old are the fastest-growing users of unlimited and free pornography.[16] Therefore, by the time boys sit through their first sex education class at school, there is a high probability that they have already viewed unhealthy sexually explicit material online. While we know that acts of masturbation are normal, healthy and can even reduce stress and anxiety temporarily, consuming high levels of online pornography can have negative effects on young men's physical health, mental health including self-esteem, confidence and their personal relationships.[17]

A growing body of research is highlighting how young men under the age of twenty-four are reporting symptoms that mimic erectile health issues.[18] Research is also finding that high levels of porn viewing alters a young person's brain.[19] Repeated exposure to heightened sexual stimuli, particularly violent and extreme pornography, increases a boy's dopamine levels, causing him to become aroused. Yet, over time, he builds a tolerance to the dopamine, prompting him to consume more extreme porn, more often, to achieve the same level of arousal. And this can become an issue when he begins forming real-life sexual relationships. This relates not only to whether these boys can provide pleasure to their real-life partner (given that porn scenes are highly manipulated, manufactured and unrealistic), but also the fact that 88 per cent of porn scenes contain acts of physical violence or aggression towards women.[20]

This means that we should educate boys on how their consumption of porn is affecting their bodies and their personal relationships. The education needs to be similar to how we, as adults, expect to be informed about the products we buy and consume. As educators, we need to inform boys about how porn is manipulated, manufactured and marketed with unhealthy and unrealistic representations of sex and sexual relationships.

HOW UNHEALTHY SEXUAL PRACTICES ARE AFFECTING YOUNG MEN'S HEALTH

Research reveals that only 43 per cent of young males always wear a condom during sex, with the two most common excuses for young people not wearing a condom being: 'I didn't want them to think I was "dirty"', and 'I didn't have one'.[21] These statistics highlight the urgent need for adults to dispel the myths associated with safe-sex practices. With one in twenty young people aged fifteen to twenty-four reported to have chlamydia,[22] teenage males are often the silent carrier, and gonorrhoea has increased by 76 per cent in teen males between 2008 and 2012.[23] With the ever increasing accessibility of the internet, mobile devices and the growing trends of hook-up cultures and sexting, young people's sexual education is being increasingly influenced by negative external sources. Sexual education is a necessary part of the development of all young people and all formal education in sex should be continually reviewed and updated to include the latest trends and emerging issues facing young men's sexual health. This also includes having consensual sexual experiences. In light of the changing cultural perception around sex and the influence of pornography, young men can be unsure of how to gain sexual consent in this evolving environment. It is imperative that we educate young people what each of these looks like and how this contributes to overall consent. This becomes even more important in lieu of statistics about porn consumption and the often non-consensual and sometimes rape-like scenes included in such content. While common messages in formal sex education promote the 'no means no' message, the Top Blokes Foundation has seen significant success in educating young men about consent and has found that these discussions don't have to be complicated. They have a simple message: teach young men that gaining consent means asking and getting a yes without pressure or coercion (and making sure that their partner is sober), not simply having their partner not say no.

A MORE INCLUSIVE UNDERSTANDING OF GENDER AND SEXUALITY

Intertwined with conversations around masculinity and stereotypes is our understanding of gender, sex and sexual orientation. One's gender identity and sexual orientation are no more a choice for the individual than their sex, and this is backed up by a growing body of research.[24] These concepts can often be difficult to grasp, particularly for those of us who have never spent much time considering our own. As mentioned earlier, there are social repercussions if boys don't align with heteronormative definitions of masculinity: they are bullied and called names such as 'faggot', 'gay' and 'pussy'. This kind of bullying reduces self-esteem and confidence, and can isolate them from their friends and peer groups. However, as educators and parents who play a key role in young people's developing of their identity and sense of self-worth, it's critical that we recognise how traditional understandings of gender can negatively impact on student wellbeing, particularly that of males. We need to help boys redefine a healthy sense of masculinity, one that helps boys be individuals, themselves and free to express their identity and personality. This includes parts of their identity such as gender and sexual orientation, as heteronormative masculinity also perpetuates binary understandings of gender and sex (for example, you are either a boy or a girl, straight or gay).

Despite your personal beliefs about gender, sex and sexuality, growing bodies of research are revealing how young people who identify as transgendered experience significantly higher rates of poor mental health and various forms of discrimination (see above). It's important to consider how we can put aside our personal bias to build an inclusive classroom, home or community environment that will improve a young person's wellbeing and overall achievement. Simple changes such as removing assumptions and altering language will give young people permission to build genuine identities and see them move more easily towards a happy and purposeful future.

OUR ROLE IN HELPING BOYS GROW INTO HEALTHY ADULT MEN

Despite all that is mentioned above, the future of boys and young men is bright. More than ever before, we have well-designed services and programmes to help young men develop the necessary tools and skills to help navigate life's challenges. Already, research indicates that traditional ideas of masculinity, like the 'indestructible male', are being challenged by young men and boys. Research shows that boys value being emotionally articulate, thoughtful and insightful when given the chance.[25] This reveals how fixed ideas of masculinity often contradict how young men and boys would like to be in reality, without the pressure of harmful, toxic and often unrealistic stereotypes.

If you are in a position where the young men in your life aren't approaching you to have these important conversations, remember to be patient as they may not want to talk to you at this time. It may well be that your role is to help build young men's support networks, made up of positive role models, friends, family members and mentors. In your conversations you will be sure to find that young men share a common hope: that their parents, teachers and mentors will give them the time of day to make their own independent (and sometimes regrettable) decisions, but will be ready to guide them back on track when things get chaotic.

When developing solutions to some of the social problems we discussed, we should involve those who are in the thick of it: boys and young men. They hold the information and insights into what can be changed from the inside. When we turn our ears towards boys and provide a safe and non-judgemental environment for them to express their opinions and experiences, we'll be pleasantly surprised with the contributions they can make. Consider how you can provide opportunities for young men to help solve some of these social issues on a local level. Help turn them into advocates and change-makers. Give them alternative ways to combat pressures around violence and alcohol consumption. Promote mental health and freedom of expression. Give them the right skills to understand their mental health and wellbeing. This may include us challenging our own biases and values as their parents, educators and mentors. In doing this, we can help build a healthy culture where young men can confidently navigate any negative social pressures without compromising their health or those around them.

Author biography

Melissa Abu-Gazaleh is the 2016 New South Wales Young Australian of the Year and CEO of the Top Blokes Foundation, a boys' mental health and wellbeing organisation that has delivered social education programmes to over 10 000 young men across Australia.

www.topblokes.org.au

www.melissaabugazaleh.com

See also:

Chapter 1: Understanding Teen Sleep and Drowsy Kids
Chapter 2: Emotions and Relationships Shape the Brains of Children
Chapter 3: Understanding the Teenage Brain
Chapter 7: Problematic Internet Use and How to Manage It
Chapter 21: Porn as a Public Health Crisis
Chapter 22: How Boys are Travelling and What They Most Need
Chapter 23: Understanding and Managing Anger and Aggression

Podcasts:

ABC Local: *Triple P Parenting*
Armin Brott: *Positive Parenting from MrDad.com*
Hyde School: *Parenting Teens: The Biggest Job We'll Ever Have*
Raising Children Network and 3RRR: *Talking Parenting*

Recommended websites:

NHS: www.nhs.uk/livewell/teenboys
Men's Health Forum: www.menshealthforum.org.uk
XY online: www.xyonline.net
Bullying UK: www.bullying.co.uk
UK Safer Internet Centre: www.saferinternet.org.uk
NHS: www.nhs.uk/livewell/youth-mental-health
Brook: www.brook.org.uk/your-life/consent

Further reading:

Carr-Gregg, M, 2010, *When to Really Worry*, Penguin, Melbourne.
Carr-Gregg, M, 2014, *Beyond Cyberbullying*, Penguin, Melbourne.
Faber, A & Mazlish, E, 2006, *How to Talk So Teens Will Listen and Listen So Teens Will Talk*, William Morrow, New York.
Hawkes, T, 2014, *Ten Conversations You Must Have with Your Son*, Hachette Australia, Sydney.
Lashlie, C, 2010, *He'll Be OK: Growing Gorgeous Boys Into Good Men*, HarperCollins, Pymble.
Manocha, R (Ed), 2017, *Growing Happy, Healthy Young Minds: Generation Next*, Hachette Australia, Sydney.

Meeker, M, 2015, *Strong Mothers, Strong Sons*, Ballantine Books, New York.

Schab, L, 2008, *Beyond the Blues: A Workbook to Help Teens Overcome Depression*, New Harbinger Publications, Oakland.

Schab, L, 2008, *The Anxiety Workbook for Teens: Activities to Help You Deal with Anxiety and Worry*, New Harbinger Publications, Oakland.

Toner, J & Freeland, C, 2016, *Depression: A Teen's Guide to Survive and Thrive*, Magination Press.

Wiseman, R, 2014, *Masterminds and Wingmen: Helping Our Boys Cope with Schoolyard Power, Locker-Room Tests, Girlfriends, and the New Rules of Boy World*, Harmony.

Zimbardo, P & Coulombe, N, 2016, *Man, Interrupted: Why Young Men are Struggling & What We Can Do About It*, Conari Press.

We also recommend the very popular companion volume **GROWING HAPPY, HEALTHY YOUNG MINDS** – resilience, bullying, depression, anxiety, body image and many more important issues.

For more online resources visit:
generationnext.com.au/handbook

ENDNOTES

1. Understanding Teen Sleep and Drowsy Kids

1. Blunden, S, Lushington, K, Lorenzen, B, Ooi, T, Fung F and Kennedy, D, 2004, 'Are Sleep Problems Under Recognised in General Practice?', *Archive of Disease in Childhood* 89 (8), pp 708-12.
2. Danner, F and Phillips, B, 2008, 'Adolescent Sleep, School Start Times, and Teen Motor Vehicle Crashes', *Journal of Clinical Sleep Medicine*, 4(6), pp 533-37.
3. 'Zurich Longitudinal Study', *Paediatrics* 3(2), 2003.
4. Tassi, P and Muzet, A, 2000, 'Sleep Inertia', *Sleep Medicine Reviews* 4(4), pp 341–353.

5. Healthy Habits for a Digital Life

1. 'Australia's Physical Activity and Sedentary Behaviour Guidelines', The Department of Health, www.health.gov.au/internet/main/publishing.nsf/content/health-pubhlth-strateg-phys-act-guidelines (accessed: 25 June 2017)
2. 'Media and Children Communication Toolkit', American Academy of Pediatrics, www.aap.org/en-us/advocacy-and-policy/aap-health-initiatives/pages/media-and-children.aspx (accessed: 25 June 2017)

6. Online Time Management

1. 'Parents, teens, and digital monitoring', 2016, www.pewinternet.org
2. 'Aussie teens and kids online', ACMA, 2016, www.acma.gov.au/theacma/engage-blogs/research-snapshots/aussie-teens-and-kids-online
3. 'Parents, teens, and digital monitoring', 2016, www.pewinternet.org
4. 'Teens and Sleep', National Sleep Foundation, 2016, www.sleepfoundation.org/sleep-topics/teens-and-sleep

7. Problematic Internet Use and How to Manage It

1. Young, K & De Abreu, C, (Eds), 2010, *Internet Addiction: A Handbook and Guide to Evaluation and Treatment*, John Wiley & Sons, New York.
2. Grusser, SM, Thalemann, R & Griffiths, MD, 2007, 'Excessive computer game playing: evidence for addiction and aggression?' *Cyberpsychology and Behaviour* 10(2), pp 290–292.
3. Tam, P & Walter G, 2013, 'Problematic Internet Use in Childhood and Youth: Evolution of a 21st Century Affliction', *Australasian Psychiatry* 21, pp 533–536.

9. Sexting – Realities and Risks

1. Marwick, A, 2013, *Status Update: Celebrity, Publicity, and Branding in the Social Media Age*, Yale University Press, Connecticut, USA

2. boyd, d, 2014, *It's Complicated: The Social Lives of Networked Teens*, Yale University Press, Connecticut, USA

11. The 'Gamblification' of Computer Games

1. Delfabbro, P, Derevensky, JL & Gainsbury, S, 2011, 'Prevalance of Youth Gambling and Problem Gambling' in *Health, Medicine and Human Development: Youth Gambling: The Hidden Addiction.*

2. Shokrizade, R, 2013, 'The Top F2P Monetization tricks', retrieved from: www.gamasutra.com/blogs/RaminShokrizade/20130626/194933/The_Top_F2P_Monetization_Tricks.php

3. King, D, Delfabbro, P & Griffiths, M, 2010, 'The Convergence of Gambling and Digital Media: Implications for Gambling in Young People', *Journal of Gambling Studies* 26 (2).

4. Sévigny, S, Cloutier, M, Pelletier, MF & Ladouceur, R, 2005, 'Internet gambling: misleading payout rates during the "demo" period', *Computers in Human Behaviour* 21 (1), pp 153–158.

5. Griffiths, MD & Wood, RTA, 2007, 'Adolescent Internet Gambling: Preliminary results of a national survey', *Education and Health* 25, pp 23–27.

6. Kim, HS, Wohl, MJA, Salmon, MM, Gupta, R & Derevensky, J, 2015, 'Do Social Casino Gamers Migrate to Online Gambling? An Assessment of Migration Rate and Potential Predictors', *Journal of Gambling Studies* 31 (4).

7. Rose, M, 2013, 'Chasing the whale: Examining the ethics of free-to-play games', retrieved from: www.gamasutra.com/view/feature/195806/chasing_the_whale_examining_the_.php

8. Shokrizade, R, 2013, loc. cit.

13. Talking to Young People about Online Porn and Sexual Images

1. Sun, C, Bridges, A, Johnson, JA & Ezzell, MB, 2016, 'Pornography and the male sexual script: An analysis of consumption and sexual relations', *Archives of Sexual Behavior* 45(4), pp 983–994.

2. Bridges, AJ, et. al., 2006, op. cit., pp 135–54.

3. Fleming, MJ, Greentree, S, Cocotti-Muller, D, Elias, KA & Morrison, S, 2006, 'Safety in cyberspace: Adolescents' safety and exposure online', *Youth and Society* 38(2), pp 135–54.

4. Bridges, AJ, Wosnitzer, R, Scharrer, E, Sun, C & Liberman, R, 2010, 'Aggression and sexual behavior in best-selling pornography videos: A content analysis update', *Violence Against Women* 16(10), pp 1065–1085.

5. Dines, G, 2016, 'Is porn immoral? That doesn't matter: It's a public health crisis', *The Washington Post.*

6. Owens, EW, Behun, RJ, Manning JC & Reid, RC, 2012, 'The Impact of Internet Pornography on Adolescents: A Review of the Research', *Sexual Addiction & Compulsivity* 19(1-2), pp 99–122.

7. APS Submission into the Senate Environment and Communications References Committee, 2016, '*Inquiry into the harm being done to Australian children through access to pornography on the internet*'.

8. Frappier, JY, Kaufman, M, Baltzer, F, Elliott, A, Lane, M, Pinzon, J & McDuff, P, 2008, 'Sex and sexual health: A survey of Canadian youth and mothers', *Paediatrics and Child Health* 13(1), p 25.

14. Advice for Parents: Be a Mentor, Not a Friend

1. Baumrind, D, 1978, 'Parental disciplinary patterns and social competence in children', *Youth & Society* 9(3), pp 239–251.

2. Nathanson, AI, 2002, 'The Unintended Effects of Parental Mediation of Television on Adolescents', *Media Psychology* 4(3), pp 207–230.

3. Buri, J, 1991, 'Parental Authority Questionnaire', *Journal of Personality Assessment* 57(1), pp 110–120.

4. Baumrind, D, 1991, 'The influence of parenting style on adolescent competence and substance use', *Journal of Early Adolescence* 11(1), pp 56–95.

5. Watabe, A & Hibard, D, 2014, 'The Influence of Authoritarian and Authoritative Parenting on Children's Academic Achievement Motivation: A Comparison between the United States and Japan', *North American Journal of Psychology* 16(2), pp 359–382.

6. Baumrind, D, 1991, 'The influence of parenting style on adolescent competence and substance use', *Journal of Early Adolescence* 11(1), p 62.

17. Dyslexia and Learning Difficulties

1. Shaywitz, S, 2005, *Overcoming Dyslexia*, Random House, New York.

2. Burden R, 2008, 'Is Dyslexia Necessarily Associated with Negative Feelings of Self-worth? A Review and Implications for Future Research', retrieved from www.interscience.wiley.com. DOI: 10.1002/dys.371. School of Education and Lifelong Learning, University of Exeter, Devon.

3. Boyes, M, Leitao, S, Claessen, M, Badcock, N & Nayton, M, 2016, 'Why Are Reading Difficulties Associated with Mental Health Problems?', *Dyslexia* 22(3), pp 263–6.

4. Le Messurier, M, 2013, 'I don't want to be here', *Generation Next*, www.youtube.com/watch?v=xqhTFuDG6KI

5. Dreikurs, R, Brunwald, B, Bronia, P & Floy, C, 1998, *Maintaining sanity in the classroom: classroom management techniques* (2nd edition), Taylor and Francis, Levittown.

6. Dyslexia International, 'The Problem', www.dyslexia-international.org/the-problem

7. Dyslexia Research Institute, www.dyslexia-add.org/issues.html

8. Allington, S, 2008, 'Why Struggling Readers Continue to Struggle', retrieved from http://ptgmedia.pearsoncmg.com

9. Alexander-Passe, N, 2007, 'The Sources and Manifestations of Stress Amongst School-aged Dyslexics, Compared with Sibling Controls', retrieved from www. interscience.wiley.com DOI: 10.1002/dys.351, November, 2016.

10. Alexander-Passe, N, 2006, 'How Dyslexic Teenagers Cope: An Investigation of Self-esteem, Coping and Depression', retrieved from www.interscience.wiley.com, DOI: 10.1002/dys.318

11. Meeks, L, Kemp, C & Stephenson, J, 2014, 'Standards in Literacy and Numeracy: Contributing Factors', *Australian Journal of Teacher Education* 39(7), retrieved from www.ro.ecu.edu.au

18. Friendship and Social Skills

1. Hattie, J, 2013, *Visible Learning for Teachers : Maximizing Impact on Learning*, Routledge, London.

2. Le Messurier, M, Nawana Parker, M, 2011, *What's the Buzz for primary age students: A social skills enrichment program*, Routledge, London; Le Messurier, M, Nawana Parker, M, 2014, *What's the Buzz for early learners: A complete social skills foundation course*, Routledge, London.

3. The Collaborative for Academic, Social, and Emotional Learning (CASEL), www.casel.org

4. Le Messurier, M; Nawana Parker, M, 2014, *Archie's Big Book of friendship adventures: A guide to solving social hitches and friendship glitches*, available: www.whatsthebuzz.net.au

5. Fabes, RA, Eisenberg, N, Hanish, LD & Spinrad, TL, 2001, 'Preschoolers spontaneous emotional vocabulary: Relations to likability', *Early Education and Development* 12, pp 11–27.

6. Nawana Parker, M, 2017, *The Resilience and Wellbeing Toolbox*, Routledge, London.

7. Siegel, DJ & Bryson, TP, 2012, *The Whole-Brain Child: 12 Revolutionary Strategies to Nurture Your Child's Developing Mind, Survive Everyday Parenting Struggles, and Help Your Family Thrive*, Bantam, USA.

19. The Commercialisation of Childhood

1. Drago, RW, Black, D & Wooden, M, 2005, 'The Existence and Persistence of Long Work Hours, IZA Discussion Paper No. 1720. available at SSRN: ssrn.com/abstract=799704

2. Humphrys, J, 2011, 'British Children: Unhappy materialists?', YouGov.UK, yougov.co.uk/news/2011/09/15/british-children-unhappy-materialists

3. Ipsos MORI Social Research Institute, 2011, 'Children's Well-being in UK, Sweden and Spain: The Role of Inequality and Materialism', www.ipsos.com/sites/default/files/publication/1177-03/sri-unicef-role-of-inequalityand-materialism-june-2011.pdf

4. Schor, J, 2004, *Born to Buy: The Commercialized Child and the New Consumer Culture*, Simon and Schuster, New York.

5. 'Committee on Communications', *Pediatrics* 118(6), 2006, available at: aappublications.org/content/118/6/2563

6. American Psychological Association, 2004, 'Report of the APA Task Force on Advertising and Children', www.apa.org/pi/families/resources/advertising-children.pdf

7. Beder, S with Varney, W & Gosden, R, 2009, *This Little Kiddy Went to Market: The Corporate Capture of Childhood*, UNSW Press, Sydney.

8. Green, L et al, 2011, 'Risks and safety for Australian children on the internet: full findings from the AU Kids Online survey of 9-16 year olds and their parents', *Edith Cowan University,* ro.ecu.edu.au/ecuworks2011/2

9. Confos, N and Davis, T, 2016, 'Young Consumer-Brand Relationship Building Potential Using Digital Marketing', *European Journal of Marketing (special issue on 'Children's Well-Being in a Digital Age')* 50(11), pp 1993–2017.

10. Tatlow-Golden, M, Boyland, E, Jewell, J, Zalnieriute, M, Handsley, E & Breda, J, 2016, 'Tackling food marketing to children in a digital world: trans-disciplinary perspectives', World Health Organization Regional Office for Europe, Copenhagen.

11. Roy Morgan Young Australians Survey, 2016, www.roymorgan.com.au/findings/5899-young-australians-saved-over-650-million-201410292227

12. Roy Morgan Understanding Young Australians Survey, July 2013 – June 2014, www.roymorganonlinestore.com/Browse/Australia/Young-Australians/Understanding-Young-Australians.aspx

13. University of Chicago Press Journals, 'In Children And Adolescents, Low Self-esteem Increases Materialism', *Science Daily*, 16 November 2007.

14. Chaplin, LN & John, DR, 2007, 'Growing up in a Material World: Age Differences in Materialism in Children and Adolescents', *Journal of Consumer Research* 34, available at: pdfs.semanticscholar.org/7671/609f151867ac3257922cbf1bf8e474122fc2.pdf

15. 'The Children's Consumer Culture Project', The University of Sussex, available at: www.sussex.ac.uk/psychology/consumercultureprojectwww.sussex.ac.uk/psychology/consumercultureproject/research/mainsurvey

16. Richins, ML & Chaplin, LN, 2015, 'Material Parenting: How the Use of Goods in Parenting Fosters Materialism in the Next Generation', *Journal of Consumer Research.*

17. Federal Trade Commission, 1981, 'In the Matter of Children's Advertising: FTC Final Staff Report and Recommendation', US Government Printing Office, Washington, DC.

18. Sherwin, A, 2011, 'Advertising ban won't stop "brand bullying", says childhood expert', *Independent,* www.independent.co.uk/news/media/advertising/advertising-ban-wont-stop-brandbullying- says-childhood-expert-2354917.html

19. Department for Communities and Local Government, 2011, 'Bailey Review of the Commercialisation and Sexualisation of Childhood: final report published', www.gov.uk/government/news/bailey-review-of-the-commercialisation-and-sexualisation-of-childhood-final-report-published

20. Department for Children, Schools and Families, 'The Impact of the Commercial World on Children's Wellbeing', webarchive.nationalarchives. gov.uk/20130401151715/http://www.education.gov.uk/publications/eOrderingDownload/00669-2009DOM-EN.pdf

21. Jacobs Foundation, 'Children's views on their lives and well-being in 15 countries', available at: www.isciweb.org/_Uploads/dbsAttachedFiles/ChildrensWorlds2015-FullReport-Final.pdf

22. Ipsos MORI Social Research Institute, 2011, 'Children's Well-being in UK, Sweden and Spain: The Role of Inequality and Materialism', available at: downloads.unicef.org.uk/wp content/uploads/2011/09/IPSOS_UNICEF_ChildWellBeingreport.pdf

23. Ibid.

24. Department for Communities and Local Government, 2011, 'Bailey Review of the Commercialisation and Sexualisation of Childhood: final report published', www.gov.uk/government/news/bailey-review-of-the-commercialisation-and-sexualisation-of-childhood-final-report-published

25. Wallman, J, 2015, *Stuffocation: Why We've Had Enough of Stuff and Need Experience More Than Ever*, Penguin Books, UK.

26. 'The Children's Consumer Culture Project', The University of Sussex, available at: www.sussex.ac.uk/psychology/consumercultureprojectwww.sussex.ac.uk/psychology/consumercultureproject/research/mainsurvey

20. Sexualisation: Why Should we be Concerned?

1. Tucci, Dr J, Generation Next, Sydney, May 2011

2. Ibid.

3. Houghton, D, 'Sex Attack Seen As "Childhood Experiment" At Queensland School', *The Courier Mail*, 12 September 2008.

4. Munro, P & Olding, R, 'It Was Terrifying', the *Sydney Morning Herald*, 20–21 August 2016

5. Hamilton, M, 2009, *What's Happening to Our Girls?*, Penguin, Melbourne, p 53.

6. Hamilton, M, op cit, p 148.

7. Hamilton, M, op cit, p 158.

8. Hamilton, M, op cit, p 148.

9. Marston, C & Lewis, R, 2014, 'Anal Heterosex Among Young People and Implications for Health Promotion: A Qualitative Study in the UK', *BMJ Open* 4(8), e004996. ISSN 2044-6055, www.researchonline.lshtm.ac.uk/1883883

10. Hamilton, M, op cit, p 145.

11. Zurbriggen, EL, et al, 2007, 'Report of the American Psychological Association Task Force on the Sexualisation of Girls', www.apa.org/pi/wpo/sexualization.html

12. Nesbitt, I, 2010, 'Adolescent Sex Offenders: A Life Sentence', *InPsych* 32(4), pp 16–17.

13. Doidge, N, 2007, *The Brain That Changes Itself: Stories of Personal Triumph from the Frontiers of Brain Science*, Penguin, London, p 103.

14. Ibid.

15. Betkowski, B, 2007, 'Study Finds Teen Boys Most Likely To Access Pornography', *Folio*, University of Alberta, www.ualberta.ca/~publicas/folio/44/13/09.html

21. Porn as a Public Health Crisis

1. Etheredge, L, 2014, 'Gender and Education Conference Paper: Is pornography colonizing young people's sexuality and normalising inequity?', www.academia.edu/12476200/Conference_Paper_Is_pornography_colonizing_young_people_s_sexuality_and_normalising_inequity

2. CNBC, 2013, 'Big Data Download: Web-based Challengers Assault Porn Industry', Yahoo Finance, www.finance.yahoo.com/blogs/big-data-download/based-challengers-assault-porn-industry-173828089.html

3. SimilarWeb, 'pornhub.com', vs xvideos.com, accessed 15 January 2017, www.similarweb.com/website/pornhub.com?competitors=xvideos.com

4. Somaiya, R, 'Nudes are Old News at Playboy', *The New York Times*, 12 October 2015. www.nytimes.com/2015/10/13/business/media/nudes-are-old-news-at-playboy.html

5. Bigelow, T, 2016, 'Futuresex and the single girl: Will sextech help or hurt your love life?' *Salon*, www.salon.com/2016/10/23/futuresex-and-the-single-girl-will-sextech-help-or-hurt-your-love-life/

6. Your Brain on Porn, 'Why shouldn't Johnny watch porn if he likes?', 18 February 2015, www.yourbrainonporn.com/why-shouldnt-johnny-watch-porn-if-he-likes

7. Doidge, N, 2007, *The Brain That Changes Itself: Stories of Personal Triumph from the Frontiers of Brain Science*, Viking, New York.

8. Wéry, A & Billieux, J, 2016, 'Online sexual activities: An exploratory study of problematic and non-problematic usage patterns in a sample of men', *Computers in Human Behavior* 56, pp 257–266. DOI: 10.1016/j.chb.2015.11.046

9. Silva, K, 'Chlamydia and gonorrhoea cases up in Queensland as doctors fear rise in unsafe sex', ABC News, 12 January 2017, www.abc.net.au/news/2017-01-13/chlamydia-and-gonorrhoea-cases-up-in-queensland-as-doctors-fear/8178730

10. Tankard Reist, M, 'Sexual pressure and degradation: This is what porn has done to every woman I know', blog comment, 8 April 2015, www.melindatankardreist.com/2015/04/sexual-pressure-coercion-degradation-this-is-what-porn-has-done-to-every-woman-i-know

11. Thege, BK, Hodgins, DC, & Wild, TC, 2016, 'Co-occurring substance-related and behavioral addiction problems: A person-centered, lay epidemiology approach', *Journal of Behavioral Addictions* 5(4), pp 614–622. DOI: 10.1556/2006.5.2016.079

12. Your Brain on Porn, Brain Studies on Porn Users, 31 July 2014, www.yourbrainonporn.com/brain-scan-studies-porn-users

13. Love, T, Laier, C, Brand, M, Hatch, L & Hajela, R, 2015, 'Neuroscience of internet pornography addiction: A review and update', *Behavioral Sciences* 5(3), pp 388-433. DOI: 10.3390/bs5030388

14. Your Brain on Porn, 'Are You Hooked On Porn? Ask ASAM', 17 September 2011, http://yourbrainonporn.com/are-you-hooked-on-porn-ask-asam

15. David, 'How Porn Nearly Killed Me', Reddit NoFap, 12 December 2014 www.reddit.com/r/NoFap/comments/2p2vs8/how_porn_nearly_killed_me

16. Owens, EW, Behun, RJ, Manning, JC & Reid, RC, 2012, 'The Impact of Internet Pornography on Adolescents: A Review of the Research. Sexual Addiction & Compulsivity', *The Journal of Treatment & Prevention* 19(1-2), pp 99–122. DOI: 10.1080/10720162.2012.660431

22. How Boys are Travelling and What They Most Need

1. Meltz, BF, 'Marketers See Babies' Noses As Pathway To Profits', *The Globe*, 19 May 2005, www.frankwbaker.com/marketers_babies_profits.htm

2. Hamilton, M, 2010, *What's Happening to Our Boys?* Penguin, Melbourne, pp 153–157.

3. op cit, pp 158–165.

4. Kohler, C, 'Red Steel Hands-On: Officially Awesome', *Game Life*, 25 October 2006, www.blog.wired.com/games/2006/10/red_steel_hands.html

5. Betkowski, B, 'Study Finds Teen Boys Most Likely To Access Pornography', *Folio*, University of Alberta, 2 March 2007, www.ualberta.ca/~publicas/folio/44/13/09.html

6. Kindlon, D & Thompson, M with Barker, T, 1999, *Raising Cain: Protecting the Emotional Life of Boys*, Ballantine Books, New York.

7. Thompson, M, et al, transcript of the panel, 'Boys to Men: Questions of Violence', Harvard Education Letter, Research Online, Forum Feature, July/August 1999, www.edletter.org/past/issues/1999-ja/forum.shtml.

8. Hyde, JS, 2014, 'Gender Similarities and Differences', *Annual Review of Psychology* 65, pp 373–398. Available at SSRN: www.ssrn.com/abstract=2376228 or www.dx.doi.org/10.1146/annurev-psych-010213-115057

9. River, JT, 'Masculinities and Men's Suicide', PhD thesis, 13 October 2014, Faculty of Education and Social Work, University of Sydney, www.hdl.handle.net/2123/12070

10. Cleary, A, 2005, 'Death Or Disclosure: Struggling To Be A Real Man', *Irish Journal of Sociology* 14(2), p 155.

11. Mayer, JD, Caruso, DR, Panter, AT & Salovey, P, 2012, 'The Growing
    Significance Of Hot Intelligences', *American Psychologist* 67(6), pp 502–3.
    DOI: 10.1037/a0029456.

23. Understanding and Managing Anger and Aggression

1. Headspace, 2016. Website accessed 22 November 2016
2. Headspace, 2016. Website accessed 22 November 2016
3. Reachout.com, 2016. Website accessed 22 November 2016
4. Suckling, A & Temple, C, 2008, *Cool Calm Kids: Resources to Help Prep to Year 2 Find
   Better Ways to Deal with Conflict and Bossy Peers*, Acer Press, Camberwell, Victoria, p 18.
5. Kids Matter, 2016, 'Anger', accessed 19 November 2016,
   www.kidsmatter.edu.au/mental-health-matters/social-and-emotional-learning/
   anger

24. Understanding Boys' Health Needs

1. Headspace, 2014, Key Statistics, www.headspace.org.au/health-professionals/
   mental-health-statistics-and-reports
2. ReachOut, 2012, Inspire Foundation Report, www.about.au.reachout.com/wp-
   content/uploads/2014/12/ReachOut-Annual-Report-2011-2012.pdf
3. Australian Bureau of Statistics, 2014, 'Causes of Death in Australia',
   www.abs.gov.au/ausstats/abs@.nsf/mf/3303.0
4. Foundation for Young Australians, 2009, 'The Impact of racism upon the Health
   and Wellbeing of Young Australians', www.fya.org.au/app/theme/default/design/
   assets/publications/Impact_of_Racism_FYA_report.pdf
5. National LGBTI Health Alliance, 2013, LGBTI People Mental Health and
   Suicide report. www.medicaldaily.com/what-it-means-beman-how-male-gender-
   stereotypes-try-fit-growing-boys-mold-and-fail-326450
6. Headspace, 2014, Key Statistics, www.headspace.org.au/health-professionals/
   mental-health-statistics-and-reports
7. The Department of Health, 2010, 'Building on the strengths of Australian
   males', http://www.health.gov.au/internet/publications/publishing.nsf/Content/
   building-strengths-males-foreword
8. Kupers, TT, 2005, 'Toxic masculinity as a barrier to mental health treatment in
   prison', *Journal of Clinical Psychology* 61(6), pp 713–724.
9. Australian Institute of Health and Welfare, 2016, www.aihw.gov.au/youth-justice
10. Bureau of Justice Statistics, 2012, www.abs.gov.au/ausstats
11. Australian Research Alliance for Children and Youth, 2010, www.aracy.org.au/
    publications-resources/command/download_file/id/122/filename/Preventing_
    Youth_Violence_-_What_does_and_doesn't_work_and_why.pdf
12. Dalton, T & Marshall, J, 2012, 'The violence tearing Australian families apart',
    The Courier-Mail, www.couriermail.com.au/news/national/the-street-violence-
    tearing-australianfamilies-apart/news-story/e6f1c465fc5a92fa686c14754699e4aa

13. Gerathy, S, Stuart & McNally, L, 2016, 'Sydney's lockout laws relaxed as part of two year trial, opinions divided on whether changes are enough', *Australia Broadcasting Corporation*, www.news.com.au/finance/business/other-industries/nsw-governments-softening-ofalcohol-lockouts-laws-criticised-as-an-insult-to-sydney/news-story/553c559e6943113a41802de169718e00

14. NSW Health Statistics, 2016, www.health.nsw.gov.au/hsnsw/Publications/chief-healthofficers-report-2016.pdf

15. Addiction.com, 2015, www.addiction.com/12159/what-happens-when-children-watchporn/

16. The Department of Health, 2010, 'Building on the strengths of Australian males', http://www.health.gov.au/internet/publications/publishing.nsf/Content/building-strengths-males-foreword

17. Bryant, C, 2009, 'Adolescence, pornography and harm', *Australian Institute of Criminology*, pp 1-6, available at: www.aic.gov.au/media_library/publications/tandi_pdf/tandi368.pdf

18. Park, BY et al, 2016, 'Is internet pornography causing sexual dysfunctions? A review with clinical reports', *Behavioural Psychology* 6(3), www.ncbi.nlm.nih.gov/pmc/articles/PMC5039517/

19. Hilton, DL & Watts, C, 2011, 'Pornography addiction: A neuroscience perspective', *Surgical Neurology International* 2(19), www.ncbi.nlm.nih.gov/pmc/articles/PMC3050060/

20. Bridges et al, 2010, 'Aggression and sexual behaviour in best-selling pornography videos: a content analysis update', *Violence Against Women* 16(10), pp 1065–1085.

21. Australian Clearing House for Youth Studies, 2014, 'Face the Facts Briefing: Young Australians and Sexual Health'.

22. Australasian Sexual Health Conference, 2013, media release: 'Chlamydia most commonly reported STI in Australia'.

23. Sexually transmitted infections in Australia, 2013, 'Annual Surveillance Report'.

24. Sanders, R et al, 2014, 'Genome-wide scan demonstrates significant linkage for male sexual orientation', *Psychological Medicine* 45(7).

25. Engebretson, K, 2006, 'Identity, Masculinity and Spirituality: A Study of Australian Teenage Boys', *Journal of Religious Education* 54(1), pp 42–57.

ESSENTIAL READING FOR PARENTS
AND PROFESSIONALS

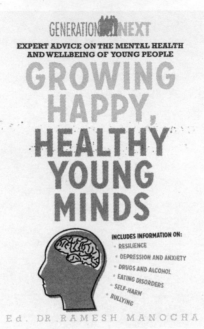

Addresses current, relevant and high-priority issues, such as bullying, depression, anxiety, drugs and alcohol, eating disorders, self-harm and resilience.

Practical and easy to read, with details on where to find unique additional resources.

A comprehensive collection from some of Australia's most respected practitioners.

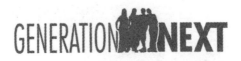